Obesity During Pregnancy in Clinical Practice

Wanda Nicholson
Kesha Baptiste-Roberts
Editors

Obesity During Pregnancy in Clinical Practice

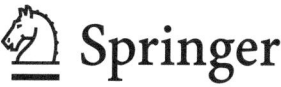

Editors
Wanda Nicholson
Department of Obstetrics
and Gynecology
Diabetes and Obesity Core
Center for Women's Health
Research
University of North Carolina
School of Medicine
Chapel Hill, NC
USA

Kesha Baptiste-Roberts
School of Nursing and
College of Medicine
Department of Public
Health Sciences
The Pennsylvania State
University
Hershey, PA
USA

ISBN 978-1-4471-2830-4   ISBN 978-1-4471-2831-1   (eBook)
DOI 10.1007/978-1-4471-2831-1
Springer London Heidelberg New York Dordrecht

Library of Congress Control Number: 2013955579

© Springer-Verlag London 2014
This work is subject to copyright. All rights are reserved by the Publisher, whether the whole or part of the material is concerned, specifically the rights of translation, reprinting, reuse of illustrations, recitation, broadcasting, reproduction on microfilms or in any other physical way, and transmission or information storage and retrieval, electronic adaptation, computer software, or by similar or dissimilar methodology now known or hereafter developed. Exempted from this legal reservation are brief excerpts in connection with reviews or scholarly analysis or material supplied specifically for the purpose of being entered and executed on a computer system, for exclusive use by the purchaser of the work. Duplication of this publication or parts thereof is permitted only under the provisions of the Copyright Law of the Publisher's location, in its current version, and permission for use must always be obtained from Springer. Permissions for use may be obtained through RightsLink at the Copyright Clearance Center. Violations are liable to prosecution under the respective Copyright Law.
The use of general descriptive names, registered names, trademarks, service marks, etc. in this publication does not imply, even in the absence of a specific statement, that such names are exempt from the relevant protective laws and regulations and therefore free for general use.
While the advice and information in this book are believed to be true and accurate at the date of publication, neither the authors nor the editors nor the publisher can accept any legal responsibility for any errors or omissions that may be made. The publisher makes no warranty, express or implied, with respect to the material contained herein.

Printed on acid-free paper

Springer is part of Springer Science+Business Media (www.springer.com)

Foreword

Obesity in the United States now constitutes a public health crisis of epidemic proportions. More than two-thirds of adults and approximately one-third of children are overweight or obese. This trend has persisted for the last decade and shows no signs of abatement. Importantly, maternal obesity is an important predictor of childhood obesity. Because of the particular concern for overweight and obesity in mothers and young children, human conception and pregnancy may represent a significant opportunity to begin to positively impact this evolving epidemic.

Nicholson and Baptiste-Roberts and their colleagues, in this concise, but complete text, provide a summary of the key evidence in the field of perinatal obesity, identify gaps in the field and provide guidance on the generation of research questions to be answered. The accomplished list of contributors to this book exemplifies the concept that perinatal obesity is complex and requires a transdisciplinary team to adequately cover the topic. The editors, Nicholson and Baptiste-Roberts, have organized the text in the order in which we clinically see perinatal obesity – starting with the influence of obesity on infertility, preconception care, challenges of transitioning the obese parturient from pregnancy to delivery, gaps in our evidence for postpartum intervention and postpartum models of care, and infant and early childhood growth. Intertwined in these core chapters are chapters that discuss the effects of body image on perinatal weight, epidemiologic trends in obesity and long-term maternal and infant outcomes, potential influence of depression on obesity in childbearing women, and gaps in evidence for family-based interventions.

This pioneering work by Wanda Nicholson and Kesha Baptiste-Roberts represents a thoughtful approach to one of the most vexing public health crisis of this generation. *Obesity During Pregnancy in Clinical Practice* provides clinicians and public health workers with a current summary of the key aspects of perinatal obesity, clinical insights on how to address this escalating public health problem and where future efforts should be targeted to break the cycle of obesity in mothers and their offspring.

Tucson, AZ   Francisco A.R. Garcia, MD, MPH, FACOG

Preface

We have had a strong passion for making a difference in the lives of adults and children through our research. Our individual careers as a clinician-researcher (Nicholson) and an epidemiologist (Baptiste-Roberts) has provided on-going and unique opportunities to influence the health of women across the lifespan. We have targeted much of our efforts on obesity and diabetes because of the underlying mechanisms linking these two conditions and the transgenerational link between mothers and their offspring. We first began to work together in 2005 when our clinical and research careers were beginning. Our partnership has led to manuscripts, grants and leadership in systematic reviews pertinent to the field of obesity and diabetes in the perinatal period. Along the way, we have met an incredible group of researchers, clinicians, and public health officials who are equally passionate about obesity in reproductive age women and who have been a strong group of interdisciplinary colleagues over the years. We have been blessed to have them participate in this endeavor.

Obesity rates continue to increase at alarming rates. More than two-thirds of women of childbearing age are either overweight or obese, contributing to persistent obesity in the expectant mother and adverse birth and childhood outcomes in the offspring. In this book, we have distilled and formulated information essential for the prevention and treatment of obesity during the perinatal period. We sought to summarize and synthesize the evidence on obesity during the perinatal period, clinical approaches and lifestyle interventions. The current state of knowledge and variety of intervention approaches allow women and their clinicians to select effective strategies best suited to an individual's personal, social and medical characteristics and requirements. Nevertheless, science is still sometimes inadequate and new hypotheses are being generated. In these situations, we have highlighted some new approaches, hypotheses currently being tested and mechanisms still under study. We hope that this book will assist clinicians, public health researchers and public health officials in obtaining a brief focused summary of the evidence and where our efforts should be targeted to reduce the burden of overweight and obesity in the perinatal period.

Chapel Hill, NC Wanda K. Nicholson
Hershey, PA Kesha Baptiste-Roberts

Acknowledgements

My thanks go out to all of the chapter authors. Despite their incredibly busy schedules, they made time to contribute to this book. I especially thank my personal team – my mother Thelma, sisters Sharon and Tammy, my nephew Brandon and my mentors. Also, I thank all of my friends and colleagues who are too numerous to mention but they know who they are – Thank you for your support.

Wanda K. Nicholson

I owe a special gratitude to people who have supported and encouraged my professional and personal development over the years. These cherished family members, friends and mentors have made a significant contribution to my life. These individuals are too numerous to mention, but they know who they are. I especially appreciate my mother Cherry, whose fearlessness and faith was instrumental in the achievement of my personal and professional goals. My father, Peter, whose dedication and expectation of the best, contributed significantly to who I am today. I am thankful for the unconditional love and support of Carlos, my husband, and our two children, Carina and Cydney. I am truly blessed. Thank you all.

Kesha Baptiste-Roberts

Contents

Part I Preconception and Pregnancy

1 Introduction: Breaking the Cycle of Obesity in Mothers and Children..................... 3
Wanda Nicholson

2 Obesity and Infertility........................ 11
Kathryn C. Calhoun

3 Preconception and Pregnancy Care in Overweight or Obese Woman................ 33
Catherine Takacs Witkop

4 Shared Decision Making and Labor Management in Parturients.................... 53
Catherine Takacs Witkop

Part II Maternal Risk Factors and Obesity

5 Epidemiologic Trends and Maternal Risk Factors Predicting Postpartum Weight Retention......... 77
Erica P. Gunderson

6 Relationship Between Depressive Mood and Maternal Obesity: Implications for Postpartum Depression.................... 99
Sarah C. Rogan, Jennifer L. Payne, and Samantha Meltzer-Brody

7 Body Image as a Contributor to Weight in Pregnancy and Postpartum: Racial Differences 121
Tiffany L. Carson, Kesha Baptiste-Roberts, and Tiffany L. Gary-Webb

Part III The Early Postpartum Period

8 Promoting a Healthy Weight After Delivery 159
Alexander Berger and Wanda Nicholson

9 Obesity and Physical Activity During Pregnancy and Postpartum: Evidence, Guidelines, and Recommendations 183
Danielle Symons Downs, Kelly R. Evenson, and Lisa Chasan-Taber

10 Maternal Obesity, Gestational Weight Gain, and Childhood Growth in the First Year of Life 229
Deborah B. Ehrenthal, Cynthia S. Minkovitz, and Donna M. Strobino

Part IV Meeting Future Challenges

11 Maternal Obesity and Implications for the Long-Term Health of the Offspring 259
Kesha Baptiste-Roberts

12 Family-Centered Interventions to Reduce Maternal and Child Obesity 297
Dianne Stanton Ward, Temitope O. Erinosho, Heather M. Wasser, and Paula M. Munoz

13 Obesity Screening Recommendations and Emerging Policies 337
Wanda Nicholson

Index 345

Contributors

Kesha Baptiste-Roberts, PhD, MPH School of Nursing and College of Medicine, Department of Public Health Sciences, The Pennsylvania State University, Hershey, PA, USA

Alexander Berger, MD, MPH Department of Obstetrics and Gynecology, Thomas Jefferson University Hospital, Philadelphia, PA, USA

Kathryn C. Calhoun, MD Reproductive Endocrinology and Infertility, The Atlanta Center for Reproductive Medicine (ACRM), Atlanta, GA, USA

Tiffany L. Carson, PhD, MPH Division of Preventive Medicine, University of Alabama at Birmingham School of Medicine, Birmingham, AL, USA

Lisa Chasan-Taber, ScD Department of Public Health, School of Public Health and Health Sciences, University of Massachusetts, Amherst, MA, USA

Danielle Symons Downs, PhD Departments of Kinesiology and OB/GYN, College of Health and Human Development, The Pennsylvania State University, University Park, PA, USA

Deborah B. Ehrenthal, MD, MPH Departments of Internal Medicine and OB/GYN, Christiana Care Health System, Newark, NJ, USA

Departments of Internal Medicine and OB/GYN, Thomas Jefferson University, Philadelphia, PA, USA

Temitope O. Erinosho, PhD Department of Nutrition, University of North Carolina at Chapel Hill, Chapel Hill, NC, USA

Kelly R. Evenson, PhD, MS Department of Epidemiology, Gillings School of Global Public Health, University of North Carolina at Chapel Hill, Chapel Hill, NC, USA

Tiffany L. Gary-Webb, PhD, MHS Department of Epidemiology, Columbia University Mailman School of Public Health, New York, NY, USA

Erica P. Gunderson, PhD Division of Research, Kaiser Permanente Northern California, Oakland, CA, USA

Samantha Meltzer-Brody, MD, MPH Department of Psychiatry, University of North Carolina at Chapel Hill, Chapel Hill, NC, USA

Cynthia S. Minkovitz, MD, MPP Department of Population, Family and Reproductive Health, Bloomberg School of Public Health, Johns Hopkins University, Baltimore, MD, USA

Paula M. Munoz Department of Nutrition, University of North Carolina at Chapel Hill, Chapel Hill, NC, USA

Wanda Nicholson, MD, MPH, MBA Department of Obstetrics and Gynecology, Diabetes and Obesity Core, Center for Women's Health Research, University of North Carolina School of Medicine, Chapel Hill, NC, USA

Jennifer L. Payne, MD Department of Psychiatry, Johns Hopkins, Baltimore, MD, USA

Sarah C. Rogan, MD, PhD Department of Obstetrics and Gynecology, University of Texas at Galveston, School of Medicine, Chapel Hill, NC, USA

Donna M. Strobino, PhD Department of Population, Family and Reproductive Health, Bloomberg School of Public Health, Johns Hopkins University, Baltimore, MD, USA

Dianne Stanton Ward, EdD Department of Nutrition, UNC School of Public Health, Chapel Hill, NC, USA

Department of Nutrition, University of North Carolina at Chapel Hill, Chapel Hill, NC, USA

Heather M. Wasser, PhD, MPH, RD Department of Nutrition, University of North Carolina at Chapel Hill, Chapel Hill, NC, USA

Catherine Takacs Witkop, MD, MPH Department of Obstetrics/Gynecology and Preventative Medicine, Uniformed Services University of the Health Sciences, Bethesda, MD, USA

Part I
Preconception and Pregnancy

Chapter 1
Introduction: Breaking the Cycle of Obesity in Mothers and Children

Wanda Nicholson

> *"The womb may be more important than the home,"* David Barker, *from the fetal and infant origins of adult disease. [1]*

Abstract Obesity in pregnancy is part of a vicious cycle that contributes to the epidemic of obesity and diabetes across generations. Breaking the cycle of *transgenerational obesity* will require a better understanding of the epidemiological and clinical aspects of obesity as well as the translation of science into standardized clinical care and targeted interventions across the life span of women and children. The objective of this book is to (1) summarize the state of the science of perinatal obesity and (2) provide clinicians with the information they need to effectively care for their patients during this important teachable moment in their lives.

Keywords Obesity • Pregnancy • Gestational diabetes • Weight loss • Transgenerational obesity • Perinatal obesity

---

W. Nicholson, MD, MPH, MBA
Department of Obstetrics and Gynecology,
Diabetes and Obesity Core, Center for Women's Health Research,
University of North Carolina School of Medicine,
Chapel Hill, NC, USA
e-mail: wanda_nicholson@med.unc.edu

W. Nicholson, K. Baptiste-Roberts (eds.),
Obesity During Pregnancy in Clinical Practice,
DOI 10.1007/978-1-4471-2831-1_1,
© Springer-Verlag London 2014

Introduction

More than two-thirds of women of childbearing age are overweight or obese [2], contributing to a vicious cycle of obesity in the expectant mother and adverse birth outcomes and obesity in her offspring (Fig. 1.1). Evidence of the pervasive concern over adult obesity is reflected in the recent American Medical Association statement that reclassified obesity as a "disease" (it was recently known as a "condition"). While some may claim that the reclassification is purely symbolic, it opens the door for clinician reimbursement for obesity counseling, prevention, and treatment with behavioral or lifestyle strategies. The change in classification represents a real paradigm shift in obesity prevention. Obesity in pregnancy is both fascinating and concerning because it involves the health of two patients – both mother and child whose partnership is intertwined from conception to delivery and beyond. As such, the mother-child dyad is at the forefront of our efforts to better understand and clinically manage obesity and to develop reasonable clinical and behavioral interventions to modify the risk of obesity in mothers and their offspring.

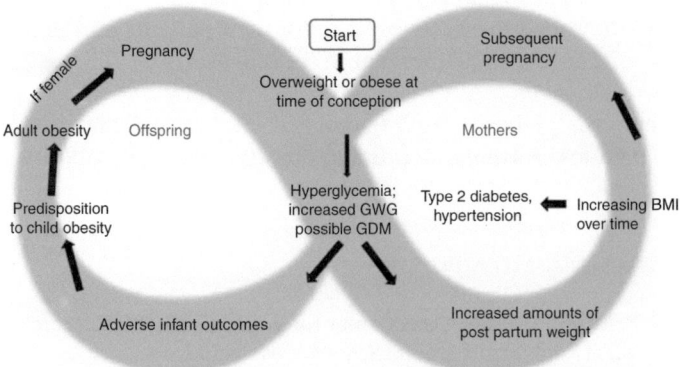

FIGURE 1.1 Transgenerational cycle of obesity for mothers and their offspring. *GWG* gestational weight gain, *GDM* gestational diabetes, *BMI* body mass index

Obesity in Pregnancy and Implications for Mother and Offspring

One of the downstream consequences of the epidemic of obesity in the USA is that more women are entering pregnancy already suffering from the burden of overweight and obesity. There are a myriad of adverse outcomes associated with a pregnancy complicated by obesity, including subfertility, preeclampsia, fetal macrosomia, and cesarean delivery. Obstetrical complications can increase as much as threefold in obese versus nonobese mothers. Obesity is a common risk factor for insulin resistance. Insulin sensitivity is already reduced by 50–60 % over the course of pregnancy, so it is not surprising that overweight or obese women who are prone to beta-cell dysfunction and glucose intolerance prior to pregnancy are at increased risk of gestational diabetes (GDM) during pregnancy (Fig. 1.1) [3, 4]. For example, in comparison to women with a normal body mass index, the risk of developing GDM rises exponentially with increasing BMI, with odds ratios (OR) of 1.97 (95 % CI 1.77–2.19), 3.01 (95 % CI 2.34–3.87), and 5.55 (95 % CI 4.27–7.21) for those who are overweight obese and morbidly obese, respectively [5]. Other markers of obesity, such as waist circumference and waist-to-hip ratio, are independently associated with a higher 2-h post-glucose response, suggesting that central obesity is an independent predictor of GDM.

Overweight and obese women are at increased risk for excessive gestational weight gain (GWG) [4–6]. The combination of pre-pregnancy overweight and obesity and excessive GWG is particularly concerning. The most recent Institute of Medicine (IOM) recommendations [7] for a smaller weight gain range for those classified as overweight (7–11.5 kg) and obese (5–9 kg) have garnered considerable attention. Longitudinal studies show a direct association between maternal obesity and infant birth weight. For women who are overweight or obese prior to conception, an increase in GWG is associated with an increase in fetal adiposity. The combination of maternal overweight or obesity and exceeding the IOM guidelines increases the risk of delivering a large-for-gestational-age infant and the associated complications of dysfunctional labor and potential cesarean delivery [8].

A growing concern, from both a clinical and public health perspective, is the intrauterine environment and the concept of *transgenerational obesity* (Fig. 1.1) [9, 10]. Obesity, GDM, and excessive weight are thought to change the intrauterine environment and contribute to increase risk of obesity in children. Early work by David Barker [1, 11] set the stage for ongoing research in fetal programming and development of adult diabetes and hypertension [12]. The Barker hypothesis postulates that nutritional insults to the fetus during critical periods of development may lead to in utero alterations in fetal metabolism or fetal programming that favors obesity-related conditions in adulthood. Of particular interest is the hypothesis that offspring of women with obesity may be predisposed to greater energy consumption and higher levels of sedentary behavior, a finding that is supported by animal models. Though outside the scope of this text, animal models have been useful in elucidating the contribution of maternal phenotypes (e.g., obesity and dietary intake) on the intrauterine environment and growth trajectories in the offspring [13]. The combination of obesity and pregnancy, inflammatory markers, adipokines, and the hormonal milieu contributes to a complex interrelation of mechanisms that with further research can broaden our understanding of the transgenerational effects of obesity.

Breaking the cycle of transgenerational obesity will require a better understanding of the epidemiological and clinical aspects of obesity as well as the translation of science into standardized clinical care and targeted interventions across the life span of women and children. To date, there are few published texts that translate the evolving state of the science of overweight and obesity from the maternal and child health perspective. The overall objectives in writing this book are to (1) translate the state of the science on overweight and obesity in the perinatal period, thus arming clinicians and public health officials that provide care to childbearing women with the knowledge necessary to communicate with their patients on the effects of obesity in this important time period; (2) communicate important clinical aspects of care that can be effectively communicated to patients by their providers in a busy practice setting; and (3) summarize the evidence for perinatal, family, and community lifestyle interventions that have been shown to be effective in promoting a healthy weight and modifying the risk of developing diabetes and obesity.

This book is our attempt to summarize the latest developments in our clinical understanding of obesity in pregnancy. Obesity is a multicomplex disease, and prevention and treatment will require transdisciplinary approaches, including clinical, research, and population-based perspectives. The content of the book differs from other textbooks on obesity because each chapter is written from a clinical and population-based perspective. Our collaborative team of experts provides important, relevant insight into each topic, emphasizing the intersection between clinical care, research, and broad dissemination of research findings. The first section provides an overview of the biological mechanisms underlying the clinical effects of obesity on the expectant mother and developing fetus. Dr. Calhoun reviews the biological pathways that account for the effect of obesity on infertility and subfertility. She summarizes the current clinical care of the overweight or obese woman and subfertility, and the lifestyle and medical options currently used to achieve conception. Both the preconception period and pregnancy represent important teachable moments in the lives of childbearing age women. Of particular concern to clinicians and public health officials is the contribution of pre-pregnancy obesity to the persistently high rates of medical complications of pregnancy (diabetes, hypertension) and adverse birth outcomes (preterm birth, low birth weight infants, and infant deaths) [14]. Dr. Witkop outlines important steps in preconception and pregnancy care in the overweight or obese women and the clinical issues to consider during this critical time period. Her chapter provides a step-by-step assessment for preconception care that can be used by multiple types of providers in diverse clinical settings. She summarizes the Institute of Medicine gestational weight gain guidelines and the role of clinicians in promoting a healthy weight before and during pregnancy. Also in this section, Dr. Witkop discusses the complex decisions faced by women and their clinicians and the important role of shared decision making in developing a labor and delivery plan that incorporates best practice and patient preferences.

In the next section, we explore complex relationships of demographics and psychosocial factors with obesity. Dr. Gunderson provides an epidemiological assessment of secular trends in maternal risk factors for postpartum weight retention. Dr. Payne and Meltzer-Brody help us to better understand the relationship of depression symptoms and obesity in the perinatal period. Drs. Cox, Baptiste-Roberts, and Gary-Webb discuss women's perception of body image and the association with weight and diabetes prevention.

Implementing diet and physical activity interventions in the periconception period takes advantage of an important "teachable moment" [15] and offers an opportunity for women to improve their health status not only to achieve a healthy pregnancy but to change the course of their long-term health. Thus, we have set the stage to discuss the current state of the science on lifestyle interventions – both diet and physical activity for mothers and their families. Dr. Nicholson summarizes the findings for the effect of combined diet and physical activity interventions on weight and adiposity in the postpartum period and outlines a research agenda to move the science forward in postpartum care for overweight or obese women. Drs. Downs, Chasen-Taber, and Evenson outline the role of physical activity in promoting a healthy weight during pregnancy and suggested guidelines for clinical counseling.

The next section focuses on the effect of maternal obesity on child growth and adiposity. Drs. Strobino, Minkovitz, and Erenthral summarize the literature on the effect of maternal pre-pregnancy body mass index (BMI), gestational weight gain on early child growth, including infant birth weight and weight and adiposity up to age 2. Dr. Baptiste-Roberts continues this discussion, providing a summary of the data on the effect on maternal obesity on child growth trajectories after the first year of life. Addressing child obesity prevention and treatment from a family perspective could be an effective strategy. Drs. Ward, Erinosho, Wasser, and Ms. Munoz discuss the findings from a comprehensive review of 19 studies of family-centered interventions to prevent or reduce or treat child obesity.

Obesity among women of childbearing age is a major public health issue warranting additional studies that investigate its impact on short- and long-term maternal and child outcomes as well as best practices for weight management during pregnancy and the postpartum period. Our book concludes with a discussion of where key organizations stand on screening for obesity and summarizes the next generation of research needed to inform clinical care.

References

1. Barker DJ. The fetal and infant origins of adult disease. BMJ. 1990;301(6761):1111.
2. Weiss JL, Malone FD, Emig D, Ball RH, Nyberg DA, Comstock CH, Saade G, Eddleman K, Carter SM, Craigo SD, Carr SR, D'Alton ME. Obesity, obstetric complications and cesarean delivery rate–a population-based screening study. Am J Obstet Gynecol. 2004;190(4):1091–7.
3. Ferrara A. Increasing prevalence of gestational diabetes mellitus: a public health perspective. Diabetes Care. 2007;30 Suppl 2:S141–6.
4. Greene MF, Solomon CG. Gestational diabetes mellitus – time to treat. N Engl J Med. 2005;352(24):2544–6.
5. Yeung EH, Hu FB, Solomon CG, Chen L, Louis GM, Schisterman E, Willett WC, Zhang C. Life-course weight characteristics and the risk of gestational diabetes. Diabetologia. 2010;53(4):668–78.
6. Baptiste-Roberts K, Barone BB, Gary TL, Golden SH, Wilson LM, Bass EB, Nicholson WK. Risk factors for type 2 diabetes among women with gestational diabetes: a systematic review. Am J Med. 2009;122(3):207–214.e4.
7. Institute of Medicine. Weight gain during pregnancy: reexamining the guidelines. Washington, DC: National Academies Press; 2009.
8. Hull HR, Thornton JC, Ji Y, Paley C, Rosenn B, Mathews P, Navder K, Yu A, Dorsey K, Gallagher D. Higher infant body fat with excessive gestational weight gain in overweight women. Am J Obstet Gynecol. 2011;205(3):211.e1–7.

9. Gluckman PD, Hanson MA, Cooper C, Thornburg KL. Effect of in utero and early-life conditions on adult health and disease. N Engl J Med. 2008;359(1):61–73.
10. Dabelea D, Hanson RL, Lindsay RS, Pettitt DJ, Imperatore G, Gabir MM, Roumain J, Bennett PH, Knowler WC. Intrauterine exposure to diabetes conveys risks for type 2 diabetes and obesity: a study of discordant sibships. Diabetes. 2000;49(12):2208–11.
11. Barker DJ. In utero programming of cardiovascular disease. Theriogenology. 2000;53(2):555–74.
12. Barker DJ, Bull AR, Osmond C, Simmonds SJ. Fetal and placental size and risk of hypertension in adult life. BMJ. 1990;301(6746):259–62.
13. Shankar K, Harrell A, Liu X, Gilchrist JM, Ronis MJ, Badger TM. Maternal obesity at conception programs obesity in the offspring. Am J Physiol Regul Integr Comp Physiol. 2008;294(2):R528–38.
14. Johnson DB, Gerstein DE, Evans AE, Woodward-Lopez G. Preventing obesity: a life cycle perspective. J Am Diet Assoc. 2006;106(1):97–102.
15. McBride CM, Emmons KM, Lipkus IM. Understanding the potential of teachable moments: the case of smoking cessation. Health Educ Res. 2003;18(2):156–70.

Chapter 2
Obesity and Infertility

Kathryn C. Calhoun

Aside from tobacco use, obesity is the most modifiable risk factor for infertility.

Abstract Elevated body weight can decrease fertility in men and women. It increases the risk of ovulatory dysfunction and insulin resistance but can also decrease chance of conception in women with regular cycles. In men, excess adipose tissue can create an unfavorable endocrine profile and decrease sperm count and quality. Obstetrical morbidity and mortality, and metabolic consequences for the next generation, increase with elevated body weight so the ideal time to optimize BMI is preconception. Strategies for weight loss should center on caloric restriction and increased physical activity, but can utilize medication and surgery as adjuncts.

Keywords Obesity • Infertility • Anovulation • PCOS • Insulin resistance • Glucose intolerance • Body mass index (BMI)

K.C. Calhoun, MD
Reproductive Endocrinology and Infertility,
The Atlanta Center for Reproductive Medicine (ACRM),
Atlanta, GA, USA
e-mail: kcalhounmd@gmail.com

Key Points
- Existing evidence suggests that elevated body weight has a detrimental effect on both male and female fertility.
- Elevated body weight exacerbates Polycystic Ovary Syndrome [1] and reduces the chance of ovulation, in both medicated and unmedicated cycles.
- Elevated body weight reduces the chance of pregnancy and live birth, in both medicated and unmedicated cycles.
- Weight loss appears to improve health, fertility, and life expectancy.
- All weight loss and weight maintenance strategies should include both diet and exercise.

Definitions

- Infertility: No conception despite 1 year of unprotected intercourse
- Body mass index (BMI): A standardized expression of body size, as determined by weight in kilograms divided by height in meters squared (kg/m^2):

   <19: Underweight
   19–24.9: Normal BMI
   25–29.9: Overweight
   30–34.5: Obesity I
   35–39.9: Obesity II
   ≥40: Obesity III

- Ovulatory dysfunction: The failure to predictably release an oocyte in a cyclic fashion (also known as "oligo-ovulation" or "anovulation")
- Insulin: Hormonal regulator of the body's use of glucose (sugar) and fat; produced by the pancreas
- Insulin resistance: Failure of the body's cells to take up glucose from the blood in response to "normal" amounts of blood insulin

- Glucose intolerance: As a result of insulin resistance (and/or inadequate insulin production by the pancreas), blood glucose levels are chronically elevated
- "Prediabetes": May refer to insulin resistance +/– glucose intolerance
- Resting metabolic rate (RMR): The number of calories consumed daily for bodily homeostasis

The Scope of the Problem

Infertility, defined as no conception after 1 year of unprotected intercourse, affects 15 % of the US population or over seven million couples [2]. In the USA, roughly 1 % of children are conceived via in vitro fertilization (IVF), with many more couples employing less aggressive medical assistance (i.e., ovulation induction medicines, intrauterine insemination) [2].

A devastating and related problem is the pandemic of obesity. Worldwide, more people are obese than starving [3]. In the USA, over 60 % of adults are above their ideal body weight; approximately 36 % of adults and 17 % of children and adolescents (<19 years old) are obese [2]. There are racial discrepancies in obesity, with 50 % of African Americans struggling with obesity. Individuals with elevated body weight suffer more illness (cardiovascular, psychological, oncologic) and earlier deaths than their counterparts who maintain an ideal body weight (CDC) [2, 4, 5]. Women who are overweight and obese have additional consequences of obstetrical and gynecologic morbidities, and both sexes have reduced fertility at elevated body weights [6, 7]. Aside from tobacco use, obesity is the most modifiable risk factor for morbidity, mortality, and infertility.

Obesity and Female Fertility

Although one large study found no significant difference in fecundity between BMI groups, the majority of the literature suggests that fecundity declines with increasing BMI [7, 8].

Decreased fertility in the obese population relates primarily to ovulatory dysfunction ("anovulation" or "oligo-ovulation"), or the failure to reliably release a mature oocyte in a cyclic fashion. In fact, BMI at age 18 has been shown to predict the risk of anovulatory infertility and nulliparity [9]. Approximately 30–47 % of overweight women have menstrual irregularities [1]. Weight loss, even modest amounts of 5–10 % of body weight, has been shown to increase the likelihood of ovulation and conception, in both medically unassisted and assisted cycles [8, 10].

There is evidence that ovulatory disorders may not be the only explanation for decreased fecundity in heavier women. Even in ovulatory women, time to conception (TTC) is more likely to be greater than 6 months in women with elevated body weight. Even after controlling for menstrual regularity, women with more visceral adiposity had a longer time to conception [11]. One study of over 3,000 ovulatory women with at least one normal tube and access to normal sperm demonstrated that pregnancy rate (PR) declined 4 % per year for every BMI unit over 29 [12]. Other factors may be involved, such as the uterus, the gamete quality, the endocrine milieu, or the presence of chronic inflammation.

Anovulation

The hypothalamic-pituitary-gonadal axis is quite vulnerable to the effects of stress, illness, and weight changes, likely reflecting an evolutionary adaptation designed to prevent increases in the population during times of starvation, conflict, or disease.

In the beginning of an ovulatory cycle, the pituitary gland responds to hypothalamic GnRH pulses with release of follicle-stimulating hormone (FSH), aimed at developing the cohort of follicles that have been recruited in the luteal phase of the previous cycle. As early as cycle day 5, a dominant follicle emerges, with superior blood flow and FSH-receptor concentrations, able to survive even when FSH secretion is attenuated in response to rising ovarian estrogen and inhibin B levels [13]. When estrogen concentrations are sustained at a threshold level (200 pg/ml) for approximately 50 h (reflecting a mature oocyte), central estrogen feedback then becomes stimulatory and pituitary luteinizing hormone (LH) is released to affect final maturation of the mature egg/follicle and, ultimately, ovulation.

There are many points in the ovulatory menstrual cycle that can be disrupted by elevated body weight/adiposity. Adipose tissue possesses aromatase and is, therefore, capable of converting peripheral androgens to estrogens (estrone). This chronic elevation of estrogen may prevent the late luteal FSH rise that is necessary to recruit a cohort of follicles for the subsequent cycle. In addition, the hypothalamic GnRH pulsatility can be altered, thereby preventing the proper ratios of FSH/LH secretion to produce a dominant follicle. Without proper stimulation and feedback loops between the brain and the ovary, the entire cohort remains immature and is not able to sustain the necessary estrogen level/duration that is necessary to trigger the LH surge for ovulation. To compound the dysfunction, the risk of insulin resistance/ hyperinsulinemia increases with excess body weight [14]. Insulin stimulates ovarian androgen production directly, but also indirectly by increasing LH secretion. Insulin also decreases hepatic production of sex hormone-binding globulin, with a net effect of increased circulating free androgens. Free androgens impair proper follicular development and can have undesired peripheral effects such as increased acne and impaired hair growth (both hirsutism and male patterned baldness). The situation further compounds itself because immature eggs/follicles eventually become atretic and join the stromal tissue of the ovary, where they begin to produce ovarian androgens and worsen the problem. Chronic elevation of LH and also leptin, a protein hormone which regulates satiety, can impair granulosa cells, and thus follicular, function [15, 16]. Insulin resistance and hyperandrogenism are arguably the central driving forces in the pathophysiology of Polycystic Ovary Syndrome (PCOS).

Polycystic Ovary Syndrome

PCOS, according to the original 1990 NIH criteria, represents a subset of anovulatory women who also suffer from hyperandrogenism [16]. The diagnosis can be made based on menstrual history and clinical or laboratory evidence of elevated androgens, after excluding other possible disorders (i.e., nonclassical congenital adrenal hyperplasia, hyperprolactinemia, hypercortisolism, thyroid dysfunction) [16]. Because these women suffer prolonged periods of anovulation, their ovaries become enlarged with excess stromal (thecal) mass from months of follicular atresia. Amongst the excess stroma, many immature follicles remain, giving the ovaries in this syndrome their "polycystic" appearance on ultrasound. As discussed above, theca cells in the increased stroma produce androgens in response to LH, and they seem to be more sensitive to LH in the ovaries of women with PCOS [14]. Though obesity is not a criterion for PCOS, adiposity contributes to anovulation, insulin resistance, and, therefore, hyperandrogenism, and a substantial majority of women with PCOS also struggle with their weight. Estimates suggest 30–80 % of women with PCOS are obese, depending on ethnicity [16]. Lean women with PCOS have more fat than non-PCOS women, matched for BMI, but they seem to have lesser degrees of hyperinsulinemia and hyperandrogenism and metabolic disturbance [14, 16]. Hyperandrogenism has been implicated in aggravation of visceral adiposity and insulin resistance [17, 18]. Hyperinsulinemia aggravates hyperandrogenism; the conditions propagate each other and the PCOS.

Significance

The importance of distinguishing women with PCOS from other women with anovulation is that PCOS women suffer greater metabolic consequences, owing to their concomitant insulin and androgen disruptions. In contrast to 1990 NIH criteria, the 2004 Rotterdam ESHRE PCOS definition requires manifestation of any two of the following three criteria: ovulatory dysfunction, hyperandrogenism, and/or polycystic ovaries on ultrasound [1]. Thus, Rotterdam criteria PCOS does not require hyperandrogenism. However, women without hyperandrogenism do not seem to manifest the same metabolic perturbations, prompting the Androgen Excess Society to reaffirm the necessity of hyperandrogenism and anovulation for inclusion in PCOS [19, 20].

Management

Due to the increased risk of metabolic consequences, women with PCOS should be screened annually with a fasting lipid panel (for hypercholesterolemia) and a 75-g, 2-h glucose tolerance test (for insulin resistance and glucose intolerance). Obese women with PCOS have 7–10 times the risk of developing insulin/glucose abnormalities as normal subjects [16]. Clearly, diet and exercise are essential to controlling cholesterol and insulin sensitivity and to combatting weight gain which increases the metabolic risks. Abdominal obesity and weight gain in the teenage years are risk factors for developing PCOS [21]. Many features of PCOS resolve following weight loss with bariatric surgery [22, 23].

In addition to diet and exercise directed at achieving and maintaining a healthy weight, therapy for women with PCOS must address their ovulatory dysfunction and hyperandrogenism. For women who are not trying to conceive, cycle regulation is best accomplished with a combined oral contraceptive pill (cOCP). In addition to cycle regulation, the estrogen in combined hormonal preparations stimulates hepatic SHBG production to decrease free androgens. For women who wish or need to avoid estrogen, progesterone-only options include cyclic progesterone administrations (not contraceptive), Implanon® (Merck Pharmaceuticals), Depo-Provera® (Pfizer), or a Mirena® (Bayer Healthcare) IUD. It is imperative that all anovulatory women avoid chronic unopposed endometrial estrogen exposure, which can lead to endometrial cancer. Progesterone-only methods prevent unopposed estrogen exposure, provide some cycle regulation, and can decrease LH-driven ovarian androgen production.

Hyperandrogenism is treated with cosmetic removal of existing hair growth and prevention of further hair follicle virilization with antiandrogen medications. As discussed above, estrogen-containing cOCPs increase SHBG to decrease free androgens. All hormonal contraceptives may decrease ovarian androgen production. Antiandrogen medications include spironolactone (a diuretic with actions against the androgen receptor) and inhibitors of 5-alpha reductase (blocks peripheral conversion of weak androgens to the more potent DHT). Antiandrogen medicines must be used in conjunction with contraception, due to their potential teratogenicity in male fetuses. Antiandrogens and cOCPs are, unfortunately, less efficacious in obese women, providing more reason to optimize weight in the treatment of PCOS [24, 25].

For women trying to conceive, anovulation is treated with oral (i.e., clomiphene citrate, letrozole) or injectable (FSH, LH) ovulation induction agents. As discussed above, antiandrogen medications are contraindicated in the periconception or pregnancy period.

The insulin-sensitizing agent, Metformin, is discussed below. It has been considered as an adjunct to ovulation induction strategies in women with PCOS, especially in women with demonstrated insulin or glucose abnormalities. Recent studies have suggested that some women with PCOS and insulin resistance have defects and/or deficiencies inositolphosphoglycan (IPG) mediators of insulin action. Myo-inositol (Pregnitude) is a supplement that has demonstrated improvements in insulin levels, cutaneous symptoms (acne, hair), and ovulation induction [26, 27].

Obesity and Male Fertility

There is concordance between partners for weight and BMI, amongst other cardiovascular risk factors [28, 29]. This finding may be due to assortative mating and/or shared environment, and two partners with excess adiposity can potentiate problems with sexuality and fertility. It is essential that research on weight/BMI and fertility include parameters for both partners.

Though frequency of sexual activity is similar in obese versus nonobese females, positional difficulties may affect frequency of intercourse in very obese women. Notably, orgasm and sexual satisfaction are negatively correlated with BMI in women and impotence and erectile dysfunction are increased in overweight and obese men [30]. Some of these effects may also be due to comorbidities, such as diabetes mellitus and depression [2].

Men with excess body weight often suffer impaired spermatogenesis. Three clinical studies have shown that obesity, as indicated by body mass index, is associated with decreased sperm concentration and motility [31–33]. Two of these studies involved males presenting with their partners for infertility treatment, and one was a study of young adult volunteers without an infertility diagnosis presenting for a routine medical examination. Significant correlations between reproductive hormone levels and BMI were observed in the study of normal volunteers [31]. From a hypothalamic-pituitary-gonadal standpoint, higher estrogen levels from adipose aromatization suppresses the LH and FSH drives to stimulate testicular testosterone and sperm production, respectively. Levels of sex hormone-binding globulin are often lowered by the estrogen so these men may demonstrate elevated free androgen levels, though testicular testosterone is suppressed, impairing spermatogenesis and, possibly, sexuality [31, 33].

At a local level, there may also be a deleterious impact from increased amounts of suprapubic and thigh fat, possibly from elevated scrotal temperatures. Improved semen quality and pregnancy rates have been reported after scrotal/suprapubic lipectomy, though this is not routinely employed [34, 35].

Similar to women, weight loss appears to benefit male fertility, with improvements in semen parameters. A 2009 study examined the relationship between BMI and reproductive hormones in obese men undergoing Roux-en-Y gastric bypass surgery and discovered that BMI correlated positively with estradiol and negatively with testosterone. Further, estradiol decreased and testosterone increased with significant postoperative weight loss. Sexual quality of life was also improved with weight loss [35]. Though one case series from Italy reported six patients who presented with secondary infertility due to nonobstructive azoospermia following Roux-en-Y gastric bypass surgery, other research studies suggest that obesity is associated with diminished sperm function and that weight loss might improve fertility [35, 36].

Infertility Treatment for the Obese Female Patient

Infertility treatment is more successful for women who are closer to their ideal body weight. For anovulatory patients, rates of both ovulation and conception with the oral ovulation induction agent clomiphene citrate are higher at lower BMIs [8]. After ovulation induction is successful, live birth rates are higher for nonobese women [8].

During in vitro fertilization (IVF) cycles, women who have elevated body weights require more medications for a longer duration and still suffer more cancellations, fewer eggs retrieved, fewer embryos transferred, lower pregnancy rates, and more miscarriages [37].

The obstetrical morbidities associated with elevated body weight are discussed elsewhere in this book but include higher rates of miscarriage, birth defects, gestational diabetes, preeclampsia, cesarean section, and still birth [37–39]. These increased risks hold true for overweight and obese women after conception with IVF [40].

Both the American Congress of Obstetricians and Gynecologists [41] and the American Society for Reproductive Medicine [1] advocate for achieving a healthy weight/BMI prior to conception [1, 41]. Advocates of the Barker hypothesis stress the impact of the in-utero environment on long-term health status and outcomes, and the lifetime consequences of obesity during pregnancy which include metabolic sequelae, that predispose the next generation to obesity and diabetes [42].

Though "normal" BMI is established as 19.5–24.9, there is no current consensus on a BMI cutoff for conception. Many independent clinics have established cutoffs for fertility treatment but, with weight problems being nearly ubiquitous, many practitioners encounter the ethical dilemma of delaying fertility treatment in a woman with dwindling ovarian reserve. As obesity and advanced maternal age may compound the risk for the same obstetrical morbidities, it seems counterintuitive to advocate pursuit of conception prior to weight loss in these women, but it may be construed as cruel to deny them an opportunity to conceive with their own oocytes.

Achieving a "normal" weight/BMI is a clear component of optimizing preconception health and should be included in any preconceptual counseling. Some women are very obese and may not ever achieve a BMI <25; in those populations, some have advocated that a BMI <35 be the target [1].

Strategies for Weight Loss

The formula for weight loss is simple: consume fewer calories than are needed to support daily activity. Operationalizing this strategy is difficult, as daily attention to caloric restriction and increased activity represents a huge life change for many individuals. Though tedious and initially awkward, it can (and must!) be done – without implementation of regular exercise, the basal metabolic rate declines with age (~2 %/decade over age 18) (acefitness.org). Everyone must incorporate diet and exercise to maintain a healthy weight; individuals who are overweight must initially restrict more aggressively to lose excess weight.

Diet

To a degree, the exact composition of the diet does not seem to be as important as the overall caloric restriction. Studies have shown low-carbohydrate and low-fat diets to achieve equivalent weight loss at 1 year and equivalent decreases in insulin, CRP, and cholesterol. One exception to this statement may be women with PCOS or individuals with insulin resistance, glucose intolerance, or "prediabetes" – in this case, a diet that pays attention to the glycemic index can be useful. The glycemic index is an objective way to measure a food's effect on blood sugar; foods with higher glycemic index scores raise blood sugar more abruptly, creating "spikes" and subsequent "crashes." Both ends of the spectrum can be unpleasant and may make a diet harder to follow. Complex carbohydrates and proteins have a lower glycemic index (under 55) meaning that they have a slower, steadier effect on blood glucose and insulin levels [43]. Low glycemic index translates into fewer blood glucose peaks and valleys, fewer surges in insulin demands, and fewer "shaky" episodes where the dieter may run to the closest vending machine for a quick glucose fix.

Sadly, most diets fail. The average weight regained by dieters is 60–85 % at 3 years and 75–120 % by 5 years [1]. The reason for this failure is that most diets are short-term plans and are not sustainable lifestyle changes. As discussed above, aging brings a predictable decrease in basal metabolic rate, making progressive caloric restriction and regular exercise vital to maintaining a healthy weight. It is essential for the individual dieter to embrace a long-term plan; extreme restriction is typically not sustainable.

A healthy rate of weight loss should not exceed 1–2 lb/week. One method to calculate daily caloric intake is to compute the resting metabolic rate (RMR) or the number of calories required to keep the body's basic functions running on a daily basis; RMR does not take into account additional exercise. Subtracting 500 cal from RMR will give an approximate daily caloric limit for losing 1–2 lb/week.

Resources permitting, it is helpful for the dieter to seek help from a nutritionist or endocrinologist. These professionals can help to design meal plans and calorie counts that take into account the individual dieter's goals, food preferences/cravings, and past experiences. Studies show that dieters in organized programs fare better [44].

Exercise

Physical activity has many benefits; not only does it reliably improve cardiovascular health but it is an essential adjunct to diet for individuals pursuing weight loss (AHA). Exercise builds upon the RMR to burn more calories and assist in weight loss. Additionally, exercise has proven effects on improving insulin sensitivity and thus glucose utilization [14]. Improvements in insulin sensitivity may well improve chances for ovulation.

The American Heart Association (AHA) recommends moderate activity for 150 min/week or vigorous activity for 75 min/week. ACOG echoes the merits of moderate exercise, even for women with uncomplicated pregnancies, recommending 30–45 min on most, if not all, days [41]. There is mounting evidence that interval training, incorporating bursts of increased exertion upon a longer period of moderate exertion, may be superior to moderate activity in improving both fitness and cardiovascular profiles [45].

As with dieting, there is an advantage to seeking out professional advice from a trainer or a staff member at a local gym/fitness center. At the very least, exercising with another person may improve compliance.

Medications

There are pharmaceutical preparations available for individuals who do not achieve adequate weight loss after 6 months of diet and exercise. Medical interventions may be reserved for those with a BMI ≥ 30 or ≥ 27 with comorbidities. On average, users demonstrate loss of an additional 2–4 kg over 7–48 weeks, representing a broad spectrum of results [46]. It must be stressed that adjunctive treatments, including medicines, must be combined with diet and regular exercise.

Sympathomimetics, i.e., Phentermine (Adipex) or Diethylpropion (Anorex, Tenuate)

These are norepinephrine stimulant and reuptake inhibitors that function as appetite suppressants. They are to be used with caution in cardiovascular disease patients and pregnancy (Class C). Patients should have regular blood pressure and weight checks. Studies have shown loss of an additional 3.6 kg/6 months vs. placebo [46].

Anti-absorptives, i.e., Orlistat (Xenical, Alli)

These are a derivative of natural inhibitor of pancreatic lipases shown to block intestinal fat absorption by 30 %. As a result, they also block the fat-soluble vitamins (ADEK). These should not be used for malabsorption or cholestasis patients. Gastrointestinal (GI) side effects, though rare, can affect the liver and kidney. Studies have shown loss of an additional 2.9 kg/12 months vs. placebo and, possibly, improved lipids and Hemoglobin A1C levels [46].

Insulin Sensitizers (Metformin/Glucophage)

This is a biguanide that inhibits hepatic glucose production and increases peripheral tissue insulin sensitivity. It often has GI side effects (diarrhea), though newer extended release preparations seem to be better tolerated. Studies have shown loss of an additional 1–2 kg more than placebo so this should not be used primarily as a weight-loss drug but more as an adjunct to exercise for patients with insulin resistance [47].

Myo-inositol (Pregnitude)

As discussed above, this medication may mediate insulin actions, thereby reducing serum insulin and testosterone levels, treating cutaneous disorders associated with hyperandrogenism (hair, acne) and enhancing ovulation [26, 27]. Though Metformin is currently the first-line medication for

PCOS patients with insulin resistance, Myo-inositol appears to be a useful alternative, particularly for patients who cannot tolerate Metformin.

Androgen-Reducing Medications

As discussed above, these may be a critical adjunct to improving insulin sensitivity in women with hyperandrogenism. Spironolactone is a diuretic with antagonistic effects on the androgen receptor. Inhibitors of 5-alpha reductase block the conversion of weak androgens to the more potent DHT, which mediates all virilizing effects on hair follicles and sebaceous units. As discussed, these must be used with contraception.

Antidepressants (SSRIs), Antiepileptics

These categories of medications have demonstrated weight loss for some patients in trials for their primary indications. However, some patients have demonstrated weight gain while on these medicines so they should not be prescribed for weight loss [1].

Ephedra/Ephedrine (Ma Huang)

Sold as an herbal supplement over the counter, this compound is a sympathomimetic that results in increased thermogenesis and acts as an appetite suppressant. Studies have shown loss of only an additional 0.6–1 kg weight per month, when compared to placebo, and this compound carries several side effect risks, including cardiovascular, GI, central nervous system, and psychiatric. It is, therefore, not recommended for weight loss [48].

Surgery

Bariatric (weight loss) surgery, first introduced in the 1960s, is recognized as the most effective treatment for Class 3 obesity [49]. It is typically reserved for patients with a BMI ≥40 or ≥35 with comorbidities, who have failed other interventions. Preoperative treatment includes intensive screening and demonstrating ability to comply with aggressive caloric restriction. There are two general categories of bariatric surgery: restrictive and malabsorptive. The former includes banding procedures and is a reversible way of decreasing the size of the stomach and increasing satiety. The latter is often a permanent anatomic alteration that results in a smaller stomach and, often, a marked reduction in absorptive intestinal surface. Both types of surgery produce dramatic weight loss postoperatively, though the malabsorptive procedures seem to result in greater total weight loss, longer sustained weight loss, and also, more nutritional deficits and considerations.

The goal of bariatric surgery is to improve obesity and related conditions. The mortality rate is less than 1 %, and it does seem to improve high blood pressure, diabetes, cholesterol, and sleep apnea. As mentioned above, the balance of evidence seems to support its role in improving both male and female fertility, including the manifestations of PCOS [1]. Eighty percent of bariatric surgery patients are female and, as the obstetrical and gynecologic community cares for more women after surgery, guidelines have been generated. Currently, it is recommended to defer pregnancy for 1 year postoperatively, as the majority of weight loss occurs during this time frame. Careful attention must be paid to iron, folate, B12, calcium, and the fat-soluble vitamins (ADEK) [49, 50]. Limited data from observational studies suggest that, after surgery-induced weight reduction, women enjoy a reduction of gestational diabetes mellitus and gestational hypertensive disorders when compared to their obese counterparts. Further research is needed on macrosomia, growth restriction, and preterm birth [50].

Future Directions

Elevated body weight affects the health, longevity, and fertility of both men and women. The burgeoning obesity pandemic threatens to shorten the life expectancy and fecundity of our species. In addition to ongoing research on the exact pathophysiology underlying obesity and its comorbid conditions, future efforts should focus on patient education and preventative health measures directed at achieving healthier body weights.

Leading medical organizations have instructed providers to assess patient weight and triage overweight and obese patients to treatment [51]. Studies have shown that patients who receive advice to lose weight are nearly three times more likely to report trying to lose weight than those who do not, thus underscoring the role of the healthcare provider as the impetus for change [52]. Unfortunately, less than half of obese adults in the USA report weight loss counseling by their care provider [52]. A recent survey found that women's healthcare providers neglect to counsel overweight and obese patients, even when they correctly recognize them as overweight/obese and acknowledge that they need counseling. The leading barrier to counseling was time constraints during the visit [53].

The United States Preventative Services Task Force concluded that physician counseling alone was only modestly effective but results could be improved by adding weight loss education and support [51]. Therefore, physicians and healthcare providers must identify women who are overweight and triage them to specialists in diet, exercise, psychological counseling, and bariatric surgery. Cultivating a lattice of physician extenders to help with weight loss will alleviate time pressures on the primary provider and improve the specialized quality of treatment and counseling. The critical step in this process is that the primary provider *must* communicate to the patient that they are overweight, identify weight loss as a priority, and provide the referral to an expert in weight reduction. If the primary provider abdicates this responsibility (and simply treats the sequelae of unchecked weight gain), the obesity epidemic will continue to claim the health and longevity of our friends and family.

It is quite possible that we need a paradigm shift towards treating obesity as an addiction, akin to other eating disorders. Intensive therapy and/or inpatient programs are likely necessary for severe and refractory cases of obesity. In addition, financial incentives have been shown to maintain weight loss group attendance so it may be helpful to institute token economies via insurance premium discounts for healthy behaviors [54–56].

Healthcare practitioners who see reproductive-aged women are the gatekeepers of maternal-fetal health. They must recognize and discuss the effects of excess body weight on reproduction and obstetrical morbidity and facilitate weight loss before pregnancy to prevent perpetuation of the obesity epidemic and its threat to fertility, wellness, and longevity.

References

1. Rotterdam ESHRE/ASRM-Sponsored PCOS Consensus Workshop Group. Revised 2003 consensus on diagnostic criteria and long-term health risks related to polycystic ovary syndrome (PCOS). Hum Reprod. 2004;19(1):41–7.
2. Centers for Disease Control and Prevention. Where are United States ART clinics located, how many ART cycles did they perform in 2009, and how many infants were born from these ART cycles? http://www.cdc.gov/art/ART2009/section1.html. Accessed on 22 Sep 2013.
3. International Red Cross. Obesity in the Background of Malnutrition. http://www.ifrc.org/. Accessed on 22 Sep 2013.
4. Manson JE, et al. Body weight and mortality among women. N Engl J Med. 1995;333(11):677–85.
5. Williamson DF, et al. Prospective study of intentional weight loss and mortality in never-smoking overweight US white women aged 40–64 years. Am J Epidemiol. 1995;141(12):1128–41.
6. Watkins ML, et al. Maternal obesity and risk for birth defects. Pediatrics. 2003;111(5 Pt 2):1152–8.
7. Howe G, et al. Effects of age, cigarette smoking, and other factors on fertility: findings in a large prospective study. Br Med J (Clin Res Ed). 1985;290(6483):1697–700.
8. Legro RS, et al. Clomiphene, metformin, or both for infertility in the polycystic ovary syndrome. N Engl J Med. 2007;356(6):551–66.
9. Rich-Edwards JW, et al. Adolescent body mass index and infertility caused by ovulatory disorder. Am J Obstet Gynecol. 1994;171(1):171–7.

10. Clark AM, et al. Weight loss results in significant improvement in pregnancy and ovulation rates in anovulatory obese women. Hum Reprod. 1995;10(10):2705–12.
11. Zaadstra BM, et al. Fat and female fecundity: prospective study of effect of body fat distribution on conception rates. BMJ. 1993;306(6876):484–7.
12. van der Steeg JW, et al. Obesity affects spontaneous pregnancy chances in subfertile, ovulatory women. Hum Reprod. 2008;23(2):324–8.
13. Chikazawa K, Araki S, Tamada T. Morphological and endocrinological studies on follicular development during the human menstrual cycle. J Clin Endocrinol Metab. 1986;62(2):305–13.
14. Legro RS. Obesity and PCOS: implications for diagnosis and treatment. Semin Reprod Med. 2012;30(6):496–506.
15. Jungheim ES, Moley KH. Current knowledge of obesity's effects in the pre- and periconceptional periods and avenues for future research. Am J Obstet Gynecol. 2010;203(6):525–30.
16. Vrbikova J, Hainer V. Obesity and polycystic ovary syndrome. Obes Facts. 2009;2(1):26–35.
17. Elbers JM, et al. Effects of sex steroids on components of the insulin resistance syndrome in transsexual subjects. Clin Endocrinol (Oxf). 2003;58(5):562–71.
18. Dahlgren E, et al. Effects of two antiandrogen treatments on hirsutism and insulin sensitivity in women with polycystic ovary syndrome. Hum Reprod. 1998;13(10):2706–11.
19. Barber TM, et al. Metabolic characteristics of women with polycystic ovaries and oligo-amenorrhoea but normal androgen levels: implications for the management of polycystic ovary syndrome. Clin Endocrinol (Oxf). 2007;66(4):513–7.
20. Azziz R, et al. Positions statement: criteria for defining polycystic ovary syndrome as a predominantly hyperandrogenic syndrome: an Androgen Excess Society guideline. J Clin Endocrinol Metab. 2006;91(11):4237–45.
21. Laitinen J, et al. Body size from birth to adulthood as a predictor of self-reported polycystic ovary syndrome symptoms. Int J Obes Relat Metab Disord. 2003;27(6):710–5.
22. Escobar-Morreale HF, et al. The polycystic ovary syndrome associated with morbid obesity may resolve after weight loss induced by bariatric surgery. J Clin Endocrinol Metab. 2005;90(12):6364–9.
23. Hezelgrave NL, Oteng-Ntim E. Pregnancy after bariatric surgery: a review. J Obes. 2011;2011:501939.
24. Koulouri O, Conway GS. A systematic review of commonly used medical treatments for hirsutism in women. Clin Endocrinol (Oxf). 2008;68(5):800–5.

25. Cibula D, Hill M, Fanta M, Sindelka G, Zivny J. Does obesity diminish the positive effect of oral contraceptive treatment on hyperandrogenism in women with polycystic ovary syndrome? Hum Reprod. 2001;16:940–4.
26. Zacche MM, et al. Efficacy of myo-inositol in the treatment of cutaneous disorders in young women with polycystic ovary syndrome. Gynecol Endocrinol. 2009;25(8):508–13.
27. Papaleo E, et al. Myo-inositol in patients with polycystic ovary syndrome: a novel method for ovulation induction. Gynecol Endocrinol. 2007;23(12):700–3.
28. Speakman JR, et al. Assortative mating for obesity. Am J Clin Nutr. 2007;86(2):316–23.
29. Di Castelnuovo A, Quacquaruccio G, Donati MB, de Gaetano G, Iacoviello L. Spousal concordance for major coronary risk factors: a systematic review and meta-analysis. Am J Epidemiol. 2009;169(1):1–8.
30. Yaylali GF, Tekekoglu S, Akin F. Sexual dysfunction in obese and overweight women. Int J Impot Res. 2010;22(4):220–6.
31. Jensen TK, et al. Body mass index in relation to semen quality and reproductive hormones among 1,558 Danish men. Fertil Steril. 2004;82(4):863–70.
32. Koloszar S, et al. Effect of body weight on sperm concentration in normozoospermic males. Arch Androl. 2005;51(4):299–304.
33. Kort HI, et al. Impact of body mass index values on sperm quantity and quality. J Androl. 2006;27(3):450–2.
34. Shafik A, Olfat S. Lipectomy in the treatment of scrotal lipomatosis. Br J Urol. 1981;53(1):55–61.
35. Hammoud A, et al. Effect of Roux-en-Y gastric bypass surgery on the sex steroids and quality of life in obese men. J Clin Endocrinol Metab. 2009;94(4):1329–32.
36. di Frega AS, et al. Secondary male factor infertility after Roux-en-Y gastric bypass for morbid obesity: case report. Hum Reprod. 2005;20(4):997–8.
37. Fedorcsak P, et al. Impact of overweight and underweight on assisted reproduction treatment. Hum Reprod. 2004;19(11):2523–8.
38. Wang JX, Davies M, Norman RJ. Body mass and probability of pregnancy during assisted reproduction treatment: retrospective study. BMJ. 2000;321(7272):1320–1.
39. Marshall NE, Spong CY. Obesity, pregnancy complications, and birth outcomes. Semin Reprod Med. 2012;30(6):465–71.
40. Dokras A, et al. Obstetric outcomes after in vitro fertilization in obese and morbidly obese women. Obstet Gynecol. 2006;108(1):61–9.
41. ACOG Committee Obstetric Practice. ACOG Committee opinion. Number 267, January 2002 exercise during pregnancy and the postpartum period. Obstet Gynecol. 2002;99(1):171–3.

42. Frias AE, Grove KL. Obesity: a transgenerational problem linked to nutrition during pregnancy. Semin Reprod Med. 2012;30(6):472–8.
43. Foster-Powell K, Holt SH, Brand-Miller JC. International table of glycemic index and glycemic load values: 2002. Am J Clin Nutr. 2002;76(1):5–56.
44. Wadden TA, Foster GD. Behavioral treatment of obesity. Med Clin North Am. 2000;84(2):441–61. vii.
45. Kessler HS, Sisson SB, Short KR. The potential for high-intensity interval training to reduce cardiometabolic disease risk. Sports Med. 2012;42(6):489–509.
46. Li Z, et al. Meta-analysis: pharmacologic treatment of obesity. Ann Intern Med. 2005;142(7):532–46.
47. Fontbonne A, et al. The effect of metformin on the metabolic abnormalities associated with upper-body fat distribution. BIGPRO Study Group. Diabetes Care. 1996;19(9):920–6.
48. Shekelle P, et al. Ephedra and ephedrine for weight loss and athletic performance enhancement: clinical efficacy and side effects. Evid Rep Technol Assess (Summ). 2003;(76):1–4.
49. American College of Obstetricians and Gynecologists. ACOG practice bulletin no. 105: bariatric surgery and pregnancy. Obstet Gynecol. 2009;113(6):1405–13.
50. Hezelgrave NL, Oteng-Ntim E. Pregnancy after bariatric surgery: a review. J Obes. 2011;2011:1–5.
51. McTigue KM, et al. Screening and interventions for obesity in adults: summary of the evidence for the U.S. Preventive Services Task Force. Ann Intern Med. 2003;139(11):933–49.
52. Galuska DA, et al. Are health care professionals advising obese patients to lose weight? JAMA. 1999;282(16):1576–8.
53. Evans-Hoeker E, Calhoun KC, Mersereau JE. Healthcare provider accuracy at estimating Women's BMI and intent to provide counseling based on appearance alone. Obesity (Expected publication, Dec 2013).
54. Sperduto WA, O'Brien RM. Effects of cash deposits on attendance and weight loss in a large-scale clinical program for obesity. Psychol Rep. 1983;52(1):261–2.
55. Petry NM, et al. A low-cost reinforcement procedure improves short-term weight loss outcomes. Am J Med. 2011;124(11):1082–5.
56. Volpp KG, et al. Financial incentive-based approaches for weight loss: a randomized trial. JAMA. 2008;300(22):2631–7.

Chapter 3
Preconception and Pregnancy Care in Overweight or Obese Woman

Catherine Takacs Witkop

> *I view preconception care as empowering women, to give them control over their pregnancy outcomes.*
> Peter M. Bernstein, Medscape July 8, 2010

Abstract Overweight and obesity are associated with multiple maternal and fetal complications, including gestational diabetes mellitus, hypertensive disorders of pregnancy, macrosomia (infant weighing more than 4,000 g), and cesarean delivery. The preconception period is a critical time frame to address overweight and obesity in reproductive-aged women. Preconception care should include education about the effect of obesity on pregnancy outcomes, long-term health of the offspring, clinical evaluation for comorbid conditions, assessment of the patient's readiness for change, and guidance on safe and effective interventions to achieve a healthy weight prior to conception. Current gaps in our knowledge include the identification of the most effective lifestyle strategies to promote a healthy weight prior to pregnancy and the

---

C.T. Witkop, MD, MPH
Department of Obstetrics/Gynecology
and Preventive Medicine, Uniformed Services University
of the Health Sciences, Bethesda, MD, USA
e-mail: cwitkop@gmail.com

W. Nicholson, K. Baptiste-Roberts (eds.),
Obesity During Pregnancy in Clinical Practice,
DOI 10.1007/978-1-4471-2831-1_3,
© Springer-Verlag London 2014

development of policies to improve the dissemination of patient-centered preconception care.

Keywords Preconception care • Overweight • Obese • Pregnancy outcomes • Lifestyle modification • Behavioral counseling

> **Key Points**
> - All reproductive-aged women should be screened for obesity by providers using body mass index (BMI).
> - Providing overweight and obese women with evidence-based lifestyle modifications can help to improve health status prior to conception.
> - Screening for obesity-related conditions including diabetes and dyslipidemia is an important step to improve a woman's health before conception.
> - Motivational interviewing, guidance on nutrition and physical activity, and patient activation tools during the preconception phase help women achieve a healthy lifestyle before pregnancy.

Introduction

Transitioning women from the preconception phase to the pregnancy phase of their lives has been an incredible challenge for providers and public health officials. The life-course model, developed by Lu and Halfon, focuses on the medical and psychosocial factors that affect a woman's health from birth until the time she conceives. The *preconception period* is an "important teachable moment" and represents a unique opportunity [1] to educate overweight and obese women about achieving a healthy weight before conception. Preconception care is defined as a set of interventions that aim to identify and modify behavioral and social risks to a woman's health or pregnancy outcomes through prevention and management [2]. If a woman is overweight or obese and contemplating pregnancy, it is incumbent upon her provider to counsel her about the potential complications of obesity on pregnancy outcomes and the health of her offspring. Such efforts can improve maternal health before pregnancy, reduce infant mortality, and lower the risk of metabolic alterations or fetal programming that can predispose to childhood obesity. In this chapter, we summarize the key clinical and behavioral components of counseling for obesity during the preconception period. These components include (1) discussion of maternal and fetal complications, (2) assessment of readiness for behavioral change, (3) guidance on safe and effective lifestyle modifications that can help women achieve weight loss prior to pregnancy, and (4) provision of information on what interventions may be necessary during pregnancy if she is overweight or obese at the time of conception. Additionally, this chapter provides insight on clinical conditions that commonly occur in the women who are overweight or obese at the time of conception, including bariatric surgery, gestational diabetes mellitus, and hypertension. The impact of obesity in polycystic ovarian syndrome and subfertility is also discussed.

Potential Risks for the Overweight or Obese Pregnant Woman

Women who are classified as obese (Table 3.1) are at increased risk for maternal and fetal complications during pregnancy [3]. Although statistics alone are not typically enough to motivate individuals to achieve significant behavioral change, it is important for women to receive accurate and timely information during the preconception visit. In a large prospective multicenter study, obese women were 2.5 times more likely than women with BMI under 30 to

Table 3.1 Institute of Medicine weight gain in pregnancy guidelines

Prepregnancy BMI	BMI (kg/m^2)	Recommended total weight gain range (lb)	Rates of weight gain (2nd and 3rd trimester) (mean range in lb/week)
Underweight	<18.5	28–40	1 (1–3)
Normal weight	18.5–24.9	25–35	1 (.8–1)
Overweight	25.0–29.9	15–25	0.6 (0.5–0.7)
Obese (includes all classes)	≥30.0	11–20	0.5 (0.4–0.6)

From Rasmussen et al. [3]

develop gestational hypertension; morbidly obese women were 3.2 times more likely [4, 5]. Obese and morbidly obese women were also 1.6 and 3.3 times, respectively, more likely to develop preeclampsia than their counterparts who were of normal weight [5]. Obese women are also at increased risk for gestational diabetes, and when obese women develop gestational diabetes, they are at increased risk for additional complications. For these reasons, women with morbid obesity are among those considered high enough risk to justify early screening for gestational diabetes (other risk factors include strong family history of type 2 diabetes, history of GDM, impaired glucose metabolism, or glucosuria) [6]. They should be screened as early as feasible and should be repeated at 24–28 weeks if the first screen is negative. Obese women are also at increased risk of labor complications, including macrosomia and cesarean delivery, which require ongoing conservations with their clinicians and shared decision-making in planning for labor and delivery (Chap. 5).

Guidelines for Perinatal Care, issued by both the American College of Obstetricians and Gynecologists

(ACOG) and the American Academy of Pediatrics (AAP), recommends that all health encounters during a woman's reproductive years include counseling to improve future pregnancy outcomes [7]. The Centers for Disease Control and Prevention (CDC) recommends that all primary care clinicians integrate preconception counseling into every health-care encounter [8]. Given the fact that overweight and obesity can have such negative impacts on the health of a woman and her child, and understanding that about 50 % of pregnancies in the USA are unplanned, preconception care should occur during every visit with an overweight or obese woman.

Approaching the Patient Who Is Overweight or Obese

Because of the social stigma attached to overweight and obesity, diagnosis and discussion may need to be handled with greater tact than a discussion about hypertension, but it does need to happen. Much research has focused on the impact of using appropriate terminology when discussing overweight and obesity with patients [9]. What appears to be consistent is that women do not respond in a consistent way to descriptors of their weight. Using terminology that describes the impact of weight on health appears to be acceptable to patients, and this approach may be the most comfortable. In the end, however, as long as derogatory language is not used, any discussion is better than ignoring the topic altogether. Cultural competency must also play a role in the discussion of weight with patients. Different cultures have varying attitudes toward overweight, so the provider may be making recommendations that are counter to a patient's perspective. Understanding the patient's background, home environment, stressors, and socioeconomic status is important before the provider embarks on recommendations to change behavior.

Clinical Assessment at the Health Visit

Body Mass Index

BMI (Table 3.1) [3] should be calculated at each health visit and reviewed as a vital sign in the same fashion as blood pressure is addressed. BMI is calculated as

$$\frac{Weight\,(kilograms)}{Height\,(meters\,squared)}$$

Electronic medical records can often be enabled to calculate BMI automatically when height and weight are entered. A standard workflow in which actual weight is measured at each visit and BMI is calculated ensures providers have this additional "vital sign."

Waist Circumference and Waist to Hip Ratio

Because central or abdominal obesity is associated with cardiovascular disease and death, waist circumference or waist to hip ratio (WHR) can be another measure to include in a preconception visit [9]. There are no specific prenatal guidelines related to these other measures of adiposity. However, these measures can provide long-term guidance about the risk of diabetes and cardiovascular disease.

Type 2 Diabetes and Lipid Screening

Screening for diabetes and dyslipidemia can be considered for the overweight or obese woman. The diagnosis of type 2 diabetes is important for pregnancy care. Type 2 diabetes is associated with a threefold increase in the prevalence of birth defects, but this risk can be reduced with proper management of diabetes before conception [10, 11]. Hemoglobin A1C levels should be in the lower range of normal (<6.1 %) prior to conception [10]. If a woman is newly diagnosed during the preconception visit, she will need a comprehensive medical evaluation with a primary care clinician or endocrinologist and referred for ophthalmic evaluation. A lipid panel would be indicated if the diagnosis of diabetes is made and may also been performed in the overweight or obese woman without diabetes. While dyslipidemia may not change obstetrical management, medications for lipid management are contraindicated in women who are attempting pregnancy, those who are currently pregnant, and lactating women. Therefore, obese women with abnormal lipids will need to be aware of the contraindications of medical therapy during the preconception and perinatal periods.

Folic Acid Supplementation

All reproductive-aged women are encouraged to take a 4 mcg daily dose of folic acid before pregnancy and at least through the first 4 weeks of pregnancy. Women who are obese have been found to have an increased risk for neural tube defects compared to women in a normal BMI range [12], but studies have not clearly demonstrated that an increased dose of folic acid would be appropriate for this population. At the very least, educating the patient about this additional risk to her offspring as a result of maternal obesity might offer additional motivation to take the recommended dose of preconception folic acid and to achieve a healthy weight before conception.

Screening for Obesity in Adults

The US Preventive Services Task Force (USPSTF) recommends screening all adults for obesity and states that clinicians should offer or refer patients with a BMI of 30 mg/m^2 or greater to intensive, multicomponent behavioral interventions [13]. The American College of Preventive Medicine

(ACPM) has also issued a practice statement about recommended counseling for overweight adults. Like most other organizations, the ACPM does not endorse any specific behavioral therapy or pharmacotherapy, but instead recommends individualized programs based on the available evidence [14]. There are two components to successful behavioral interventions. The first is to understand the relative effectiveness of different programs and recommend the intervention most likely to be successful for a given patient. The second is to engage the patient in a manner that will most likely lead to an activated patient who is likely to change her behavior.

Interventions for Lifestyle Modifications

Interventions for lifestyle modification have been shown time and again to be successful in reaching clinically relevant outcomes in diverse groups of women. For example, three large randomized controlled clinical trials of primary prevention of type 2 diabetes in three different countries have all demonstrated that maintenance of 3–5 kg (7–10 lb) of weight loss through diet and physical activity reduced the incidence of type 2 diabetes in high-risk individuals by 40–60 % over 3–4 years [15–17]. The largest study randomized over 3,000 patients to control, use of metformin, or lifestyle intervention (achieve and maintain 7 % or greater weight loss through a low-calorie, low-fat diet and at least 150 min of moderate physical activity per week) [17]. Over 3 years, the lifestyle intervention group lost an average of 5.6 kg, and the incidence of diabetes was reduced by 58 % [17]. While the outcomes in these studies were focused on prevention of diabetes, they demonstrated that lifestyle modification was indeed a worthwhile intervention in high-risk women. In a systematic review, Powell et al. reviewed and identified nine lifestyle modification trials. In the successful trials, weekly interventions resulted in the greatest weight reduction among participants, but after the initial intensive phase, monthly or bimonthly contact appeared to maintain 60–80 % of the initial weight loss [18].

The evidence does demonstrate that lifestyle modification works, but it is certainly not without significant challenges. It is important, therefore, to utilize tools that have been demonstrated to facilitate behavioral change. Understanding models of behavior change and implementing patient activation tools can help women's health providers as they care for overweight and obese women.

Models of Behavioral Change

Providers of women's health care can apply social cognitive theory (SCT) to behavioral change counseling. SCT has been employed as the theoretical basis for a multitude of behavioral interventions. It supposes that three factors—environment, person, and behavior—interact and a change in one affects the other two [19]. A provider may be limited in the ability to alter the patient's physical or social environment, but can make recommendations on how the patient can modify her surroundings or with whom she interacts. The "person" variables include behavioral capability (knowledge and skills to engage in the behavior), outcomes expectancies, observational learning, and perceived self-efficacy. Having the patient set realistic weight loss goals can increase perceived self-efficacy early on in the process. The transtheoretical model is the foundation of many of the behavioral interventions used in clinical medicine, and it assumes that all individuals transition through five stages of change in the process of altering a behavior: *precontemplation, contemplation, preparation, action, and maintenance* (Table 3.2) [20]. These models are important and useful, but successful behavioral change also requires activated patients. Motivational interviewing is one tool to achieve that goal.

Motivational Interviewing

The goal of motivational interviewing (MI), first described by William Miller in 1983, is to use reflective listening and other tools to allow the patient to move through stages of change as described in the TTP [21]. The following are the key points of motivational interviewing [22]:

TABLE 3.2 Applying the transtheoretical model (TTM)

Stage of change	Description of patient	Ways to assist patient
Precontemplation	No plans to change behavior(s)	Motivational interviewing (can be used throughout)
	Does not believe behavior leads to adverse health outcomes	Ask patient's permission to discuss behavior/issues
Contemplation	May begin to understand relationship between behavior and adverse consequences on her health	Ensure patient has knowledge and skills to change behavior
		Address doubts in self-efficacy
Preparation	Commits to behavior change	Encourage family/friend involvement
	Makes concrete, actionable plans	Help her recognize potential obstacles
		Advise her that relapses may occur
Action	Makes change in lifestyle or acquires healthy new behaviors	Provide encouragement
		If relapse, identify ways to reduce risk of future relapse (avoid unhealthy triggers)
Maintenance	Continues to implement lifestyle change	Ongoing evaluation, though less frequent
	Works to prevent relapse	Provide encouragement
		Demonstrate empathy

Modified from Prochaska and Velicer [20]

1. Motivation to change is elicited from the client.
2. It is the patient's task to articulate and resolve her ambivalence about the behavior.

3. Direct persuasion is not an effective method for resolving the ambivalence.
4. The counseling style is quiet and eliciting.
5. The provider is directive in helping the patient examine and resolve ambivalence.
6. Readiness to change is a fluctuating product of interpersonal interaction.
7. The therapeutic relationship is more like a partnership than expert/recipient roles.

The key skills can be summarized by the OARS acronym: (1) open-ended questions, (2) affirm, (3) reflect, and (4) summarize.

In a meta-analysis of 72 RCTs, motivational interviewing had a significant and clinically relevant effect in changing behaviors in about 75 % of the studies [23]. MI has been shown to be effective in studies of smoking cessation, unhealthy alcohol and drug use, and high-risk sexual behaviors [24]. It has also been studied in overweight and obesity. In an observational study of 40 primary care physicians, examining 461 of their provider-patient encounters, investigators found that use of motivational interviewing techniques during recorded patient visits was associated with statistically significant increases in amount of weight lost 3 months after the encounter [25]. Such techniques included verbalizing an understanding of the patient's perspective, understanding motivation or lack of motivation, helping patients to find their own solutions and their own internal motivation to change, and assuring the patient that he or she has freedom to change. Other behaviors consistent with MI included praising, collaborating, and evoking "change statements" from patients [25].

These studies are promising, but future studies evaluating the use of motivational interviewing and other techniques that actively engage patients are needed [26]. Training providers in the use of MI and other such patient activation techniques and studying the effects via prospective randomized controlled trials can help determine if such provider tools improve effectiveness of lifestyle modification counseling. ACOG has recommended that providers understand and utilize MI with their patients in the appropriate clinical settings [27]. Not only is MI effective in certain scenarios but it also is very likely to improve the patient-provider relationship and provide useful insight into a patient's successes and obstacles related to behavioral change.

Providing Tools for Preconception Weight Loss in Clinical Practice

Successful weight loss programs include setting of goals, monitoring, modification of the environment, cognitive restructuring, and setting plans to avoid relapse [28]. Referring the patient for individual or small group behavioral treatment may be helpful to enforce the behavioral modification [29]. Modification of lifestyle typically includes change in diet and increase in physical activity. The basic principle of weight loss is that energy intake must be less than energy expenditure. Overall, consumption of approximately 500 fewer kcal per day will allow loss of about 1 lb (0.45 kg) per week. Weight loss goals need to be realistic, and the means by which a patient is planning on reaching those goals need to be feasible. Loss of 5–10 % of current body weight (or 2 BMI units) over 6 months is a reasonable goal. Involvement of a dietician has been shown to facilitate weight loss in the office setting, supporting the notion of the importance of knowledge and tools for any behavioral change [30]. Dietary counseling is time-consuming if done well, and obstetrics providers may not have the time in a preconception visit to do a thorough assessment of a patient's food intake and make effective recommendations. The provider's main goal in preconception counseling should be to help identify realistic goals for the patient and provide a referral to a dietician to work through the details necessary to realize those goals. Another option that would likely ease the burden on the patient would be to provide nutritional guidance within the office setting. Having personnel on staff who fully realize the importance of a multidisciplinary approach to health and diet can lead to greater success for patients.

Low-fat diets traditionally restrict dietary fat intake to less than 30 % of total calories, and very-low-fat diets restrict to less than 15 % of total calories from fat. Weight loss does occur with low-fat diets, but very-low-fat diets may be difficult to maintain. In most studies, low-carbohydrate diets have demonstrated more weight loss than low-fat diets, at least in the first 12 months [29]. One potential side effect may be an increase in LDL cholesterol, which in the population of overweight or obese patients could be detrimental in the long run. Other commercial diets are also popular. Two recent randomized controlled trials comparing several different commercial diets found similar weight loss within the first 6–12 months in all diets [31, 32].

A large meta-analysis demonstrated that increases in physical activity combined with caloric restriction result in greater weight reduction and fat mass versus lean mass balance than either alone [33]. Physical activity in particular does rely heavily on environmental factors. Many women, with one or more jobs, children, and other life stressors, will find it challenging to fit in physical activity. Furthermore, many women live in areas where it may not be safe to exercise outside and may not have access to other exercise options. Again, motivational interviewing may be beneficial in identifying the barriers to increased physical activity and some of the patient's own feelings about exercise. Without identifying and addressing both personal and environmental factors that are playing a role in a sedentary lifestyle, the provider will not be able to adequately promote behavior change.

Depending on a woman's readiness for change, the provider may want to recommend delaying pregnancy until the woman can achieve a healthy weight. If she is not using effective contraception, the provider should recommend contraceptive options that will not make weight loss more difficult and that are easily reversible when pregnancy is desired. One type of contraception that may be less desirable is depot medroxyprogesterone acetate (DMPA) which could result in weight gain and may result in longer time to ovulation when conception is desired. Pharmaceutical management of obesity is outside the scope of this chapter, but lifestyle modification is also critical to the success of patients who are undergoing such treatment.

Bariatric Surgery

Bariatric surgery may be recommended for women with BMI of 40 kg/m^2 and above or for women with BMI over 35 kg/m^2 when comorbidities (such as diabetes, coronary artery disease, or severe sleep apnea) are present [34]. In general, women who undergo bariatric surgery demonstrate improvement in measures related to medical comorbidities as well as quality of life. Providers should counsel patients to avoid pregnancy for at least 12–18 months after surgery, and if conception should occur, pregnancy should be monitored more closely for potential complications. Patients should take vitamin B12, at least 400 µg/day of folic acid, and iron supplementation. Patients should be monitored for bowel obstruction, stricture, and nutritional deficiencies.

A systematic review of cohort studies evaluating the effect of bariatric surgery on pregnancy outcomes concluded that rates of adverse maternal and neonatal outcomes may be lower in obese women who have undergone bariatric surgery before conception [35]. A recent retrospective study showed a decreased risk in gestational diabetes in women who underwent bariatric surgery as compared with obese and morbidly obese controls who did not have bariatric surgery, but there was also a 17.4 % rate of small for gestational age (SGA) infants in the surgery group as compared to the control group (5.0 %) [36].

Providing Guidance for Weight Gain During Pregnancy

The ideal time for all of the above interventions is before pregnancy. However, if an overweight or obese patient presents in early pregnancy, most of the aforementioned recommendations are still appropriate [37, 38]. In addition, gestational weight gain (GWG) needs to be discussed at the first prenatal visit. In 2009, the IOM released its revised recommendations for gestational weight gain lowering the total weight gain recommended for women who are classified as obese at the time of conception (Table 3.1) [3, 39]. These weight gain recommendations are applicable to adult and adolescent mothers. Providers should discuss the GWG recommendations at length with patients, and GWG should be assessed at each visit. For women of short stature (<157 cm), the recommendation is to maintain the GWG at the lower end of what is recommended for prepregnancy BMI [40–43].

The American Congress of Obstetricians and Gynecologists has outlined recommended practices when managing pregnancy in a woman who is overweight or obese [3, 44]. First, similar to caring for women during preconception, it is critical to treat BMI as a vital sign in the newly gravid woman. The provider should clearly convey the diagnosis and show her the BMI value on a BMI chart. The provider should explain the risks associated with being obese in pregnancy and recommend a specific range of GWG based on IOM recommendations [5]. Finally the provider should discuss physical activity and diet during pregnancy. Although small studies examining effects of exercise on pregnancy outcomes have reported inconsistent findings, ACOG recommends 30 min or more of moderate exercise on most days of the week for pregnant women [45–49]. Using the same techniques described above, it is important to identify the patient's readiness to change and use her current situation to help motivate her. The provider should give detailed information about resources available, including nutrition counseling, exercise-related materials, and how to access those resources. Some additional ideas to implement in practice that may help make weight loss more feasible for patients include providing patients with a pedometer, partnering with a local gym to provide discounts, or utilizing other community resources. Actual weight should be documented at each prenatal visit and appropriate feedback provided to the patient based on recommended GWG.

Lifestyle modification during pregnancy has not been studied quite as extensively as in the nongravid woman. Two recent systematic reviews assessing the evidence found no statistically significant difference in maternal or neonatal outcomes between women randomized to antenatal lifestyle intervention and those who received usual care [46, 47]. However, many of the included studies were limited by sample size, unclear randomization procedures, and attrition.

Research Gaps and the Next Generation of Research

Gaps in clinical practice for preconception care were outlined clearly in the CDC/ATSDR Preconception Care Work Group in 2006 [5]. The recommendations made at that time remain timely and relevant to current practice: (1) Individual responsibility across the lifespan: each woman, man, and couple should be encouraged to have a reproductive life plan; (2) Consumer awareness: increase public awareness of the importance of preconception health behaviors and preconception care services; (3) Preventive visits: risk assessment and educational and health promotion counseling should be part of every primary care visit for women of childbearing age to improve pregnancy outcomes; and (4) Interventions for identified risks: increase the proportion of women who receive interventions, in particular those with evidence of effectiveness.

The fourth recommendation captures the highest priority research gap for preconception care of the overweight and obese woman. There is limited evidence to guide providers and public health officials to the most effective interventions for weight loss in overweight and obese women who are considering pregnancy. Clinical trials of lifestyle interventions that target women considering pregnancy are critical to improving the long-term health of women regardless of their preferences or plans for childbearing [50, 51].

Conclusion

Our ability to confidently provide guidance on appropriate preconception interventions for overweight or obese women is limited by few clinical trials focusing on this particularly important time frame in the life of reproductive age women. Providers and public health officials should take advantage of the preconception period, which is an important teachable moment in the life of women.

References

1. McBride CM, Emmons KM, Lipkus IM. Understanding the potential of teachable moments: the case of smoking cessation. Health Educ Res. 2003;18(2):156–70.
2. Centers for Disease Control and Prevention. Preconception health and healthcare. http://www.cdc.gov/preconception/index.html. Accessed on 12 Sep 2013.
3. Rasmussen KM, Yaktine AL, editors. Weight gain during pregnancy: reexamining the guidelines. Institute of Medicine (US) and National Research Council (US) Committee to Reexamine IOM Pregnancy Weight Guidelines. Washington, DC: National Academies Press; 2009.
4. American College of Obstetricians and Gynecologists. Obesity in pregnancy. ACOG Committee opinion no. 315. Obstet Gynecol. 2005;106:671–5.
5. Weiss JL, Malone FD, Emig D, Ball RH, Nyberg DA, Comstock CH, et al. Obesity, obstetric complications and cesarean delivery rate: a population based screening study. Am J Obstet Gynecol. 2004;190:1091–7.
6. International Association of Diabetes and Pregnancy Study Groups Consensus Panel, Metzer BE, Gabbe SG, Persson B, Buchanan TA, Catalano PA, et al. International association of diabetes and pregnancy study group's recommendations on the diagnosis and classification of hyperglycemia in pregnancy. Diabetes Care. 2010;33:676–82.
7. American College of Obstetricians and Gynecologists. Guidelines for perinatal care. 7th ed. Elk Grove Village, IL: American Academy of Pediatrics; 2012.
8. Johnson K, Posner SF, Blerman J, Cordero JF, Atrash HK, Parker CS, CDC/ATSDR Preconception Care Work Group: Select Panel on Preconception Care, et al. Recommendations to improve preconception health and health care—United States. MMWR Recomm Rep. 2006;55(RR-6):1–23.

9. Shaw KA, Caughey AB, Edelman AB. Obesity epidemic: how to make a difference in a busy OB/GYN practice. Obstet Gynecol Surv. 2012;67(6):365–73.
10. American Diabetes Association. Preconception care of women with diabetes. Diabetes Care. 2004;27 Suppl 1:S76–8.
11. Roland JM, Murphy HR, Ball V, Northcote-Wright J, Temple RC. The pregnancies of women with type 2 diabetes: poor outcomes but opportunities for improvement. Diabet Med. 2005;22(12):1774–7.
12. Rasmussen SA, Chu SY, Kim SY, Schmid CH, Lau J. Maternal obesity and risk of neural tube defects: a meta-analysis. Am J Obstet Gynecol. 2008;198(6):611–9.
13. Moyer VA. Screening for and management of obesity in adults: U.S. Preventive services task force. Ann Intern Med. 2012;157(5):373–8.
14. Nawaz H, Katz DL. American College of Preventive Medicine Policy statement. Weight management counseling of overweight adults. Am J Prev Med. 2001;21(1):73–8.
15. Pan XR, Li GW, Hu YH, Wang JX, Yang WY, An ZX, et al. Effects of diet and exercise in preventing NIDDM in people with impaired glucose tolerance. The Da Qing IGT and Diabetes Study. Diabetes Care. 1997;20(4):537–44.
16. Tuomilehto J, Lindstrom J, Eriksson JG, Valle TT, Ilanne-Parikka P, et al. Prevention of type 2 diabetes mellitus by changes in lifestyle among subjects with impaired glucose tolerance. N Engl J Med. 2001;344(18):1343–50.
17. Knowler WC, Barrett-Connor E, Fowler SE, Hamman RF, Lachin JM, Walker EA, et al. Reduction in the incidence of type 2 diabetes with lifestyle intervention or metformin. N Engl J Med. 2002;346(6):393–403.
18. Powell LH, Calvin III JE, Calvin Jr JE. Effective obesity treatments. Am Psychol. 2007;62(3):234–46.
19. Bandura A. Human agency in social cognitive theory. Am Psychol. 1989;44(9):1175–84.
20. Prochaska JO, Velicer WF. The transtheoretical model of behavior change. Am J Health Promot. 1997;12(1):38–48.
21. Rollnick S, Miller WR. What is motivational interviewing? Behav Cogn Psychother. 1995;23:325–34.
22. Miller WR, Zweben A, DiClemente CC, Rychtarik RG. Motivational Enhancement Therapy Manual. Washington, DC: National Institute on Alcohol Abuse and Alcoholism. 1992. http://motivationalinterviewing.org/content/motivational-enhancement-therapy-manual. Accessed on 13 Sep 2013.
23. Rubak S, Sandbaek A, Lauritzen T, Christensen B. Motivational interviewing: a systematic review and meta-analysis. Br J Gen Pract. 2005;55:305–12.
24. Lai DTC, Cahill K, Qin Y, Tang J-L. Motivational interviewing for smoking cessation. Cochrane Database Syst Rev. 2010;(1):CD006936. doi:10.1002/14651858.CD006936.pub2.

25. Pollak KI, Alexander SC, Coffman CJ, Tulsky JA, Lyna P, Dolor RJ, James IE, Brouwer RJN, Manusov JRE, Ostbye T. Physician communication techniques and weight loss in adults: project CHAT. Am J Prev Med. 2010;39(4):321–8.
26. West DS, Dilillo V, Bursac Z, Gore SA, Greene PG. Motivational interviewing improves weight loss in women with type 2 diabetes. Diabetes Care. 2007;30:1081–7.
27. American College of Obstetricians and Gynecologists. Motivational interviewing: a tool for behavior change. ACOG Committee opinion no. 423. Obstet Gynecol. 2009;113:243–6.
28. Poston II WS, Foreyt JP. Successful management of the obese patient. Am Fam Physician. 2000;61(12):3615–22.
29. Eckel RH. Nonsurgical management of obesity in adults. N Engl J Med. 2008;358:1941–50.
30. Ashley JM, St Jeor ST, Schrage JP, Perumean-Chaney SE, Gilbertson MC, McCAll NL, Bovee V. Weight control in the physician's office. Arch Intern Med. 2001;161(3):1599–604.
31. Dansinger ML, Gleason JA, Griffith JL, Selker HP, Shaefer EJ. Comparison of the Atkins, Ornish, weight watchers, and Zone diets for weight loss and heart disease reduction: a randomized trial. JAMA. 2005;293(1):43–53.
32. Truby H, Baic S, de Looy A, Fox KR, Livingstone MB, Logan CM, et al. Randomised controlled trial of four commercial weight loss programmes in the UK: initial findings from the BBC "diet trials". BMJ. 2006;332(7553):1309–14.
33. Miller WC, Koceja DM, Hamilton EJ. A meta-analysis of the past 25 years of weight loss research using diet, exercise or diet plus exercise intervention. Int J Obes Relat Metab Disord. 1997;21(10):941–7.
34. American College of Obstetricians and Gynecologists (ACOG). ACOG practice bulletin no. 105: bariatric surgery and pregnancy. Obstet Gynecol. 2009;113(6):1405–13.
35. Maggard MA, Yermilov I, Li Z, Maglione M, Newberry S, Suttorp M, et al. Pregnancy and fertility following bariatric surgery: a systematic review. JAMA. 2008;300(19):2286–96.
36. Lesko J, Peaceman A. Pregnancy outcomes in women after bariatric surgery compared with obese and morbidly obese controls. Obstet Gynecol. 2012;119(3):547–54.
37. Santoro N, Lasley B, McConnell D, Allsworth J, Crawford S, Gold EB. Body size and ethnicity are associated with menstrual cycle alterations in women in the early menopausal transition: the Study of Women's Health Across the Nation (SWAN) daily hormone study. J Clin Endocrinol Metab. 2004;89(6):2622–31.
38. Henshaw SK. Unintended pregnancy in the United States. Fam Plann Perspect. 1998;30(1):24–9, 46.
39. Jungheim ES, Moley KH. Current knowledge of obesity's effects in the pre- and periconceptional periods and avenues for future research. Am J Obstet Gynecol. 2010;203(6):525–30. Epub 2010 Aug 24.

40. Gunderson EP, Abrams B, Selvin S. The relative importance of gestational gain and maternal characteristics associated with the risk of becoming overweight after pregnancy. Int J Obes Relat Metab Disord. 2000;24(12):1660–8.
41. Siega-Riz AM, Herring AH, Carrier K, Evenson KR, Dole N, Deierlein A. Sociodemographic, perinatal, behavioral, and psychosocial predictors of weight retention at 3 and 12 months postpartum. Obesity (Silver Spring). 2010;18(10):1996–2003. Epub 2009 Dec 24.
42. Stotland NE, Cheng YW, Hopkins LM, Caughey AB. Gestational weight gain and adverse neonatal outcome among term infants. Obstet Gynecol. 2006;108(3 Pt 1):635–43.
43. Nohr EA, Bech BH, Vaeth M, Rasmussen KM, Henriksen TB, Olsen J. Obesity, gestational weight gain and preterm birth: a study within the Danish National Birth Cohort. Paediatr Perinat Epidemiol. 2007;21(1):5–14.
44. Catalano PM. Management of obesity in pregnancy. Obstet Gynecol. 2007;109(2 Pt 1):419–33.
45. Herring SJ, Platek DN, Elliott P, Riley LE, Stuebe AM, Oken E. Addressing obesity in pregnancy: what do obstetric providers recommend? J Womens Health (Larchmt). 2010;19(1):65–70.
46. Dodd JM, Grivell RM, Robinson JS. Antenatal interventions for overweight or obese pregnant women: a systematic review of randomised trials. BJOG. 2010;117(11):1316–26.
47. Oteng-Ntim E, Varma R, Croker H, Poston L, Doyle P. Lifestyle interventions for overweight and obese pregnant women to improve pregnancy outcome: systematic review and meta-analysis. BMC Med. 2012;10:47.
48. Asbee SM, Jenkins TR, Butler JR, White J, Elliott M, Rutledge A. Preventing excessive weight gain during pregnancy through dietary and lifestyle counseling: a randomized controlled trial. Obstet Gynecol. 2009;113(2 Pt 1):305–12.
49. ACOG Committee Obstetric Practice. ACOG Committee opinion. Number 267, January 2002: exercise during pregnancy and the postpartum period. American College of Obstetricians and Gynecologists. Obstet Gynecol. 2002;99(1):171–3.
50. Kramer MS, McDonald SW. Aerobic exercise for women during pregnancy. Cochrane Database Syst Rev. 2006;(3):CD000180.
51. Quinlivan J, Julania S, Lam L. Antenatal dietary interventions in obese pregnant women to restrict gestational weight gain to Institute of Medicine recommendations: a meta-analysis. Obstet Gynecol. 2011;118(6):1395–401.

Chapter 4
Shared Decision Making and Labor Management in Parturients

Catherine Takacs Witkop

> *"Pregnancy presents an opportunity for women to develop skills to be engaged, savvy, knowledgeable consumers …"Amy Romano, "The First National Maternity Care Shared Decision Making Initiative," (www. Informedmedicaldecisions.org)*

Abstract Overweight and obesity are risk factors for several labor and postpartum complications, including macrosomia, shoulder dystocia, and cesarean delivery. Anesthesia and surgical intervention also present unique challenges, but research has provided new insights on how to reduce complications in these two areas. Providers can use currently available evidence to counsel patients, and this conversation should begin during the prenatal period. Further research is needed to address the gaps in our understanding of the most effective methods of delivery and postpartum care for overweight and obese women.

Keywords Overweight • Obese • Pregnancy outcomes • Labor • Delivery • Cesarean delivery

---

C.T. Witkop, MD, MPH
Department of Obstetrics/Gynecology
and Preventive Medicine, Uniformed Services University
of the Health Sciences, Bethesda, MD, USA
e-mail: cwitkop@gmail.com

W. Nicholson, K. Baptiste-Roberts (eds.),
Obesity During Pregnancy in Clinical Practice,
DOI 10.1007/978-1-4471-2831-1_4,
© Springer-Verlag London 2014

Key Points
- Overweight and obesity increase the risk of maternal and newborn complications during labor, delivery, and the immediate postpartum period.
- Shared decision making acknowledges that a woman's values and preferences will influence her decisions for care during labor and assist in assessing the balance of benefits and harms of treatment decisions.
- Labor patterns in overweight and obese women differ from patterns in normal-weight women and may account for the higher incidence of cesarean delivery in overweight and obese women.
- Overweight and obese women are at increased risk for anesthetic complications, but adequate anesthesia is critical during labor, given the increased chance of cesarean delivery.
- Cesarean delivery in the obese parturient can pose unique surgical challenges for the obstetrician, but some preventive measures have been shown to help reduce complications.

Introduction

Overweight and obese women face a number of potential complications in labor that are directly or, in some cases, indirectly related to their weight. Studies have demonstrated that not only are there more adverse outcomes in overweight and obese women but that the risks increase proportionately with extent of overweight [1]. When considering the entire population of overweight and obese women, potential complications can include an increased risk of preeclampsia, gestational diabetes, large for gestational age (LGA) or macrosomic infants, antepartum stillbirth, instrumental delivery, shoulder dystocia, cesarean delivery, intraoperative and postoperative complications, difficulty with anesthesia, meconium aspiration, fetal distress, and early neonatal death [1–4].

Information about these risks is best shared with reproductive-aged women during preconception counseling appointments. If an overweight or obese woman conceives, the next intervention opportunity is during her prenatal care, preferably during the first trimester. However, as seen in the previous chapter, antenatal interventions to limit gestational weight gain within the recommended range are often challenging to implement. Even if the patient does not gain excessive weight during pregnancy, it appears many of the complications are associated with prepregnancy weight. That leaves the obstetric provider with the complex task of managing labor and delivery in a patient who is vulnerable to a number of complications. As will become clear, the evidence demonstrates that there is not a straightforward algorithm for labor management in overweight or obese patients. A decision to avoid one set of potential complications leads to the possibility of a host of others.

Shared decision making is an approach that is being used increasingly in many areas of clinical medicine, in particular, for complex decisions about screening or treatment options. One goal of shared decision making is to provide the patient with the information and tools to help her understand the state of the evidence related to the topic. Even more importantly, this approach acknowledges that a patient's values and preferences will impact her decisions during her pregnancy, especially when risks and benefits are such that significant uncertainty about outcomes remains.

Because of the twenty-first-century nature of this problem, the medical literature is not replete with prospective studies on management of labor and delivery in the obese patient. But the obesity epidemic is not going away. And until high-quality prospective studies help inform appropriate prenatal or intrapartum interventions, management will rely primarily on available evidence from observational studies, which are unfortunately limited in scope.

Risks of Labor Complications

Overweight and obese women, even those who have normal glucose tolerance, have an increased risk of delivering an infant that is macrosomic [4]. This introduces a number of potential complications during labor and delivery including increased incidence of cesarean or instrumental delivery and increased risk of shoulder dystocia, perineal lacerations (in particular, third- and fourth-degree lacerations), and postpartum hemorrhage.

What is the risk of macrosomia in overweight or obese women? In a prospective, multicenter database study of 16,102 patients, the incidence of macrosomia (as defined as birth weight over 4,000 g) was 14.6 % in morbidly obese women and 13.3 % in obese women as compared to 8.3 % in women with BMI less than 30 kg/m^2 [4]. Teasing out the independent risk of obesity versus gestational diabetes, which is more likely in obese women, can be a challenge, but has been attempted. The risk of a macrosomic or large for gestational age (LGA) infant (newborn weight greater than the 90th percentile for gestational age at the institution where the study was performed) was higher in women with pregestational diabetes (OR 4.4), but the risk in nondiabetic obese women was still significant (OR 1.6) in multivariate analysis [5]. In another study of nondiabetic women, prepregnancy weight had the strongest correlation with neonatal fat and body fat percentage in the infant, regardless of glucose tolerance [6]. Based on these and several other studies, it does appear that obesity is independently associated with macrosomia.

Obese women also have a higher risk of shoulder dystocia and birth trauma than normal-weight women, but, again, whether obesity is an independent predictor of shoulder dystocia has been debated. In one study of 9,667 vaginal deliveries, obese women still had a 2.7-fold risk of shoulder dystocia, even after adjustment for macrosomia and diabetes [7]. The most significant risk factors for shoulder dystocia were, however, noted to be macrosomia and diabetes. Cedergren et al. also demonstrated that obesity was an independent risk factor for shoulder dystocia [1].

Chapter 4. Shared Decision Making

Since a study over 25 years ago, many have held that a certain threshold of estimated fetal weight provides sufficient support to perform an elective cesarean delivery [8]. In that study by Spellacy et al., women with macrosomic infants (over 4,500 g) were more likely to have cesarean delivery, and the infants had more birth trauma and shoulder dystocia, lower Apgar scores, and higher death rates [8]. In the group with the triad of obesity, diabetes, and postdates, the macrosomia frequency was 5–14 %. Shoulder dystocia occurred significantly more frequently in patients with fetal weight of 4,500–4,999 g (7.3 %) and those over 5,000 g (14.6 %). In that paper, the authors recommended that "women at risk should be screened for macrosomic infants, and if found, they should be delivered electively by cesarean section" [8]. A second study by Lipscomb and colleagues demonstrated an 18.5 % incidence of shoulder dystocia in macrosomic (4,500 g) vaginal deliveries, and women with diabetes had a significantly higher incidence (50 %) than nondiabetic women (13.3 %) [9]. Based primarily on this evidence, the American College of Obstetricians and Gynecologists (ACOG) has recommended that cesarean delivery be considered for pregnancies without diabetes but with a fetus with an estimated fetal weight greater than 5,000 g. Women with gestational diabetes and an estimated fetal weight of >4,500 g should also discuss cesarean delivery with their providers [10].

This recommendation is complicated by the fact that estimating fetal weight in general is a difficult task. Ultrasound is the primary modality to estimate fetal weight, but concerns about using ultrasound to estimate fetal weight arose partly because of studies that showed decreased visualization of fetal structures in obese women. In one study, in patients with BMI in the 97.5th percentile (BMI of 49.4 kg/m^2), only 63 % of anatomic structures were visualized [11]. Visualization was slightly better (79.3 %) in women with BMI above 90th percentile (BMI of 36.21 kg/m^2) but was still significantly worse than that in normal-weight women and that in women with BMI less than the 10th percentile. In the thinnest women, 90.2 % of the anatomic structures could be visualized [11].

However, in a more recent study, the accuracy of clinical estimation of fetal weight was evaluated across BMI categories

[12]. The sensitivity and specificity were 9.7 and 96.6 % for predicting neonatal birth weight greater than the 90th percentile and were not affected by maternal BMI. It would appear that using ultrasound to estimate fetal weight in overweight and obese women can be supported by current evidence, but providers and patients need to understand the risks in making decisions based on estimated fetal weight.

Delivery decisions in the setting of suspected macrosomia can be among the most complex that will be made in the prenatal period. The counseling should occur during the prenatal period, with adequate time to answer questions and allow for the patient to make an informed decision with which she is comfortable. Decision tools are now available that outline questions for the patient to ask herself and her provider regarding the options when complex decisions are to be made. Management of suspected macrosomia is one such situation where providing the patient with such tools could be helpful. For example, induction of labor is not indicated for macrosomia, but patients may come to prenatal appointments requesting induction. Extensive counseling with an informed patient (i.e., one who has received relevant evidence-based information beforehand) is also recommended before making a decision about performing an elective cesarean delivery in the setting of suspected macrosomia. This discussion should not be delayed until the patient is in labor.

Walking a patient through the uncertainty that exists for these decisions and understanding her values and preferences optimizes the decision-making process. She needs to know that some cesarean deliveries will be performed needlessly and vaginal delivery may still result in shoulder dystocia. Furthermore, there is currently no evidence-based recommendation for elective cesarean delivery *specifically* for obese women.

Labor Management

Management of labor in the overweight or obese patient needs to be undertaken with a great deal of preparation. One author recommends that obstetric units that care for extremely obese pregnant patients develop a "bariatric protocol" and ensure appropriate beds, intraoperative equipment, and supplies are available [13]. ACOG also recommends specific resources, including additional blood products, a large operating table, and enough personnel to assist with the potential complications that may ensue [2]. Given the current obesity epidemic, it is prudent for most obstetric wards to have such a protocol. Table 4.1 provides a reasonable checklist, compiled from several sources, for a labor and delivery suite where obese patients may deliver. This checklist can be modified,

TABLE 4.1 Checklist for equipment to support obese pregnant patients [2, 13, 14]

Bariatric bed (600–1,000 lb capacity; 42–54 in width), with frame and trapeze for mobility

Chairs in room without sides

Bariatric operating table (600–1,000 lb capacity)

Larger belt or straps for securing legs to table

Toilet capable of accommodating 500+ pounds

Inflatable mattress

Extra-wide wheelchairs (400–700 lb capacity; 20–30 in width)

Extra-large inflatable sequential pneumatic compression devices

Bariatric surgical tray (for BMI >40 kg/m^2)

    Extra-long surgical instruments

    Bookwalter self-retaining retractor

    Long clamps

Appropriate size blood pressure cuff (or thigh cuff)

Ability to achieved central venous access if peripheral IV not feasible

Ability to place arterial line

Access to blood products (blood typed and crossed for transfusion)

Appropriate gown sizes

Extra personnel in delivery room

depending on the practice environment and patient population. For example, accommodating the extremely obese patient can pose additional challenges. Some of the issues related to this population are discussed later in the chapter.

Labor in obese women has been shown to vary from that of normal-weight women, so standard provider expectations for cervical dilation and the threshold for cesarean delivery may need to be adjusted. In one observational study of 509 nulliparous patients, the rate of cervical dilation was inversely proportional to maternal weight [15]. In another study of nulliparous women, duration of labor was significantly longer for overweight and obese women than for normal-weight women, even when adjusting for other potential confounders, such as induction, oxytocin use, epidural analgesia, maternal weight gain, and fetal size [16]. In that study, the median duration of labor from 4 to 10 cm was 7.9 h for obese women, 7.5 h for overweight women, and 6.2 h for normal-weight women [16]. The etiology of the longer labor is not clear but does not appear to be the strength of uterine contractions. When intrauterine pressure was measured in 71 women during the second stage of labor, there was no difference in uterine contractility between three groups of women (normal, overweight, and obese women), although obese women labored longer during the active phase and a BMI greater than 25 kg/m^2 was associated with a higher frequency of the need for oxytocin augmentation [17]. Future studies should examine reasons for the difference in labor patterns between women of different weight classifications. One hypothesis relates to increased soft tissue deposits in the pelvis of obese women, but this has not been demonstrated.

For practical purposes, however, clinicians need to understand that labor patterns may be dissimilar in overweight and obese women and thresholds for interventions (or lack of interventions) may need to be adjusted accordingly. An individualized approach to the overweight and obese parturient may result in fewer cesarean deliveries and the complications that might result. Additional challenges that may be encountered when an overweight or obese patient is laboring, include difficulty in monitoring the fetus and the contractions. A fetal scalp electrode and intrauterine pressure catheter may be needed to help guide labor management, especially in a patient with other complications during labor. Cardiovascular issues are also more common in obese women, and more intensive monitoring may be required than with normal-weight women.

Induction of Labor

With an increase in rates of labor induction for both medical and nonmedical indications, the risk-benefit ratio of induction specifically found in the overweight and obese population must be examined. The concepts of shared decision making discussed above are also applicable here. In situations where a medical indication exists for induction of labor, the benefits likely exceed the risks. However, elective induction of labor should not be undertaken without a candid discussion with the patient about risks and benefits, in a way she understands.

In a secondary analysis of a study in which women randomly received cervical ripening with 10 mg dinoprostone, 50 µg misoprostol, or 100 µg misoprostol, the median dose and duration of oxytocin required before delivery (3.5 units and 7.7 h) were significantly greater in obese women and extremely obese women (5.0 units and 8.5 h) as compared to the dose and duration (2.6 units and 6.5 h) in "lean" women (BMI less than 30 kg/m^2) [18]. Furthermore, median time to delivery (27.0 h) was significantly longer in the extremely obese group (BMI over 40 kg/m^2) than the "lean" group (22.7 h) [18].

The relationship is not clear-cut, however. In another retrospective cohort study of 29,224 women with prolonged pregnancy (defined as 41 and 3/7 weeks' gestation or longer), there was no association of in length of labor, incidence of postpartum hemorrhage, shoulder dystocia, and neonatal outcomes with weight [19]. Obese women did have a significantly higher rate of cesarean delivery. For women undergoing their first delivery, the cesarean delivery rate was 38.7 % in obese women versus 23.8 % in normal-weight women. Future studies should also continue to examine labor patterns in overweight and obese women and how they differ from normal-weight women, so that abnormal labor can be better characterized and recommendations made for management of labor. Until then, providers should help the patient understand the evidence that exists and help her make an informed decision about undertaking elective induction of labor.

Cesarean Delivery

Given the growing epidemic of obesity and the increasing cesarean delivery rate, it is important to understand the relationship between obesity and risk of cesarean delivery. Both obesity and cesarean deliveries impact the public health. In a systematic review of 11 cohort studies specifically focused on nulliparous patients, the risk of cesarean delivery was increased by 50 % in women with BMI between 25 and 30 kg/m^2, and the risk in women with BMI over 30 kg/m^2 was more than twice that in women with normal BMI [3]. Although not included in that systematic review, a large population-based study reflected the findings from the review: in the population of nulliparous patients, the rate of cesarean delivery was 20.7 % for the normal BMI group, 33.8 % in the obese group, and 47.4 % for morbidly obese patients ($\geq$35 kg/m^2) [4]. In another prospective, population-based cohort study, 3,480 women with body mass index (BMI) over 40 kg/m^2 had an increased risk of cesarean delivery, and women with BMI between 35.1 and 40 kg/m^2 also demonstrated similar associations, but to a slightly lesser extent [1].

With the rapidly increasing numbers of obese and morbidly obese women, another population is growing in size, the extremely obese women (BMI $\geq$50 kg/m^2). In a retrospective cohort study of 64,272 obese women, extremely obese women were found to have a number of worse outcomes, including higher risk of preeclampsia, macrosomia, cesarean delivery, neonatal hypoglycemia, neonatal length of stay greater than 5 days, and worse composite neonatal score [20]. Interestingly, in this population, 49.1 % of extremely obese women delivered by cesarean delivery (33.8 % of the extremely obese women had scheduled primary cesarean). The indications for the scheduled primary cesarean sections were not clear from this study, and the authors recommended further study to evaluate reasons for such high rates of elective cesarean delivery.

Anesthesia

Providers caring for overweight and obese women need to address potential anesthetic concerns, preferably before labor ensues. It should be standard practice to obtain an anesthetic consultation before planned cesarean section in an obese woman, and it is highly recommended in all obese women during the prenatal period, even if cesarean delivery is not scheduled. This is to account both for pain management during labor as well as to evaluate the patient to prepare for a possible difficult airway in the event of the need for general anesthesia.

In general, regional anesthesia is recommended for the overweight or obese patient in labor or for cesarean delivery. The identification of the epidural space in pregnant women, and particularly in overweight and obese women, can be extremely difficult. Even in the most controlled circumstance, for example in preparation for a scheduled cesarean delivery, complications are a possibility. In a cohort study of women undergoing elective scheduled cesarean delivery, women with BMI 50 kg/m^2 or greater were most likely to have complications: 4 % had insufficient duration, 6 % required general anesthesia, and 3 % demonstrated intraoperative hypotension [21]. Overall anesthetic complications were 8.4 % in the extremely obese population as compared to 0 % in the normal-weight women [21]. It is important to counsel patients that such complications can also occur in a controlled, non-emergent situation, such as for an elective cesarean delivery. Decisions to perform elective procedures should not be made lightly.

Although not specifically focused on obese women, studies by Grau on the use of ultrasound to assist in skin-epidural space detection may be of utility in patients with difficult landmarks [22]. In one randomized controlled study of 300 parturients, women in the study group (who underwent ultrasonography for the identification of intervertebral structures and to determine depth and angle for placement of Tuohy needle) had fewer puncture attempts and were more likely to have complete analgesia and lower VAS (visual analog scale) pain score than those in the control group (typical placement without ultrasound). Ultrasound added 75 s to the mean preparation time. The rate of side effects (also including postpartum headache and backache) was lower, and patient acceptance was higher in the study group [22].

Ultrasound guidance is not without risk, as measurements may differ by millimeters between the image and actual depth. Anesthetic providers should still use standard procedures (e.g., loss of resistance (LOR) technique) to assist in placement of the epidural catheter. Obstetric providers may wish to discuss the option of ultrasound-guided epidural placement with anesthesia colleagues, especially for care of overweight and obese patients in their practices.

Regardless of the method used, discussing the benefits of epidural placement early in labor is worthwhile. Given the significantly increased risks of general anesthesia, such as difficult endotracheal intubation and intraoperative respiratory events, it is highly recommended that regional anesthesia is performed in a controlled setting without time pressures [2]. An obese patient without an epidural who requires an emergency cesarean delivery will likely require general anesthesia, resulting in potential further morbidity. Combined spinal-epidural is an ideal solution in an obese patient in labor, or spinal alone can be considered for the patient preparing for cesarean delivery.

Surgical Issues

Overweight and obese women may have an increased risk of intrapartum and postpartum hemorrhage, longer operative times, thromboembolic complications, postpartum endometritis, and wound infection [2]. Obese women undergoing cesarean delivery, whether elective, indicated, or emergency, are at increased risk for infectious complications [23]. Obese patients in one study were more likely to develop endomyometritis and wound infection, even if they received prophylactic antibiotics [23]. BMI and maternal obesity, in addition to length of labor and number of digital cervical examinations, remained significantly associated with infectious morbidity, even after multivariate analysis [23]. Based on their data, the authors recommend providers attempt to shorten labor to less than 10 h and perform fewer than four digital exams in obese and overweight women to reduce risk of infection.

A broad-spectrum antibiotic, such as a first-generation cephalosporin, should be administered within 60 min preceding the skin incision. One consideration in extremely obese women is whether there is adequate tissue penetration. There have been no adequate studies in pregnant women to determine the correct dosing for overweight or obese women, but a recent study estimating the adequacy of antimicrobial activity of preoperative antibiotics found that cefazolin concentrations within adipose tissue obtained at skin incision were inversely proportional to maternal BMI [24]. Furthermore, in this study of women undergoing scheduled cesarean delivery who received 2 g of cefazolin at least 30 min before skin incision, a significant proportion of obese and extremely obese women did not have minimal inhibitory concentrations in adipose tissue when sampled at opening and closing of the incision [24]. Common practice is to administer 2 g of cefazolin in obese women (e.g., when BMI is >30 kg/m^2) [2]. More studies are clearly needed to determine adequate dosing of antibiotics or the utility of adding a second antibiotic in this high-risk population.

Performing a cesarean delivery on an obese woman requires a clear understanding of anatomic relationships and a skilled surgeon to reduce operative complications. Obese women will often have a significant panniculus that needs to be taken into account in order to effectively deliver the infant in a safe and expeditious manner. Furthermore, obese women who undergo cesarean delivery are more likely than their normal-weight counterparts to have increased likelihood of wound breakdown and infection. There are differing opinions about the benefits of vertical versus horizontal skin incision, but there have been no prospective randomized trials to guide surgeons in this decision. The traditionally stated disadvantage to Pfannenstiel is reduced exposure and potentially more difficulty in delivering a macrosomic infant and difficulty in managing wound breakdown or infection after Pfannenstiel incision.

Several retrospective studies have attempted to answer this question. The incidence of wound complications was 12 % in one retrospective study, and the incidence of wound complications was greater (35 % vs. 9 %) in women with vertical skin incisions [25]. In another smaller case–control study, however, there were no differences in infections or other complications between women undergoing supraumbilical versus Pfannenstiel incisions [26]. In a large multicenter cohort study that examined only emergency cesarean deliveries (2,498 women in all), a vertical incision was found to reduce delivery incision-to-delivery interval by 1 min for primary and by 2 min for repeat cesarean but was associated with more frequent endometritis and postpartum transfusion [27].

Based on the evidence that is available, Pfannenstiel incision can be recommended in most cases, and an incision in the lower abdomen below the panniculus appears to be the ideal approach [29]. The panniculus needs to be retracted cephalad and held in place to ensure visualization, but close attention must be paid to ensure this does not cause respiratory compromise [13]. The other option is to make a higher transverse periumbilical (either supra- or infraumbilically, depending on the body habitus) incision above the panniculus which can be retracted inferiorly if needed. This approach has the advantage of creating the incision where there is the least amount of subcutaneous adipose tissue [25, 27]. Regardless of the approach, a vacuum extractor should be available in the room in the event of difficult delivery of the vertex in an obese woman with limited visualization.

Studies have also focused on closure techniques that could reduce postoperative complications such as wound dehiscence and infection. Closure of the fascia should follow routine procedures, using no. 1 or no. 2 delayed monofilament suture [e.g., polydioxanone (PDS)]. Some experts recommend a Smead-Jones "mass" closure if a vertical incision has been made [13]. The use of a subcutaneous stitch has been more controversial but can be recommended based on a meta-analysis of six studies on this topic that showed there was a significant decrease in wound disruption (which seems to be as a result of decrease in wound seromas) [28, 30]. Moreover, in women with subcutaneous adipose tissue thickness of greater than 2 cm, there was a 34 % (RR 0.66) (risk reduction of 6.2 %) decrease in risk of wound disruption in women [28, 30]. There are no known risks to placing a subcutaneous stitch, other than prolonging operating time, and therefore should be considered in overweight and obese women. The placement of drains has been similarly studied. Research has not demonstrated a clear advantage to using a drain to reduce infectious morbidity [30, 31], nor have studies adequately demonstrated any significant risks with the placement of such a drain. This decision should be left up to the surgeon, although there is not clear evidence indicating its use.

Postoperative and Postpartum Complications

Overweight and obese women are at increased risk for thromboembolic complications. As a result, consideration should be given to preventive measures, especially in women who have undergone a surgical procedure that will reduce postpartum ambulation. Options include pharmacologic interventions and physical measures such as compression stockings and intermittent pneumatic compression. Given the increased risk of venous thromboembolism in this population, all overweight or obese women should have pneumatic compression devices placed before surgery (unless already receiving pharmacologic prophylaxis) [2]. The more difficult question is: when to use pharmaceutical thromboprophylaxis? A systematic review of 13 trials, involving 1,774 women, examined a range of methods of thromboprophylaxis in pregnant women [31, 32]. Unfortunately, the authors concluded that there is insufficient evidence on which to base recommendations. A 2006 consensus panel of experts also reviewed the evidence and determined that, although obese women have a higher incidence of complications in pregnancy, the evidence cannot currently support prescribing heparin or low-dose aspirin to high-risk obese patients who have not had a venous thromboembolism [32, 33]. The panel did suggest that, because multiple studies have demonstrated a possible impact on prothrombotic risk, providers may consider screening obese women for common thrombophilic mutations [32, 33]. There are currently no data supporting this practice. However, providers should keep in mind that obese women are at increased risk and this association might tip the balance toward thromboprophylaxis, especially when another risk factor is present.

It is critical to remember that dosing of thromboprophylactic medications (and also when used for therapeutic purposes) is impacted by weight. Therefore, for appropriate care of overweight and obese patients who require thromboprophylaxis for other indications, providers need to be familiar with weight-based dosing of these medications.

Vaginal Birth After Cesarean (VBAC)

With cesarean deliveries making up 32.8 % of all deliveries in the USA, the issue of delivery management in obese women with previous cesarean delivery is one of great public health importance [33, 34]. Complications of both vaginal delivery and cesarean delivery are higher in overweight and obese women than in normal-weight women, so deciding on the appropriate mode of delivery can be a challenge. Providers have a vital role in educating patients about the risks and benefits of each route and assisting patients in their decisions. In a prospective observational study of obese women (defined as over 300 lb) with history of cesarean delivery, the success rate of vaginal birth after cesarean (VBAC) among the 30 women who underwent trial of labor (TOL) was 13 % (due to arrest of labor, "fetal distress," and failed induction) as compared to the overall rate of TOL success of 65 % in the institution where the study was conducted [34, 35]. Furthermore, endometritis rates were higher in the trial of labor group [34, 35]. In a subsequent, retrospective study of VBAC success by weight class, examining data in the same institution, the TOL success rate was only 13.3 % in the heaviest women (over 300 lb), which was significantly different from the 81.8 % success rate in the group of women who were less than 200 lb at delivery [35, 36]. Infectious morbidity (including both endometritis and wound infection) was also significantly more common in the group of women over 300 lb. These studies, however, may not be representative of the overall population. In larger, prospective, multicenter study, the VBAC rates were higher, 70 %, but still lower than that in nonobese women, in whom 85 % were successful [36, 37]. And in women with BMI of 40 kg/m^2 or higher, success was only 61 %. Furthermore, the investigators noted higher rates of uterine scar dehiscence, composite morbidity, and neonatal injury rates in the obese and morbidly obese women [36, 37]. In a study of extremely obese women, there were no differences in VBAC success rate between different obesity groups, although the success rates were low in all groups [20].

While these statistics might sway some to recommend repeat cesarean delivery over attempted VBAC, the surgical risks in overweight and obese women discussed earlier need to be considered. In a facility with adequate support, a trial of labor can certainly be attempted and should be considered. Again, adequate counseling during the prenatal period, not when the patient presents in labor, is ideal.

Special Considerations

As has been mentioned throughout this chapter, gestational diabetes mellitus (GDM) poses additional risk for the overweight and obese patient. Accurate diagnosis in this population is particularly important, given the implications for the fetus as well as for management of labor and delivery. In the recent Hyperglycemia and Adverse Pregnancy Outcome (HAPO) study, risk of birth weight over the 90th percentile was significantly increased when both GDM and obesity were present (OR 3.62) as compared to GDM alone (OR 2.19) or obesity alone (OR 1.73) [37, 38]. And although obesity alone is a risk factor for preeclampsia, GDM in addition to obesity was associated with an even greater risk of preeclampsia than either factor alone (OR 5.98) [37, 38]. Unfortunately, the ideal delivery management in patients with both GDM and obesity is not clear. Although there is no clear evidence to support the practice, some experts recommend individualizing care and considering cesarean delivery when estimated fetal weight is 4,000–4,500 g in GDM patients [38, 39]. Others have recommended earlier induction of labor in women with GDM [39, 40]. A recent systematic review, however, found that further research is necessary to inform timed delivery in patients with GDM [14, 40]. Furthermore, caution must be advised in patients with both GDM and obesity, as management in that population has not been as extensively studied.

Future Research

Clinical research on appropriate interventions in the overweight and obese population has not kept up with the gaps in our understanding. Several opportunities for research have already been mentioned. For example, a well-designed prospective study to characterize labor patterns in women of different weight classifications could inform guidelines and practice patterns. Such research would need to take into account the use of cervical ripening agents, amniotomy, and oxytocin. The use of intrauterine pressure catheters during such a study might also help inform the possible etiology of differences in labor curves. Because of the desire to avoid cesarean delivery in overweight and obese women, studies to examine the best policies and practices for induction of labor (or expectant management) in this population (with and without gestational diabetes) would also be extremely helpful to clinicians. For example, studies looking at characteristics of women with successful induction of labor can help clarify what factors should be considered when making such decisions. The management of patients with comorbid conditions, such as GDM and obesity, is another area that requires further research to determine recommended intrapartum management.

Another area where further research is needed is in the intraoperative and postoperative care of obese women who deliver by cesarean delivery. What is an adequate dose of antibiotics to adequately cover obese and super-obese women? Prospective studies should also look at prevention of thromboembolic disease, which is more likely in obese women and which remains one of the most significant causes of maternal mortality.

Throughout this chapter, we have recommended the implementation of shared decision making to help pregnant women with complicated decisions that may arise during the prenatal period. While engaging the expectant women might seem to be an easily attainable task, the art and science of shared decision making has not been extensively studied in the obstetrical patient. Patient and provider communication is critical in order to fully inform the patient of her choices and to integrate her values and preferences into her final decisions for care. Future studies looking at both perinatal outcomes and patient satisfaction with care would help inform how shared decision making can best be used during pregnancy.

References

1. Cedergren MI. Maternal morbid obesity and the risk of adverse pregnancy outcomes. Obstet Gynecol. 2004;103(2):219–24.
2. American College of Obstetricians and Gynecologists. Obesity in pregnancy. ACOG committee opinion No. 549. Obstet Gynecol. 2013;121(1):213–7.
3. Poobalan AS, Aucott LS, Gurung T, Smith WC, Bhattacharya S. Obesity as an independent risk factor for elective and emergency caesarean delivery in nulliparous women – systematic review and meta-analysis of cohort studies. Obes Rev. 2009;10(1):28–35.
4. Weiss JL, Malone FD, Emig D, Ball RH, Nyberg DA, Comstock CH, et al. Obesity, obstetric complications and cesarean delivery rate – a population-based screening study. FASTER Research Consortium. Am J Obstet Gynecol. 2004;190(4):1091–7.
5. Ehrenberg HM, Mercer BM, Catalano PM. The influence of obesity and diabetes on the prevalence of macrosomia. Am J Obstet Gynecol. 2004;191(3):964–8.
6. Sewell MF, Huston-Presley L, Super DM, Catalano PM. Increased neonatal fat mass, and not lean body mass, is associated with maternal obesity. Am J Obstet Gynecol. 2006;195(4):1100–3.
7. Mazouni C, Porcu G, Cohen-Solal E, et al. Maternal and anthropomorphic risk factors for shoulder dystocia. Acta Obstet Gynecol Scand. 2006;85(5):567–70.
8. Spellacy WN, Miller S, Winegar A, Peterson PQ. Macrosomia – maternal characteristics and infant complications. Obstet Gynecol. 1985;66(2):158–61.
9. Lipscomb KR, Gregory K, Shaw K. The outcome of macrosomic infants weighing at least 4500 grams: Los Angeles County and University of Southern California experience. Obstet Gynecol. 1995;85(4):558–64.
10. American College of Obstetricians and Gynecologists Shoulder dystocia. ACOG practice bulletin 40. Obstet Gynecol. 2002;100(5 Pt 1):1045–50.
11. Wolfe HM, Gross TL, Sokol RJ, et al. Maternal obesity: a potential source of error in sonographic prenatal diagnosis. Obstet Gynecol. 1990;76(3 Pt 1):339–42.
12. Goetzinger KR, Tuuli MG, Odibo AO, Roehl KA, Macones GA, Cahill AG. Screening for fetal growth disorders by clinical exam in the era of obesity. J Perinatol. 2012. doi:10.1038/jp.2012.130.
13. Gunatilake RP, Perlow JH. Obesity and pregnancy: clinical management of the obese gravida. Am J Obstet Gynecol. 2011;204(2):106–19.
14. Johnson D. Management of cesarean delivery in the morbidly obese woman. From http://contemporaryobgyn.modernmedicine.com/contemporary-obgyn/news/modernmedicine/modern-medicine-feature-articles/management-cesarean-delivery. Retrieved 10 Jan 2013.

15. Nuthalapaty FS, Rouse DJ, Owen J. The association of maternal weight with cesarean risk, labor duration, and cervical dilation rate during labor induction. Obstet Gynecol. 2004;103(5 Pt 1):452–6.
16. Vahratian A, Zhang J, Troendle JF, Savitz DA, Siega-Riz AM. Maternal prepregnancy overweight and obesity and the pattern of labor progression in term nulliparous women. Obstet Gynecol. 2004;104(5):943–51.
17. Buhimschi CS, Buhimschi IA, MAlinow AM, Weiner CP. Intrauterine pressure during the second stage of labor in obese women. Obstet Gynecol. 2004;103(2):225–30.
18. Pevzner L, Powers BL, Rayburn WF, Rumney P, Wing DA. Effects of maternal obesity on duration and outcomes of prostaglandin cervical ripening and labor induction. Obstet Gynecol. 2009;114(6):1315–21.
19. Arrowsmith S, Wray S, Quenby S. Maternal obesity and labour complications following induction of labour in prolonged pregnancy. BJOG. 2011;118(5):578–88.
20. Marshall NE, Guild C, Cheng Y, Caughey AB, Halloran DR. Maternal superobesity and perinatal outcomes. Am J Obstet Gynecol. 2012;206(5):417.e1–6. doi:10.1016/j.ajog.2012.02.037. Epub 2012 Mar 7.
21. Vricella LK, Lois JM, Mercer BM, Bolden N. Anesthesia complications during scheduled cesarean delivery for morbidly obese women. Am J Obstet Gynecol. 2010;203(3):276.e1–5. doi:10.1016/j.ajog.2010.06.022. Epub 2010 Jul 31.
22. Grau T, Leipold RW, Conradi R, et al. Efficacy of ultrasound imaging in obstetric epidural anesthesia. J Clin Anesth. 2002;14(3):169–75.
23. Myles TD, Gooch J, Santolaya J. Obesity as an independent risk factor for infectious morbidity in patients who undergo cesarean delivery. Obstet Gynecol. 2002;100:959–64.
24. Pevzner L, Swank M, Krepel C, Wing DA, Chan K, Edmison Jr CE. Effects of maternal obesity on tissue concentrations of prophylactic cefazolin during cesarean delivery. Obstet Gynecol. 2011;117(4):877–82.
25. Wall PD, Deucy EE, Glantz JC, Pressman EK. Vertical skin incisions and wound complications in the obese parturient. Obstet Gynecol. 2003;102(5 pt 1):952–6.
26. Houston MC, Raynor BD. Postoperative morbidity in the morbidly obese parturient woman: supraumbilical and low transverse abdominal approaches. Am J Obstet Gynecol. 2000;182(5):1033–5.
27. Wylie BJ, Gilbert S, Landon MB, Spong CY, Rouse DJ, Leveno KJ, et al. Eunice Kennedy Shriver National Institute of Child Health and Human Development (NICHD) Maternal-Fetal Medicine Units Network (MFMU). Comparison of transverse and vertical skin incision for emergency cesarean delivery. Obstet Gynecol. 2010;115(6):1134–40.

28. Chelmow D, Rodriguez EJ, Sabatini MM. Suture closure of subcutaneous fat and wound disruption after cesarean delivery: a meta-analysis. Obstet Gynecol. 2004;103(5 Pt 1):974–80.
29. Catalano PM. Management of obesity in pregnancy. Obstet Gynecol. 2007;109(2 pt 1):419–33.
30. Ramsey PS, White AM, Guinn DA, Lu GC, Ramin SM, Davies JK, et al. Subcutaneous tissue reapproximation, alone or in combination with drain, in obese women undergoing cesarean delivery. Obstet Gynecol. 2005;105(5 Pt 1):967–73.
31. Tooher R, Gates S, Dowswell T, Davis LJ. Prophylaxis for venous thromboembolic disease in pregnancy and the early postnatal period. Cochrane Database Syst Rev. 2010;12(5):CD001689. doi:10.1002/14651858.CD001689.pub2.
32. Duhl AJ, Paidas MJ, Ural SH, Branch W, Casele H, Cox-Gill J, et al. Antithrombotic therapy and pregnancy: consensus report and recommendations for prevention and treatment of venous thromboembolism and adverse pregnancy outcomes. Am J Obstet Gynecol. 2007;197(5):457.e1–21.
33. Martin JA, Hamilton BE, Ventura SJ, Osterman MJK, Wilson EC, Mathews TJ. Births: final data for 2010. National vital statistics reports, vol. 61 no 1. Hyattsville: National Center for Health Statistics; 2012.
34. Chauhan SP, Magann EF, Carroll CS, Barrilleaux PS, Scardo JA, Martin JN. Mode of delivery for the morbidly obese patient with prior cesarean delivery; vaginal versus repeat cesarean section. Am J Obstet Gynecol. 2001;185(2):349–54.
35. Carroll CS, Magann EF, Chauhan SP, Klauser CK, Morrison JC. Vaginal birth after cesarean section versus elective repeat cesarean delivery: weight-based outcomes. Am J Obstet Gynecol. 2003;188(6):1516–22.
36. Hibbard JU, Gilbert S, Landon MB, Hauth JC, Leveno KJ, Spong CY, et al. Trial of labor or repeat cesarean delivery in women with morbid obesity and previous cesarean delivery. Obstet Gynecol. 2006;108(1):125–33.
37. Catalano PM, McIntyre HD, Cruickshank JK, McCance DR, Dyer AR, Metzger BE, et al. The hyperglycemia and adverse pregnancy outcome study: associations of GDM and obesity with pregnancy outcomes. Diabetes Care. 2012;35(4):780–6.
38. Landon MB, Gabbe SG. Gestational diabetes mellitus. Obstet Gynecol. 2011;118(6):1379–93.
39. Kjos S, Henry O, Montoro M, Buchanan TA, Mestman JH. Insulin-requiring diabetes in pregnancy: a randomized trial of active induction of labor and expectant management. Am J Obstet Gynecol. 1993;169(3):611–5.
40. Witkop CT, Neale D, Wilson LM, Bass EB, Nicholson WK. Active compared with expectant delivery management in women with gestational diabetes: a systematic review. Obstet Gynecol. 2009;113(1):206–17.

Part II
Maternal Risk Factors and Obesity

Chapter 5
Epidemiologic Trends and Maternal Risk Factors Predicting Postpartum Weight Retention

Erica P. Gunderson

Abstract Over the past decade, women have become heavier at the time of conception, gain more weight during pregnancy, and are a greater risk of postpartum weight retention. Excessive weight gain during pregnancy is a key predictor of postpartum weight retention. Characterizing trends in postpartum weight retention can help to identify high-risk women who are susceptible to substantial weight retention postpartum and accelerated weight gain trajectories in midlife. Understanding postpartum weight trajectories can inform our efforts for primary prevention of obesity and help to reduce long-term obesity and its associated consequences.

Keywords Gestational diabetes mellitus • Atherosclerosis • Cardiovascular disease • Prospective cohort studies • Diabetes • Glucose tolerance • Epidemiology • Pregnancy • Women

E.P. Gunderson, PhD
Division of Research, Kaiser Permanente
Northern California, 2000 Broadway,
Oakland, CA 94612, USA
e-mail: erica.gunderson@kp.org

W. Nicholson, K. Baptiste-Roberts (eds.),
Obesity During Pregnancy in Clinical Practice,
DOI 10.1007/978-1-4471-2831-1_5,
© Springer-Verlag London 2014

Key Points
- Women are starting pregnancy heavier than ever before.
- Women have higher average weight gains during pregnancy than in past generations.
- The strongest predictors of postpartum weight retention are high maternal body size before pregnancy, excessive gestational weight gain, young age at menarche, and excessive gestational weight gain.

Introduction

Weight gain and becoming overweight during the reproductive years are strong independent predictors of cardiovascular disease morbidity and mortality, particularly among women [1–4]. The hormonal adaptations to pregnancy promote gestational weight gain and fat accumulation to support fetal growth and development, as well as provide energy stores for lactation [5]. Yet, in modern societies, the abundant food supplies and sedentary lifestyles are likely to result in gestational weight gain exceeding optimal levels. Pregnancy's physiological adaptations may predispose susceptible women to marked postpartum weight retention as triggers for the development of overweight or obesity [6]. Excessive gestational weight gain not only increases the risk of some pregnancy complications (i.e., gestational diabetes mellitus, hypertensive disorders, C-section delivery) but can have lasting adverse effects on women's health including greater risk of developing the metabolic syndrome, type 2 diabetes, and/or cardiovascular disease in mid- or late life [4, 7, 8]. Moreover, shortened duration of lactation and formula supplementation may compromise postpartum cardiometabolic profiles and increase disease risk [9–12].

Women are starting pregnancy heavier than ever and are gaining more weight during pregnancy than in past generations.

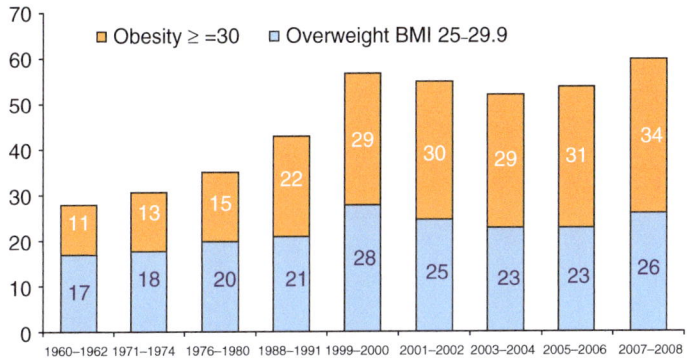

FIGURE 5.1 US trends in overweight and obesity in women 1960–2008 (age 20–44 or 20–39 years)

Both maternal body mass index (BMI) and gestational weight gain have increased for the general US population during the past three decades. Recent estimates show that 60 % of all US women are overweight or obese (BMI ≥25) and that at least one-third are obese (BMI ≥30) [13]. The secular trends for increasing overweight and obesity prevalence are highest among women aged 35–44 years [13]. From 1960 to 2008, the prevalence of overweight (BMI 25–29.9) and obesity (BMI ≥30) in women of reproductive age increased from 28 to 60 % (Fig. 5.1) [14]. Within the past 20 years, the proportion of women exceeding gestational weight gain recommendations has increased significantly. Excessive gestational weight gain [i.e., above the levels recommended by the Institute of Medicine (IOM) for their BMI category] [15] was reported by 43 % of pregnant women in 2008 compared to 33 % in 1988 (Fig. 5.2) [14]. The increasing proportion of US women who are overweight or obese before pregnancy combined with higher gestational weight gain during pregnancy and more sedentary lifestyle behaviors and short duration of breastfeeding are key contributors to increasing postpartum weight retention and obesity risk among young women.

Maternal overweight or obesity before pregnancy is the most common high-risk obstetric condition [16] and is associ-

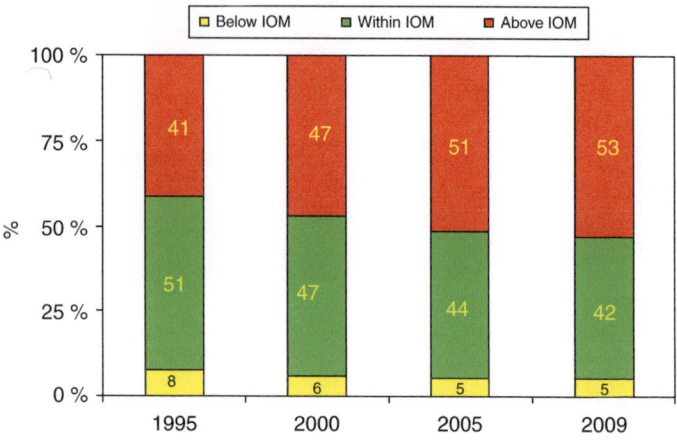

FIGURE 5.2 Secular trends in gestational weight gain from 1995 to 2009; US Pregnancy Nutrition Surveillance, CDC

ated with greater maternal and infant morbidity, including gestational diabetes and hypertension disorders in the woman as well as neural tube defects, macrosomia, and perinatal mortality in the newborn [17, 18]. Women who are already overweight or obese before pregnancy tend to retain more weight postpartum than those not overweight [19, 20], despite having lower gestational weight gain and larger newborns [21].

Weight gain trajectories before pregnancy may exert a significant influence on the weight gain related to pregnancy, as age at reproductive maturation and genetic characteristics may influence the tendency to retain weight after pregnancy. The American College of Obstetrics and Gynecology (ACOG) recommends modification of maternal weight before conception as well as advice and monitoring of gestational weight gain during pregnancy as measures that may prevent pregnancy complications and adverse long-term outcomes for women and their children [18]. Characterization of the trends in postpartum weight retention and identification of high-risk women who are susceptible to substantial weight retention postpartum and accelerated weight gain trajectories in midlife are important to our understanding of targets for primary prevention of obesity and future chronic disease in young women.

Pregnancy Cohort Studies and Postpartum Weight Retention

A meta-analysis of early and late postpartum weight retention estimated that postpartum weight retention (as measured by BMI) averages 2.5 kg/m^2 (about 6 kg) at 6 weeks, 1.25 kg/m^2 (about 3 kg) at 6 months, and 0.5 kg/m^2 (about 1.25 kg) at 1 year [22]. A major limitation of practically all pregnancy cohort design studies is that they rely on maternal recall of body weight before conception and/or early first trimester weight measurements. Self-report of prepregnancy weight is biased toward underreporting to a greater extent in overweight or obese women and thereby inflate the estimates of postpartum weight retention for high-BMI groups. Pregnancy cohort studies based on self-reported pregravid weight may introduce substantial bias because high-BMI groups underreport body weight by about 5 kg versus 1 kg for other groups [23, 24]. Therefore, reporting bias affects estimates of gestational weight gain and postpartum weight retention to a greater extent for high- than low-BMI groups. An underestimate of 5 kg may overestimate gestational weight gain by almost 50 % for obese women, and an error of 1 kg may overestimate postpartum weight change by more than 100–200 %.

Furthermore, postpartum weight retention may be overestimated in the high-BMI groups due to the higher trajectory of weight gain established before conception that may continue at the similar accelerated pace after pregnancy. Thus, weight retention at 1–2 years postpartum may not be due to retention of gestational gain but weight gain after delivery. Previous studies with serial postpartum weight measurements have distinguished between weight retention and subsequent weight gain by prepregnancy body size [20].

Childbearing Cohorts and Pregnancy-Related Weight Gain

Longitudinal cohort studies focusing on the natural history of childbearing among women of reproductive age suggest that a first birth has adverse effects on overall adiposity, while increasing number of births (parity) has cumulative effects on central adiposity. In CARDIA women, waist circumference increased with each subsequent birth controlling for prepregnancy measurements [25], while body weight increased primarily after the first birth [25, 26]. The findings suggest that the greatest impact on overall fat stores is after the first birth but subsequent births increase central obesity. The Coronary Artery Risk Development in Young Adults (CARDIA) study estimated pregnancy-related weight gain from before to after pregnancy controlling for secular trends in weight gain and to assess differences within prepregnancy BMI (overweight or obese) and parity groups (primiparas) [25]. The unique strengths of this study include the longitudinal design, standardized research measurements of body weight from before to after pregnancy (3- to 5-year intervals), and high retention rates. The large sample size enabled investigators to determine that pregnancy-related weight gain depended on the first birth (primiparity) and by maternal prepregnancy overweight. In CARDIA, postpartum weight retention averaged 1 kg for women who were not overweight before pregnancy (BMI <25) and about 3–6 kg for women who were already overweight or obese before pregnancy (BMI ≥25) controlling for sociodemographics, prepregnancy BMI, and lifestyle factors [25, 27]. Being overweight before pregnancy signifies the predisposition for weight gain, and pregnancy may exacerbate this tendency for many women. The CARDIA study provides most accurate estimates of long-term weight gain due to pregnancy and its aftermath, by accounting for secular trends in weight gain during the same period among women who did not bear children.

Certain lifestyle behaviors are also likely to influence women's risk of becoming overweight or obesity in midlife [6, 28]. For example, among nonsmokers in CARDIA, giving birth was associated with a twofold greater risk of becoming overweight within several years versus not giving birth [6]. Yet, among smokers, women who had given birth were half as likely to become overweight as those who had never given birth; OR=0.41(95 % CI: 0.17,0.96) for women delivering one birth only and 0.36 (95 % CI: 0.08,1.65) for women delivering two or more births [6]. Other modifiable risk factors include postpartum sleep, dietary practices, and physical activity, although biological risk factors such age at menarche and primiparity also appear to play key roles.

Pregnancy Cohorts and Estimates of Average Postpartum Weight Retention

A 2011 meta-analysis examined average postpartum weight retention with several time periods [29]. On average, at 6 months or less postpartum, women who experienced gestational weight gain above IOM recommendations retained an average of 4 kg more than those gaining within recommendations. By 6–12 months postpartum, the weight retention averaged 2.5 kg in the group with excessive gestational weight gain. By 3 years postpartum, the retention was estimated to be 3 kg greater. However, these estimates are based on very few studies, in which serial measurements of postpartum weights were not available, and had variable sample characteristics which may explain the higher "retention" for the longer period of follow-up. The variability in estimates of average postpartum weight retention may be related to maternal characteristics such as race, sociodemographics and economic status, age, smoking, and levels of gestational weight gain.

Pregnancy Cohorts and Risk of Substantial Postpartum Weight Retention

Large pregnancy cohort studies ($n > 400$) generally report that 13–20 % of pregnant women (Table 5.1) experience substantial weight retention by 1 year postpartum (defined as body weight of 5 kg above preconception weight). Substantial postpartum weight retention has been reported

TABLE 5.1 Prepregnancy high BMI (%), excessive GWG (%), and substantial postpartum weight retention (PPWR) (%) at 1–2 years postpartum from cohort studies ($n > 400$) from 1988 to 2011

Author, year Country (years data collected)	Sample size (n)	Age range (years)	Time of postpartum measurement	Overweight or obese before pregnancy (%)	Substantial PPWR ≥5 kg (%)
Ohlin, 1990 [48] Sweden (1971–1984)	1,423	17–49	12 months	7[c]	14
Keppel, 1993[a] [44] USA (1988)	2,944	>15	10–18 months	10[b]	>20
Greene, 1988[a] [46] USA (1959–1965)	7,116	23 ± 11	Variable (between 2 pregnancies)	24[d]	~20
Gunderson, 2001 [20] USA (1980–1990)	1,300	18–41 (mean 27)	Variable (between 2 pregnancies)	13[b]	>20
Olson, 2003 [33] USA (not stated)	540	18 to >40	12 months	41[b]	~20

Gunderson, 2008 [34] USA (1999–2003)	940	33 ± 5	12 months	25[b]	13
Siega-Riz, 2010 [31] USA (2001–2005)	550	31 ± 5	3, 12 months	33[b]	~40
Rothberg, 2011[a] [32] USA (2001–2004)	427	14–25	12 months	52	~50
Rode, 2012 [30] Denmark (1996–1999)	1,840	<25 to >36	12 months	20	13

Substantial PPWR defined as ≥5 kg above prepregnancy weight
[a]Sample includes teenagers
[b]Defined as BMI ≥26 kg/m^2
[c]Defined as BMI ≥24 kg/m^2
[d]Defined as >120 % of ideal body weight for height

among 7–52 % of women at 1 year postpartum when studies including special populations, such as low-income groups and pregnant adolescents, are included. However, the percentages with substantial postpartum weight retention correlate closely with the prevalence of prepregnancy overweight and obesity for the specific cohort. For example, northern European and US cohorts with lower rates of maternal prepregnancy overweight or obesity (7–25 %) reported lower proportion of women with substantial weight retention (10–20 %). The US cohorts that focused largely on women from low socioeconomic groups reported much higher rates of maternal prepregnancy overweight or obesity (24–52 %) and reported the highest proportions of women experiencing substantial postpartum weight retention (20–50 %) [6, 28, 30–33].

Correlates of substantial postpartum weight retention based on epidemiologic studies include high gestational gain, pregravid overweight, primiparity, black race, low socioeconomic status, smoking cessation, and fewer than 5 h of sleep per day [19, 33, 34]. The strongest predictors of postpartum weight retention include maternal overweight or obesity before pregnancy, excessive gestational weight gain exceeding the IOM recommendations, and primiparity [27, 35, 36]. Maternal characteristics associated with a two- to threefold higher risk of becoming overweight after pregnancy independent of gestational weight gain include young age at menarche (less than 12 years), short interval (less than 8 years) from menarche to first birth, maternal age 24–30 years [28], and short sleep duration (<5 h per 24 h period) at 6 months postpartum [34]. These risk factors may indirectly represent either genetic or biologic influences on adult body weight prior to pregnancy, socioeconomic differences in maternal age when childbearing begins, and/or postpartum behavior changes. Although the strength of associations with postpartum weight retention for these traits is similar to total gestational weight gain, for some risk factors, their lower prevalence in a population may result in relatively lower attributable risk for postpartum weight retention than gestational weight gain or maternal body size.

Risk of Becoming Overweight or Obese After Pregnancy

A two- to threefold greater risk of becoming overweight after pregnancy has been associated with reproductive factors such as excessive gestational weight gain, young age at menarche (<12 years), and pregnancy within 8 years of menarche [28]. Very few studies have examined the risk of becoming overweight due to pregnancy, although some have linked gestational weight gain to weight status more than a decade later [37, 38]. These data suggest that weight gain trajectories may be influenced by genetic factors influencing reproductive maturation and that pregnancy at a young age exacerbates the risk of becoming overweight to the same extent as excessive gestational weight gain.

Evidence from childbearing cohorts and pregnancy cohorts suggests that a first birth and maternal prepregnancy body size are key predictors of long-term weight retention and that gestational weight gain is likely to mediate these associations. The next sections critically examine these risk factors and their impact on weight changes after pregnancy.

Prepregnancy Body Size

Although gestational weight gain is linked to postpartum weight retention, primiparity and larger body size before pregnancy exert important influences that modify these relationships. Evidence that prepregnancy BMI influences weight retention has varied by attributes of the populations studied and the inadequate sample size to assess effect modification by prepregnancy BMI categories in the gestational weight gain and postpartum weight association. Women who are overweight or obese before pregnancy are generally more likely to have excessive as well as inadequate gestational weight gains [21, 39]. Excessive gestational weight gain increases the risk of postpartum weight retention, but the effect may depend on prepregnancy body size, maternal age, and primiparity. Yet, very few studies have addressed the joint effects of these key risk factors. Weight retention or gain following delivery may also be highly variable and strongly influenced by both the weight gain trajectory that preceded pregnancy (i.e., high prepregnancy BMI) and excessive gestational weight gain.

Gestational Weight Gain

In the USA, at least 43 % of all pregnant women [14] and two-thirds of overweight women exceed the recommended amount of weight gain during pregnancy, while one-third of obese women gain more than 25 lb [39–42]. Specifically, overweight and obese women are two to six times more likely to exceed the weight gain recommendations during pregnancy [39, 42, 43] than other BMI groups. They are also predisposed to higher postpartum weight gain and retention after pregnancy [44].

Gestational weight gain is strongly, positively correlated with maternal weight change from preconception to beyond 6 months postpartum and exerts long-term effects on maternal body weight [45–49]. In multiple linear regression models, total gestational gain has accounted for 20–35 % of the variability in the weight change [19, 45, 48, 49]. In the NMIHS cohort, Parker and Abrams found that high gestational gain was associated with a twofold increase in risk of substantial weight gain (above 9 kg) from preconception to 10–18 months postpartum among women who were underweight and normal weight prior to pregnancy [50] but high body size was also directly associated with postpartum weight. Gunderson et al. reported that gestational gain above the recommended levels was associated with a threefold higher risk of becoming overweight after pregnancy (BMI ≥26) among women who were under- or average weight before pregnancy in large, multiethnic cohort [28].

Reproductive Maturation and Timing of Pregnancy

Reproductive maturation, including young age at menarche (<12 years) and pregnancy onset within 8 years of menarche, may increase a woman's risk of weight retention or becoming overweight after pregnancy [28]. Weight gain trajectories after pregnancy may be influenced by genetic factors or other biological influences from early childhood. These risk factors appear to influence postpartum weight retention as strongly as excessive gestational weight gain and should be incorporated into future studies as a way of refining subgroups for whom weight control during pregnancy has the greatest impact in reducing weight retention.

Pregnancy Weight Gain Triggering Maternal Obesity

The impact of gestational weight gain on risk of substantial postpartum weight retention (>5 kg) and risk of becoming overweight after pregnancy has been reported in only a few studies [28, 48, 51]. Overall, average weight gain related to childbearing among women who became overweight after pregnancy was about 10 kg [28]. Yet, the risk of becoming overweight or obesity due to childbearing is an important outcome to assess the impact on health risk for young women of childbearing age. Specifically, excessive gestational weight gain not only adversely affects perinatal health outcomes but may be the first trigger of obesity in young women [25, 37]. As a potentially modifiable risk factor, gestational weight gain may provide the critical opportunity for slowing the weight gain trajectory in young women that results in midlife obesity.

Fat Accumulation and Body Composition Changes Due to Pregnancy

Total gestational gain is highly variable resulting in large variation between individuals in postpartum weight retention and body fat distribution. During pregnancy about 30 % of gestational weight gain is comprised of fat, with deposition preferentially in the femoral and abdominal regions producing a more gynecoid body fat distribution.

Longitudinal studies of body fat deposition from prepregnancy to postpartum have found differences in body fat deposition by maternal body size. Obese women showed a tendency to develop more central obesity at 6 months postpartum [52]. In 557 healthy women, subcutaneous body fat (skinfold thicknesses) measured from before, during, and 6 weeks after pregnancy reported that central body fat gains in the subscapular area were relatively high during pregnancy and that primiparas gained more fat at both thigh and subscapular locations than other women [53]. Moreover, fat stores in the triceps and thigh regions were utilized to a greater extent within the first 6 weeks postpartum.

A study of 15 women using magnetic resonance imaging (tomographs) to measure subcutaneous and non-subcutaneous adipose tissue from before pregnancy and at four intervals postpartum reported that 68 % of gestational fat gain was deposited in the trunk and that excess fat gain remaining at 1 year postpartum tended to be localized centrally [54]. Data from large, population-based studies are consistent with these findings. Parity has been correlated with higher abdominal girth many years after childbearing with larger waist-hip ratios (WHR) [55–57], and longitudinal studies of childbearing age women found cumulative increases in WHR [26] and waist circumference changes from before to after pregnancies in CARDIA women [25].

Pregnancy and Visceral Fat Changes

Some evidence suggests that pregnancy increases visceral adiposity. In a longitudinal study of 122 premenopausal CARDIA women (50 black, 72 white), adipose tissue (visceral and subcutaneous) compartments were measured via computed tomography from before pregnancy (1995–1996) and again 5 years later (1999–2000). We identified 14 women who gave birth once during the 5-year interval and had adipose tissue measured before and after the birth as well as in 108 women who did not give birth during this same time interval [58]. In multiple linear regression models adjusted for age, race, and changes in total and subcutaneous adiposity, the visceral adipose tissue levels increased by 40 and 14 % above initial levels for the parous and nonparous groups, respectively; group mean difference (95 % Confidence Interval) in visceral fat levels was 18.0 cm^2 (4.8, 31.2) controlling for gain in total body fat and covariates, $p<0.01$. There was also a borderline greater group difference in mean (95 % CI) waist girth of 2.3 cm (0, 4.5), $p=0.05$, that represented an absolute mean increase of 6.3 cm (4.1, 8.5) versus 4.0 cm (3.2, 4.8) for parous versus nonparous group. Thus, pregnancy is associated with preferential accumulation of adipose tissue in the visceral compartment for similar gains in total body fat. Thus, childbearing increases central adiposity to a greater extent than overall adiposity. These findings are important because chronic disease risk is better predicted by central obesity, particularly visceral adiposity, even among nonobese individuals.

Conclusions

Weight gain before, during, and after pregnancy may not only affect maternal and fetal health for current and subsequent pregnancies but may be a primary contributor to future development of obesity in women during midlife and beyond [6, 37, 59]. Identification of high-risk women who may benefit from preconception and prenatal interventions to avoid the accelerated gestational weight gain is the key to prevention of pregnancy-related weight gain and long-term obesity-related chronic disease in women of reproductive age. More information regarding the influence of socioeconomic factors and culture practices, smoking cessation, lactation, and other behaviors on weight changes both during and after pregnancy is also needed.

High prepregnancy body size may be the most important risk factor for pregnancy-related weight retention. Women who are moderately overweight before a first pregnancy may benefit from weight loss several months before pregnancy as well as require additional support during early pregnancy to carefully control gestational weight gain within IOM recommendations. Overweight and obese women who succeed in achieving gestational weight gain within the recommended ranges need additional support for lactation and to promote postpartum weight loss to below preconception weight. Women who begin pregnancy in the normal range, but have excessive gestational weight gain or other risk factors (i.e., gestational diabetes, young age, primiparity, or depression), may benefit from weight control programs during the first year postpartum to reduce weight retention.

Accelerated prepregnancy weight gain trajectories, pregnancy complications, medical conditions, and/or other behaviors among women may predispose them to substantial weight gain and obesity during midlife. Risk assessment is needed to identify the subgroup of women who are predisposed to greater risk of substantial postpartum weight retention or to becoming overweight or obese after pregnancy. Weight gain and development of overweight during the reproductive years are an increasing problem and confer excess risk of cardiovascular disease morbidity and mortality, particularly among women [1–4]. During the life span, cumulative weight gain may eventually lead to development of the metabolic syndrome, type 2 diabetes, and/or cardiovascular disease [4, 7, 8]. As modifiable risk factors, prevention of excessive gestational weight gain and substantial postpartum weight retention during the reproductive years provides a critical opportunity for early obesity and chronic disease prevention efforts among women.

Grant and Acknowledgment Funding is provided by the National Institute of Diabetes and Digestive and Kidney Diseases (K01 DK059944 and R01 DK090047).

References

1. Hubert HB, Feinleib M, McNamara PM, Castelli WP. Obesity as an independent risk factor for cardiovascular disease: a 26-year follow-up of participants in the Framingham Heart Study. Circulation. 1983;67(5):968–77.
2. Manson JE, Colditz GA, Stampfer MJ, et al. A prospective study of obesity and risk of coronary heart disease in women. N Engl J Med. 1990;322(13):882–9.
3. Manson JE, Willett WC, Stampfer MJ, et al. Body weight and mortality among women. N Engl J Med. 1995;333(11):677–85.
4. Willett WC, Manson JE, Stampfer MJ, et al. Weight, weight change, and coronary heart disease in women. Risk within the 'normal' weight range. JAMA. 1995;273(6):461–5.
5. Hytten FE, Leitch I. The physiology of pregnancy. 2nd ed. Oxford/London/Edinburgh: Blackwell Scientific Publications; 1971.
6. Gunderson EP, Quesenberry Jr CP, Lewis CE, et al. Development of overweight associated with childbearing depends on smoking habit: the Coronary Artery Risk Development in Young Adults (CARDIA) Study. Obes Res. 2004;12(12):2041–53.
7. Gunderson EP, Jacobs Jr DR, Chiang V, et al. Childbearing is associated with higher incidence of the metabolic syndrome among women of reproductive age controlling for measurements before pregnancy: the CARDIA study. Am J Obstet Gynecol. 2009;201(2):177.e1–9.
8. Colditz GA, Willett WC, Stampfer MJ, Rosner B, Speizer FE, Hennekens CH. A prospective study of age at menarche, parity, age at first birth, and coronary heart disease in women. Am J Epidemiol. 1987;126(5):861–70.
9. Stuebe AM, Rich-Edwards JW, Willett WC, Manson JE, Michels KB. Duration of lactation and incidence of type 2 diabetes. JAMA. 2005;294(20):2601–10.
10. Gunderson EP, Lewis CE, Wei GS, Whitmer RA, Quesenberry CP, Sidney S. Lactation and changes in maternal metabolic risk factors. Obstet Gynecol. 2007;109(3):729–38.

11. Gunderson EP, Jacobs Jr DR, Chiang V, et al. Duration of lactation and incidence of the metabolic syndrome in women of reproductive age according to gestational diabetes mellitus status: a 20-year prospective study in CARDIA (Coronary Artery Risk Development in Young Adults). Diabetes. 2010;59(2):495–504.
12. Gunderson EP, Hedderson MM, Chiang V, et al. Lactation intensity and postpartum maternal glucose tolerance and insulin resistance in women with recent GDM: the SWIFT cohort. Diabetes Care. 2012;35(1):50–6.
13. Flegal KM, Carroll MD, Kit BK, Ogden CL. Prevalence of obesity and trends in the distribution of body mass index among US adults, 1999–2010. JAMA. 2012;307(5):491–7. doi: 10.1001/jama.2012.39. Epub 2012 Jan 17. PubMed PMID: 22253363.
14. Center for Disease Control & Prevention. Pediatric & pregnancy nutrition surveillance system. 2011, http://www.cdc.gov/pednss/pnss_tables/tables_numeric.htm.
15. Institute of Medicine (US) and National Research Council (US) Committee to Reexamine IOM Pregnancy Weight Guidelines. Weight gain during pregnancy: reexamining the guidelines. Washington, DC: National Academies Press (US); 2009.
16. Catalano PM. Increasing maternal obesity and weight gain during pregnancy: the obstetric problems of plentitude. Obstet Gynecol. 2007;110(4):743–4.
17. Galtier-Dereure F, Boegner C, Bringer J. Obesity and pregnancy: complications and cost. Am J Clin Nutr. 2000;71(5 Suppl):1242S–8.
18. American College of Obstetricians and Gynecologists. ACOG Committee Opinion number 315, September 2005. Obesity in pregnancy. Obstet Gynecol. 2005;106(3):671–5.
19. Gunderson EP, Abrams B. Epidemiology of gestational weight gain and body weight changes after pregnancy. Epidemiol Rev. 1999;21(2):261–75.
20. Gunderson EP, Abrams B, Selvin S. Does the pattern of postpartum weight change differ according to pregravid body size? Int J Obes Relat Metab Disord. 2001;25(6):853–62.
21. Institute of Medicine. Nutrition during pregnancy. Washington, DC: National Academy of Sciences; 1990.
22. Schmitt NM, Nicholson WK, Schmitt J. The association of pregnancy and the development of obesity – results of a systematic review and meta-analysis on the natural history of postpartum weight retention. Int J Obes (Lond). 2007;31(11):1642–51.
23. Stevens-Simon C, Roghmann KJ, McAnarney ER. Relationship of self-reported prepregnant weight and weight gain during pregnancy to maternal body habitus and age. J Am Diet Assoc. 1992;92(1):85–7.
24. Rowland ML. Self-reported weight and height. Am J Clin Nutr. 1990;52(6):1125–33.

25. Gunderson EP, Murtaugh MA, Lewis CE, Quesenberry CP, West DS, Sidney S. Excess gains in weight and waist circumference associated with childbearing: the Coronary Artery Risk Development in Young Adults Study (CARDIA). Int J Obes Relat Metab Disord. 2004;28(4):525–35.
26. Smith DE, Lewis CE, Caveny JL, Perkins LL, Burke GL, Bild DE. Longitudinal changes in adiposity associated with pregnancy. The CARDIA Study. Coronary Artery Risk Development in Young Adults Study. JAMA. 1994;271(22):1747–51.
27. Rosenberg L, Palmer JR, Wise LA, Horton NJ, Kumanyika SK, Adams-Campbell LL. A prospective study of the effect of childbearing on weight gain in African-American women. Obes Res. 2003;11(12):1526–35.
28. Gunderson EP, Abrams B, Selvin S. The relative importance of gestational gain and maternal characteristics associated with the risk of becoming overweight after pregnancy. Int J Obes Relat Metab Disord. 2000;24(12):1660–8.
29. Nehring I, Schmoll S, Beyerlein A, Hauner H, von KR. Gestational weight gain and long-term postpartum weight retention: a meta-analysis. Am J Clin Nutr. 2011;94(5):1225–31.
30. Rode L, Kjaergaard H, Ottesen B, Damm P, Hegaard HK. Association between gestational weight gain according to body mass index and postpartum weight in a large cohort of Danish women. Matern Child Health J. 2012;16(2):406–13.
31. Siega-Riz AM, Herring AH, Carrier K, Evenson KR, Dole N, Deierlein A. Sociodemographic, perinatal, behavioral, and psychosocial predictors of weight retention at 3 and 12 months postpartum. Obesity (Silver Spring). 2010;18(10):1996–2003.
32. Gould Rothberg BE, Magriples U, Kershaw TS, Rising SS, Ickovics JR. Gestational weight gain and subsequent postpartum weight loss among young, low-income, ethnic minority women. Am J Obstet Gynecol. 2011;204(1):52.e1–11.
33. Olson CM, Strawderman MS, Hinton PS, Pearson TA. Gestational weight gain and postpartum behaviors associated with weight change from early pregnancy to 1 y postpartum. Int J Obes Relat Metab Disord. 2003;27(1):117–27.
34. Gunderson EP, Rifas-Shiman SL, Oken E, et al. Association of fewer hours of sleep at 6 months postpartum with substantial weight retention at 1 year postpartum. Am J Epidemiol. 2008;167(2):178–87.
35. Gunderson EP. Childbearing and obesity in women: weight before, during, and after pregnancy. Obstet Gynecol Clin North Am. 2009;36(2):317–32; ix.
36. Linne Y, Rossner S. Interrelationships between weight development and weight retention in subsequent pregnancies: the SPAWN study. Acta Obstet Gynecol Scand. 2003;82(4):318–25.

37. Rooney BL, Schauberger CW, Mathiason MA. Impact of perinatal weight change on long-term obesity and obesity-related illnesses. Obstet Gynecol. 2005;106(6):1349–56.
38. Amorim AR, Rossner S, Neovius M, Lourenco PM, Linne Y. Does excess pregnancy weight gain constitute a major risk for increasing long-term BMI? Obesity (Silver Spring). 2007;15(5):1278–86.
39. Brawarsky P, Stotland NE, Jackson RA, et al. Pre-pregnancy and pregnancy-related factors and the risk of excessive or inadequate gestational weight gain. Int J Gynaecol Obstet. 2005;91(2):125–31.
40. Taffel SM, Keppel KG, Jones GK. Medical advice on maternal weight gain and actual weight gain. Results from the 1988 National Maternal and Infant Health Survey. Ann N Y Acad Sci. 1993; 678:293–305.
41. Cogswell ME, Serdula MK, Hungerford DW, Yip R. Gestational weight gain among average-weight and overweight women–what is excessive? Am J Obstet Gynecol. 1995;172(2 Pt 1):705–12.
42. Wells CS, Schwalberg R, Noonan G, Gabor V. Factors influencing inadequate and excessive weight gain in pregnancy: Colorado, 2000-2002. Matern Child Health J. 2006;10(1):55–62.
43. Chasan-Taber L, Schmidt MD, Pekow P, Sternfeld B, Solomon CG, Markenson G. Predictors of excessive and inadequate gestational weight gain in Hispanic women. Obesity (Silver Spring). 2008;16(7): 1657–66.
44. Keppel KG, Taffel SM. Pregnancy-Related Weight Gain and Retention: Implications of the 1990 Institute of Medicine Guidelines. Am J Public Health. 1993;83(8):1100–1103.
45. Boardley DJ, Sargent RG, Coker AL, Hussey JR, Sharpe PA. The relationship between diet, activity, and other factors, and postpartum weight change by race. Obstet Gynecol. 1995;86(5):834–8.
46. Greene GW, Smiciklas-Wright H, Scholl TO, Karp RJ. Postpartum weight change: how much of the weight gained in pregnancy will be lost after delivery? Obstet Gynecol. 1988;71(5):701–7.
47. Schauberger CW, Rooney BL, Brimer LM. Factors that influence weight loss in the puerperium. Obstet Gynecol. 1992;79(3):424–9.
48. Ohlin A, Rossner S. Maternal body weight development after pregnancy. Int J Obes. 1990;14(2):159–73.
49. Kac G, Benicio MH, Velasquez-Melendez G, Valente JG, Struchiner CJ. Gestational weight gain and prepregnancy weight influence postpartum weight retention in a cohort of Brazilian women. J Nutr. 2004;134(3):661–6.
50. Parker JD, Abrams B. Differences in postpartum weight retention between black and white mothers. Obstet Gynecol. 1993;81(5 (Pt 1)): 768–74.
51. Mamun AA, Kinarivala M, O'Callaghan MJ, Williams GM, Najman JM, Callaway LK. Associations of excess weight gain during pregnancy with long-term maternal overweight and obesity: evidence

from 21 y postpartum follow-up. Am J Clin Nutr. 2010;91(5): 1336–41.
52. Soltani H, Fraser RB. A longitudinal study of maternal anthropometric changes in normal weight, overweight and obese women during pregnancy and postpartum. Br J Nutr. 2000;84(1):95–101.
53. Sidebottom AC, Brown JE, Jacobs Jr DR. Pregnancy-related changes in body fat. Eur J Obstet Gynecol Reprod Biol. 2001;94(2):216–23.
54. Sohlstrom A, Forsum E. Changes in adipose tissue volume and distribution during reproduction in Swedish women as assessed by magnetic resonance imaging. Am J Clin Nutr. 1995;61(2):287–95.
55. Troisi RJ, Wolf AM, Mason JE, Klingler KM, Colditz GA. Relation of body fat distribution to reproductive factors in pre- and postmenopausal women. Obes Res. 1995;3(2):143–51.
56. den Tonkelaar I, Seidell JC, van Noord PA, Baanders-van Halewijn EA, Ouwehand IJ. Fat distribution in relation to age, degree of obesity, smoking habits, parity and estrogen use: a cross-sectional study in 11,825 Dutch women participating in the DOM-project. Int J Obes. 1990;14(9):753–61.
57. Kaye SA, Folsom AR, Prineas RJ, Potter JD, Gapstur SM. The association of body fat distribution with lifestyle and reproductive factors in a population study of postmenopausal women. Int J Obes. 1990;14(7):583–91.
58. Gunderson EP, Sternfeld B, Wellons MF, et al. Childbearing may increase visceral adipose tissue independent of overall increase in body fat. Obesity (Silver Spring). 2008;16(5):1078–84.
59. Linne Y, Dye L, Barkeling B, Rossner S. Weight development over time in parous women–the SPAWN study–15 years follow-up. Int J Obes Relat Metab Disord. 2003;27(12):1516–22.

Chapter 6
Relationship Between Depressive Mood and Maternal Obesity: Implications for Postpartum Depression

Sarah C. Rogan, Jennifer L. Payne, and Samantha Meltzer-Brody

> *Feeling fat lasts nine months, but the joy of becoming a mom lasts forever – Nikki Dalton*

Abstract Depression in the perinatal period (PND) is common and can have devastating consequences for the mother and child. Obesity and depression have a bidirectional relationship, with each being a causal factor for the other. Here, we review the literature examining the associations

---

S.C. Rogan, MD, PhD (✉)
Department of Obstetrics and Gynecology,
University of Texas at Galveston,
School of Medicine, Chapel Hill, NC, USA

J.L. Payne, MD
Department of Psychiatry, Johns Hopkins, Baltimore, MD, USA

S. Meltzer-Brody, MD, MPH
Department of Psychiatry,
University of North Carolina at Chapel Hill,
Chapel Hill, NC, USA
e-mail: meltzerb@med.unc.edu

between PND, obesity, and postpartum weight retention. The literature is limited but supports a greater incidence of PND among obese women. Universal screening for PND should be part of comprehensive perinatal care, as identification of PND can lead to referral and treatment. Future work should elucidate markers for both obesity and PND to facilitate early identification and intervention.

Keywords Perinatal depression • Antenatal depression • Postpartum depression • Obesity • Overweight • Prepregnancy weight • Weight loss

> **Key Points**
> - There is a bidirectional relationship between depression and obesity.
> - It is likely that biological factors, lifestyle changes, and psychosocial factors contribute to both depression and obesity in the perinatal period.
> - There is modest evidence that obesity and postpartum weight retention increase the risk for postpartum depression. The relationship between obesity and antenatal depression is less clear.
> - The literature examining the relationship between obesity and perinatal depression has many limitations and more prospective and larger studies are needed.

Perinatal Depression

Major depressive disorders occurring during pregnancy and postpartum depression (PPD), collectively known as perinatal depression (PND), have a prevalence of 10–15 % in adult women [1–3] and are associated with significant morbidity to the mother, the newborn, and her family [4–7]. The prevalence of PND is significantly higher than both gestational diabetes mellitus and hypertension and incurs significant maternal/fetal morbidity and mortality. Depression during pregnancy is the single greatest risk factor for PPD [1, 8–11]. The point prevalence of major and minor depression occurring during pregnancy ranges from 8.5 % to 11.0 %, with data suggesting incidence rates of major or minor depression to be approximately 14.5 % [12]. Moreover, it is estimated that more than 60 % of PPD cases begin during pregnancy [8].

The literature consistently documents that maternal PND has multiple adverse consequences including maternal suicide and infanticide [13]. Depressed pregnant women are much less likely to engage in appropriate prenatal and postpartum care [14] and are more likely to engage in unhealthy lifestyle behaviors such as smoking and substance abuse and to make worse dietary choices [14–16]. In the postpartum period, maternal depression is associated with poorer maternal-infant attachment [13, 17] and parenting behavior that can have long-lasting adverse psychological consequences in the offspring [6, 7].

Screening for PND during pregnancy and postpartum can be readily accomplished with the use of a validated screening instrument. Table 6.1 describes commonly used instruments. One example is the Edinburgh Postnatal Depression Scale (EPDS), which is among the most commonly used and widely studied perinatal depression screening instruments in the world [12, 18, 23, 24]. The EPDS was specifically developed to assess PND and minimizes confounding of the somatic symptoms of MDD with parenting an infant (e.g., insomnia) [18]. Other depression screening instruments that have been used in the perinatal period include the Postpartum Depression Screening Scale (PDSS) [19], the Patient Health Questionnaire 9-item [20], the Beck Depression Scale (BDI) [21], and the Center for Epidemiological Studies Depression Scale (CES-D) [22].

However, despite the significant public health impact of PND, many risk factors have not been well described, including the relationship of maternal obesity and depression during pregnancy and postpartum. Obesity in the perinatal

TABLE 6.1 Description of commonly used screening instruments for perinatal depression

Name of depression screening instrument	Author of scale	Type of assessment	Number of items	Time to complete scale (min)	Time period assessed
Edinburgh Postnatal Depression Scale (EPDS)	Cox et al. [18]	Self-report	10	<5	In the past 7 days
Postpartum Depression Screening Scale (PDSS)	Beck et al. [19]	Self-report	35	5–10	Over the past 2 weeks
Patient Health Questionnaire (9 items)	Kroenke et al. [20]	Self-report	9	<5	Over the past 2 weeks
Beck Depression Scale	Beck et al. [21]	Clinician-rated	21	5–10	Over the past week
Center for Epidemiological Studies Depression Scale (CES-D)	Radloff [22]	Self-report	20	<5	Past 7 days

period is a complicated topic as there are a variety of clinical presentations. For example, some women come into the pregnancy already overweight or obese, while other women gain weight during the pregnancy that they are unable to shed in the postpartum period. In this chapter, we first review the literature on obesity and depression occurring outside of the perinatal period followed by a discussion of the studies investigating obesity and depression during the perinatal period.

Obesity and Major Depression: A Two-Way Street

Both major depressive disorder (MDD) and obesity are common public health concerns with up to 65 % of Americans meeting criteria for being overweight or obese [25] and 10 % of the general population meeting criteria for MDD [26]. Both of these conditions carry a high disease burden and increase the risk for mortality including via cardiovascular disease [27]. The question of whether MDD leads to an increased risk of obesity and, conversely, whether obesity leads to an increased risk of MDD is an important one as identification of high-risk populations for both of these conditions could lead to earlier and more targeted interventions and improved outcomes.

Over the past decade, research has provided more and more evidence of a link between the two conditions [28–33]. Cross-sectional studies provide a "snapshot" of the study population at one time point and allow determination of the risk for a condition in the setting of another. A systematic review of cross-sectional studies found "weak evidence supporting the hypothesis that obesity increases the incidence of depression outcomes" [34] and concluded that more prospective and longitudinal studies needed to be done. A more recent meta-analysis of community-based studies examined 17 studies with a total of more than 200,000 participants and found an odds ratio of 1.18, indicating that individuals with obesity were more likely to have depressive symptoms [35]. Interestingly, sex acted as a moderating factor, and the association was found only in women.

Cross-sectional studies do not allow insight into the direction of the relationship between two conditions. Longitudinal studies, on the other hand, though more difficult to conduct, allow researchers to determine if one condition leads to another and can provide insight into the mechanisms underlying the risk. A recent systematic review and meta-analysis of longitudinal studies on the relationship between depression, obesity, and being overweight confirmed a reciprocal link between depression and obesity [28]. They found that obesity at baseline increased the risk of the onset of MDD at follow-up with an unadjusted odds ratio of 1.55 (CI 1.22–1.98, $P<0.001$) and that being overweight at baseline increases the risk for MDD with an unadjusted odds ratio of 1.27 (CI 1.07–1.51, $P<0.01$). Thus, there appears to be a "dose–response relationship" in that the risk for MDD was larger in those who were obese as compared to those who were overweight. In contrast, baseline MDD did not increase the risk of being overweight over time, but increased the odds of being obese (OR 1.58, CI 1.33–1.87, $P<0.001$) [28]. In contrast to the meta-analysis of cross-sectional studies, sex was not a moderator of the association.

There are several proposed mechanisms for the reciprocal relationship between obesity and MDD. MDD might increase the risk for obesity in several ways. People with MDD are more likely to engage in unhealthy lifestyles including smoking, unhealthy eating habits, and decreased exercise. MDD is also associated with dysregulation of the stress system [36, 37] that can lead to weight gain. Moreover, common symptoms of MDD predispose a person to gaining weight. For example, one of the specific criteria for the diagnosis of MDD is an altered appetite that can take the form of an increased appetite and overeating. In addition, MDD is often associated with decreased energy that can lead to decreased exercise and activity. Finally, most antidepressant medications are associated with some weight gain.

There are also several ways that obesity might increase the risk of MDD including both biological and psychological mechanisms. The hypothalamic-pituitary-adrenal axis (HPA axis) is dysregulated in both MDD [38, 39] and obesity [40, 41]; thus, dysregulation induced by obesity might trigger MDD. Weight gain and obesity have been shown to activate inflammatory pathways [42, 43], and inflammation is thought to play a role in MDD [44–46]. Obesity increases the risk for diabetes and insulin resistance, which could affect the brain in such a way as to increase the risk for MDD [28]. From a psychological perspective, obesity tends to be associated with decreased self-esteem, adverse childhood experiences, and teasing [36], which might increase the risk of MDD.

Regardless of the mechanism, it is becoming increasingly clear that the relationship between obesity and MDD is bidirectional in that obesity and depression are each causal factors for the other [28, 47]. Given the strength of this association, one would expect that obesity is a risk factor for PND and that depression during or after pregnancy would be associated with obesity or difficulty losing gestational weight gain. As the perinatal period represents a highly vulnerable time in a woman's life, it is critical to understand other risk factors for maternal depression, including maternal obesity.

The Link Between Obesity and Perinatal Depression: A Conceptual Model

There are a number of factors that likely interact to influence the association between obesity and depression during the perinatal time. These factors include biological changes such as inflammation, HPA axis dysregulation, and the hormonal changes that are associated with pregnancy, labor, and delivery. Psychosocial factors including poor body image and poor self-esteem might also influence the risk of both obesity and depression. Previous research has demonstrated that there are very different attitudes towards eating behaviors and weight gain during pregnancy compared to postpartum [44].

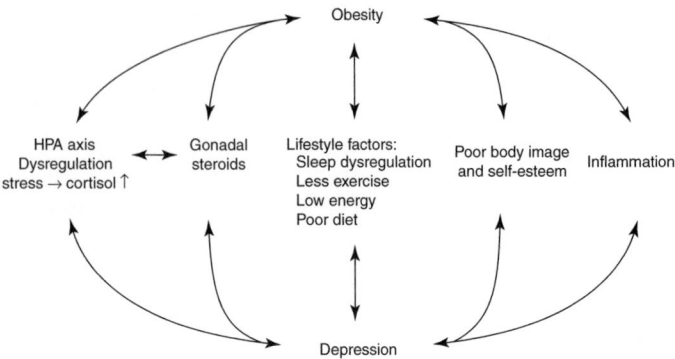

FIG. 6.1 A conceptual model of the relationships between obesity and depression in the perinatal period

Negative self-directed cognitions concerning eating, weight, and shape seem to be less pervasive during pregnancy and might be less likely to impact mood or anxiety [44]. Women might feel justified eating more during pregnancy, and weight gain is associated with nurturing a developing infant. In contrast, women are expected to lose weight during the postpartum period, and a failure to do so, coupled with a changed physique, could lead to negative cognitions that predisposes one to the development of depression. Lifestyle factors also play a role as many women decrease activity and have lower energy during pregnancy and postpartum. Sleep is often dysregulated, both during and after pregnancy, and a poor diet due to food cravings or the stress of becoming a mother can increase the risks for obesity and depression. A conceptual model of the relationships between obesity and depression in the perinatal period is depicted in Fig. 6.1.

Obesity and Perinatal Depression

The literature examining obesity and antenatal depression is small, and three studies document that obesity is not associated with antenatal depression [44, 48, 49]. In contrast,

Bodnar et al. [50] reported a strong, positive dose–response association between prepregnancy obesity (based on BMI) and the likelihood of antenatal MDD. A major strength of this study compared to the previous literature, which generally assessed depressive symptoms, is the use of a structured clinical interview (the Structured Clinical Interview for DSM-IV Diagnoses or SCID), which allows a diagnosis of MDD to be made. The association of prepregnancy obesity with antenatal MDD remained after controlling for confounders and suggests that overweight mothers' antenatal mood may be unaffected by the absolute amount of weight gained but is more robustly associated with the mother's weight at the time of conception [50]. One possibility is that prepregnancy obesity leads to body image dissatisfaction or biological factors (inflammation, HPA axis dysregulation) that increase the risk of depression during pregnancy.

The literature assessing the risk of PPD among women who were overweight or obese prepregnancy is larger than that for antenatal depression. Most of these studies are small cross-sectional or longitudinal analyses [51]. Studies from Jenkin and Tiggemann [52] and Carter et al. [44] assessed depressive affect in the third trimester and again in the postpartum period, and both studies found significant associations between obesity and PPD. In contrast, a cross-sectional analysis from Vernon et al. [53] found no direct association between BMI and depression, but subjects with lower levels of physical activity tended to weigh more and to have more depressive symptoms, suggesting an indirect relationship between weight and depression.

Two studies from Lacoursiere et al. have also found significant associations between obesity and PPD [54, 55]. In an initial study of over 700 subjects [54], researchers examined depressive symptoms using the question "In the months after your delivery, would you say that you were not depressed at all, a little depressed, moderately depressed, very depressed, or very depressed and had to get help?" Patients who responded with "not depressed at all" or "a little depressed" were classified as not depressed, and those with any other responses were classified as depressed. Normal-weight women reported the lowest rate of moderate or stronger depressive symptoms (22.8 %), compared to underweight (27.7 %), overweight (24.8 %), and obese (30.8 %) women. The adjusted odds ratio for moderate or greater depressive symptoms among obese women was 1.53 (95 %, CI 1.15–2.02), and overweight and obese women were more likely to seek assistance for their depression than underweight or normal-weight women. In a follow-up study, Lacoursiere et al. [55] used a more rigorous and well-validated measure of depression, namely, the EPDS. They enrolled 1,027 women immediately postpartum and followed them for 6–8 weeks to determine whether prepregnancy BMI is associated with a positive PPD screen. Overall, the authors reported the lowest rate of depression among normal-weight subjects (14.4 %). Underweight (BMI <18.5), pre-obese (BMI 25–29.9), and class 1 obese (BMI 30–34.9) women had insignificantly higher rates of positive EPDS screens (18, 18.5 and 18.8 %, respectively). In contrast, significantly higher rates of depression were measured among obese class 2 (32.4 %, BMI 35–39.9) and obese class 3 (40.0 %, BMI 35–39.9) women. Consistent with previously described research linking obesity and major depression, prepregnancy BMI correlated with a history of depression. Additionally, the authors reported an association between BMI and a history of PPD, suggesting that obese women had an increased baseline risk for a positive EPDS, but a multiple logistic regression showed prepregnancy BMI to be an independent risk factor for PPD. Interestingly, women with a lower prepregnancy BMI were more likely to complete the study. Depressed women might be less likely to complete and return the EPDS. Therefore, the study results could underestimate the prevalence of depression among overweight and obese women.

In the largest study of which we are aware, Sundaram et al. [56] investigated the association between prepregnancy BMI and PPD. The authors extracted data on 45,285 women from the Pregnancy Risk Assessment Monitoring System, a national population-based survey. The authors assessed depression using a two-item questionnaire modeled on the PHQ-2, which is a brief clinical test to assess depressive symptoms. Their initial results indicated a 1.15-fold increase in the prevalence of PPD among obese (BMI ≥30) women (95 %, CI 1.023–1.302), but that effect was no longer significant after the authors controlled for maternal variables such as age, race, education, income, and pregnancy complications. Additionally, the authors found no differences in rates of PPD among under-, normal-, and overweight women (Table 6.2).

Perinatal Intervention Studies to Address Obesity

Several studies have attempted to directly examine the relationship between gestational weight gain and PPD in the setting of interventions to minimize weight gain, but none have found a significant associations. These studies have typically used behavioral modification techniques to minimize gestational weight gain or intensify postpartum weight loss and have assessed affective symptoms in intervention and control subjects. Krause et al. [69] investigated PPD rates among 491 overweight or obese women who enrolled in a randomized control behavioral intervention designed to encourage postpartum weight loss. The authors administered the EPDS to subjects 6 weeks postpartum. The authors failed to find an association between PPD and BMI.

In a similar study, a Swedish group investigated whether participation in a validated [70] weight restriction program during pregnancy impacted measures of depression or anxiety among 151 obese women [71]. Investigators administered the Beck Anxiety Inventory (BAI) and the EPDS to assess anxiety and depression, respectively, at 15 and 35 weeks' gestation and 11 weeks postpartum. With respect to either anxiety or depression, they found no significant differences between the control and intervention groups at any of the time points, nor did they find an association between anxiety

TABLE 6.2 Summary of research investigating obesity and postpartum depression

Study	Study type	N	Findings
Obesity and postpartum depression			
Carter et al. [44]	Longitudinal	64	Y: overweight women had more depressive symptoms
Jenkin and Tiggemann [52]	Longitudinal	115	Y: depressive affect correlated with weight gain
Lacoursiere et al. [57]	Population-based survey	716	Y: prepregnancy BMI correlated with PPD symptoms
Lacoursiere et al. [58]	Cross-sectional	1,053	Y: prepregnancy obesity correlated with positive EPDS screen
Sundaram et al. [59]	Retrospective cohort	45,285	Y: 1.15-fold increase in PPD symptoms among obese women, but effect not significant after controlling for maternal variables
Vernon et al. [60]	Cross-sectional	51	N: BMI not associated with depression, but low physical activity correlated with obesity and depression
Intervention studies			
Boury et al. [61]	Cross-sectional analysis of randomized trial	151	N: body weight did not correlate with depression
Claesson et al. [62]	Control trial	151	N: weight control intervention did not decrease depression or anxiety symptoms
Krause et al. [63]	Cross-sectional	491	N: BMI did not correlate with PPD

Postpartum depression and weight retention

Harris et al. [64]	Retrospective cohort	74	N: depression not associated with weight retention
Herring et al. [48]	Longitudinal	850	Y: PPD doubled risk of postpartum weight retention
Huang et al. [65]	Longitudinal	602	Y: normal-weight women with depression retained less weight postpartum
Pedersen et al. [66]	Longitudinal	37,127	Y: depression and anxiety increase risk of postpartum weight retention
Siega-Riz et al. [67]	Longitudinal	688,550	N: depression not associated with BMI or weight retention
Walker [68]	Longitudinal	149	Y: depression correlated with increased weight gain

BMI body mass index, *PPD* postpartum depression, *Y* yes a significant association was found, *N* no significant association or depressive symptoms and weight gain. However, the intervention was unsuccessful as there was no difference in weight gain between the intervention and control groups. The authors did conduct a secondary analysis comparing patients within each group who had limited weight gain with those who did not and again found no differences in BAI or EPDS scores, but the study was not designed to detect such within-group differences.

In a third intervention study, body weight again did not relate to depressive symptoms. Boury et al. [61] examined women in a randomized clinical trial for weight management. Their cohort consisted of 151 women with children under 2 years of age. While the postpartum time differed greatly among subjects, 55 % were 6 months or fewer postpartum, 31 % were 6–12 months postpartum, and 14 % were 12–24 months postpartum. Researchers used the Beck Depression Inventory (BDI) and found that 51 % of the sample had some degree of depression but that BMI did not correlate with BDI scores. They also failed to find an association between weight gain during pregnancy or waist circumference and depression.

Postpartum Depression and Weight Retention

Postpartum weight retention is a significant contributor to adult obesity and increases maternal and fetal morbidity in future pregnancies. Thus, identifying risk factors for excess weigh retention is important. Several studies have investigated the link between PPD and postpartum weight retention.

One study assessed weight retention and depression among 230 women who were 1 year postpartum and found that more women who retained ≥5 kg reported depressive symptoms than women who retained <5 kg (53 % vs. 28 %) [68]. Similarly, Herring et al. [48] found that PPD resulted in a 2.5-fold increase in the risk of retaining ≥5 kg at 1 year postpartum, even after controlling for prepregnancy BMI, gestational weight gain, parity, and maternal sociodemographics (OR 2.54, 95 %, CI 1.06–6.09). When the authors controlled for postpartum behaviors such as sleep, walking, trans-fat intake, and television watching, the effect of PPD on weight retention was insignificant (OR 2.38, 95 %, CI 0.96–5.88) suggesting that the lack of sleep and the physical inactivity that often accompany depression partially account for the weight retention. On the other hand, antenatal depression, either alone or in combination with PPD, did not increase the risk of weight retention.

Pedersen et al. [72] conducted one of the largest studies, a prospective cohort study of >37,000 Danish women, to examine psychosocial risk factors for postpartum weight retention. They found that women with symptoms of depression and/or anxiety during pregnancy had higher weight retention at both 6 and 18 months postpartum. Women who also had depressive or anxious symptoms postpartum had an even higher risk of weight retention.

By contrast, a Taiwanese study [73] found that 6 months postpartum, normal-weight, depressed women retained less weight than their nondepressed counterparts. The authors speculated that the sleep disturbances and loss of appetite that often accompany depression contributed to the decrease in post-pregnancy weight gain. Additionally, several studies have failed to find a correlation between postpartum weight retention and maternal depression [64, 74]. Many variables contribute to postpartum weight retention including diet, physical activity, prepregnancy BMI, gestational weight gain, social support, and socioeconomic factors. It is likely that when models control for all of these variables, small studies are inadequately powered to assess the direct effect of PPD and weight retention on each other.

Conclusions

In summary, there is modest evidence that obesity and postpartum weight retention increase the risk for PPD. The relationship between obesity and antenatal depression is less clear. Overall, the existing evidence does not provide strong support for a link between obesity and PND, but several flaws in the current literature preclude drawing definitive conclusions. First, studies have assessed depression using a variety of methods. While the EPDS and BDI are well-validated tools with documented cutoff scores consistent with a diagnosis of MDD, several studies [52–54, 56] used other methods of assessing depressive symptoms that might not be correlated to a clinical diagnosis of MDD. In addition to the unknown validity of such depression measures, it is difficult to compare findings among studies when each uses a different method of assessing depression. Moreover, the presence of depressive symptoms in the postpartum period does not imply a diagnosis of PPD; thus, the true prevalence of PPD in several of the studies is unknown. Second, each study assessed PPD at different postpartum intervals ranging from 4 weeks to 2 years. With respect to the cross-sectional studies in particular, none of which has found an association between obesity and depression [8], the prevalence of depression could be underestimated, depending on whether the timing of assessment correlated with the presence and severity of PPD symptoms. Third, all of these studies are subject to a selection bias, as women who respond to study advertisements are probably less likely to be depressed. In particular for those studies with a behavioral intervention targeting weight loss, the responding population is likely more motivated to lose weight than the general population. Fourth, many of the studies have small sample sizes; with an expected PPD prevalence of 10–15 %, many of the studies do not have an adequate number of depressed patients to draw significant conclusions regarding the association between obesity and PPD. Future studies will require longitudinal assessment of women recruited prepregnancy and followed through the postpartum period using a valid and reliable assessment of PND and tracking weight and BMI with large sample sizes, so that studies are adequately powered.

Perinatal depression is a critical cause of perinatal morbidity and has important effects on the entire family, including the newborn. While the current evidence linking obesity and PND is mixed, and as obesity becomes a greater public health problem, further research will likely better define the relationship between obesity and PPD. The association between obesity and both PND and MDD outside of the perinatal period likely reflects overlapping mechanisms and risk factors. However, it is important that we clinically identify those people at risk.

The perinatal period represents a time of high contact with health-care providers. Therefore, universal screening for PND should be part of comprehensive perinatal care, as identification of PND can lead to referral and treatment. The literature demonstrates that PPD is associated with increased risk of weight retention, so treatment of PPD might lessen the incidence of postpartum obesity. As posited by Shelton and Miller [31], obesity and depression are part of a vicious cycle whereby obesity predisposes one to depression, contributing to inactivity and dietary changes, which worsens obesity. In the postpartum period, sleep disturbances, fatigue, and the constant demands of caring for a newborn likely exacerbate this cycle, enhancing an already precarious relationship. Therefore, recognition and treatment of PPD remains an important aspect of postpartum care for all women. Moreover, future work should concentrate on identifying clinical markers of the population of people at risk for developing both obesity and PND and exploring methods of early intervention in order to decrease risks associated with both of these serious conditions.

References

1. Yonkers KA, Ramin SM, Rush AJ, Navarrete CA, Carmody T, March D, et al. Onset and persistence of postpartum depression in an inner-city maternal health clinic system. Am J Psychiatry. 2001;158(11):1856–63.
2. Gavin NI, Gaynes BN, Lohr KN, Meltzer-Brody S, Gartlehner G, Swinson T. Perinatal depression: a systematic review of prevalence and incidence. Obstet Gynecol. 2005;106(5 Pt 1):1071–83.

3. O'Hara MW, Swain AM. Rates and risk of postpartum depression-A meta-analysis. Int Rev Psychiatry. 1996;8(1):37–54.
4. Leahy-Warren P, McCarthy G. Postnatal depression: prevalence, mothers' perspectives, and treatments. Arch Psychiatr Nurs. 2007;21(2):91–100.
5. Murray L, Stein A. The effects of postnatal depression on the infant. Baillieres Clin Obstet Gynaecol. 1989;3(4):921–33.
6. Marmorstein NR, Malone SM, Iacono WG. Psychiatric disorders among offspring of depressed mothers: associations with paternal psychopathology. Am J Psychiatry. 2004;161(9):1588–94.
7. Flynn HA, Davis M, Marcus SM, Cunningham R, Blow FC. Rates of maternal depression in pediatric emergency department and relationship to child service utilization. Gen Hosp Psychiatry. 2004;26(4):316–22.
8. Munk-Olsen T, Laursen TM, Pedersen CB, Mors O, Mortensen PB. New parents and mental disorders: a population-based register study. JAMA. 2006;296(21):2582–9.
9. Milgrom J, Gemmill AW, Bilszta JL, Hayes B, Barnett B, Brooks J, et al. Antenatal risk factors for postnatal depression: a large prospective study. J Affect Disord. 2008;108(1–2):147–57.
10. Robertson E, Grace S, Wallington T, Stewart DE. Antenatal risk factors for postpartum depression: a synthesis of recent literature. Gen Hosp Psychiatry. 2004;26(4):289–95.
11. Wisner KL, Chambers C, Sit DK. Postpartum depression: a major public health problem. JAMA. 2006;296(21):2616–8.
12. Gaynes BN, Gavin N, Meltzer-Brody S, Lohr KN, Swinson T, Gartlehner G, et al. Perinatal depression: prevalence, screening accuracy, and screening outcomes. Evid Rep Technol Assess (Summ). 2005;119:1–8.
13. Lindahl V, Pearson JL, Colpe L. Prevalence of suicidality during pregnancy and the postpartum. Arch Womens Ment Health. 2005;8(2):77–87.
14. Zuckerman B, Amaro H, Bauchner H, Cabral H. Depressive symptoms during pregnancy: relationship to poor health behaviors. Am J Obstet Gynecol. 1989;160(5 Pt 1):1107–11.
15. Chittleborough CR, Lawlor DA, Lynch JW. Prenatal prediction of poor maternal and offspring outcomes: implications for selection into intensive parent support programs. Matern Child Health J. 2012;16(4):909–20. Research Support, Non-U.S. Gov't.
16. Newport DJ, Ji S, Long Q, Knight BT, Zach EB, Smith EN, et al. Maternal depression and anxiety differentially impact fetal exposures during pregnancy. J Clin Psychiatry. 2012;73(2):247–51. Research Support, N.I.H., Extramural.
17. Stein A, Gath DH, Bucher J, Bond A, Day A, Cooper PJ. The relationship between post-natal depression and mother-child interaction. Br J Psychiatry. 1991;158:46–52.

18. Cox JL, Holden JM, Sagovsky R. Detection of postnatal depression. Development of the 10-item Edinburgh Postnatal Depression Scale. Br J Psychiatry. 1987;150:782–6.
19. Beck CT, Gable RK. Further validation of the Postpartum Depression Screening Scale. Nurs Res. 2001;50(3):155–64.
20. Kroenke K, Spitzer RL, Williams JB. The PHQ-9: validity of a brief depression severity measure. J Gen Intern Med. 2001;16(9):606–13.
21. Beck AT, Ward CH, Mendelson M, Mock J, Erbaugh J. An inventory for measuring depression. Arch Gen Psychiatry. 1961;4:561–71.
22. Radloff LS. The CES-D scale: a self-report depression scale for research in the general population. Appl Psychol Meas. 1977;1:385–401.
23. Boyd RC, Le HN, Somberg R. Review of screening instruments for postpartum depression. Arch Womens Ment Health. 2005;8(3):141–53.
24. Hewitt CE, Gilbody SM. Is it clinically and cost effective to screen for postnatal depression: a systematic review of controlled clinical trials and economic evidence. BJOG. 2009;116(8):1019–27.
25. Flegal KM, Carroll MD, Ogden CL, Johnson CL. Prevalence and trends in obesity among US adults, 1999–2000. JAMA. 2002;288(14):1723–7.
26. Kessler RC, McGonagle KA, Zhao S, Nelson CB, Hughes M, Eshleman S, et al. Lifetime and 12-month prevalence of DSM-III-R psychiatric disorders in the United States. Results from the National Comorbidity Survey. Arch Gen Psychiatry. 1994;51(1):8–19.
27. Penninx BW, Beekman AT, Honig A, Deeg DJ, Schoevers RA, van Eijk JT, et al. Depression and cardiac mortality: results from a community-based longitudinal study. Arch Gen Psychiatry. 2001;58(3):221–7.
28. Luppino FS, de Wit LM, Bouvy PF, Stijnen T, Cuijpers P, Penninx BW, et al. Overweight, obesity, and depression: a systematic review and meta-analysis of longitudinal studies. Arch Gen Psychiatry. 2010;67(3):220–9.
29. Cizza G. Major depressive disorder is a risk factor for low bone mass, central obesity, and other medical conditions. Dialogues Clin Neurosci. 2011;13(1):73–87.
30. Cizza G, Ronsaville DS, Kleitz H, Eskandari F, Mistry S, Torvik S, et al. Clinical subtypes of depression are associated with specific metabolic parameters and circadian endocrine profiles in women: the power study. PLoS One. 2012;7(1):e28912.
31. Shelton RC, Miller AH. Inflammation in depression: is adiposity a cause? Dialogues Clin Neurosci. 2011;13(1):41–53.
32. Pickering RP, Grant BF, Chou SP, Compton WM. Are overweight, obesity, and extreme obesity associated with psychopathology? Results from the national epidemiologic survey on alcohol and related conditions. J Clin Psychiatry. 2007;68(7):998–1009.
33. Simon GE, Von Korff M, Saunders K, Miglioretti DL, Crane PK, van Belle G, et al. Association between obesity and psychiatric disorders in the US adult population. Arch Gen Psychiatry. 2006;63(7):824–30.

34. Atlantis E, Baker M. Obesity effects on depression: systematic review of epidemiological studies. Int J Obes (Lond). 2008;32(6):881–91.
35. de Wit L, Luppino F, van Straten A, Penninx B, Zitman F, Cuijpers P. Depression and obesity: a meta-analysis of community-based studies. Psychiatry Res. 2010;178(2):230–5.
36. Stunkard AJ, Faith MS, Allison KC. Depression and obesity. Biol Psychiatry. 2003;54(3):330–7.
37. Bornstein SR, Schuppenies A, Wong ML, Licinio J. Approaching the shared biology of obesity and depression: the stress axis as the locus of gene-environment interactions. Mol Psychiatry. 2006;11(10):892–902.
38. Belanoff JK, Kalehzan M, Sund B, Fleming Ficek SK, Schatzberg AF. Cortisol activity and cognitive changes in psychotic major depression. Am J Psychiatry. 2001;158(10):1612–6.
39. Holsboer F. The corticosteroid receptor hypothesis of depression. Neuropsychopharmacology. 2000;23(5):477–501.
40. Pasquali R, Vicennati V. Activity of the hypothalamic-pituitary-adrenal axis in different obesity phenotypes. Int J Obes Relat Metab Disord. 2000;24 Suppl 2:S47–9.
41. Walker BR. Activation of the hypothalamic-pituitary-adrenal axis in obesity: cause or consequence? Growth Horm IGF Res. 2001;11(Suppl A):S91–5.
42. Emery CF, Fondow MD, Schneider CM, Christofi FL, Hunt C, Busby AK, et al. Gastric bypass surgery is associated with reduced inflammation and less depression: a preliminary investigation. Obes Surg. 2007;17(6):759–63.
43. Shoelson SE, Herrero L, Naaz A. Obesity, inflammation, and insulin resistance. Gastroenterology. 2007;132(6):2169–80.
44. Carter AS, Baker CW, Brownell KD. Body mass index, eating attitudes, and symptoms of depression and anxiety in pregnancy and the postpartum period. Psychosom Med. 2000;62(2):264–70.
45. Bremmer MA, Beekman AT, Deeg DJ, Penninx BW, Dik MG, Hack CE, et al. Inflammatory markers in late-life depression: results from a population-based study. J Affect Disord. 2008;106(3):249–55.
46. Milaneschi Y, Corsi AM, Penninx BW, Bandinelli S, Guralnik JM, Ferrucci L. Interleukin-1 receptor antagonist and incident depressive symptoms over 6 years in older persons: the InCHIANTI study. Biol Psychiatry. 2009;65(11):973–8.
47. Miller GE, Freedland KE, Carney RM, Stetler CA, Banks WA. Pathways linking depression, adiposity, and inflammatory markers in healthy young adults. Brain Behav Immun. 2003;17(4):276–85.
48. Herring SJ, Rich-Edwards JW, Oken E, Rifas-Shiman SL, Kleinman KP, Gillman MW. Association of postpartum depression with weight retention 1 year after childbirth. Obesity (Silver Spring). 2008;16(6):1296–301.
49. Walker LO, Kim M. Psychosocial thriving during late pregnancy: relationship to ethnicity, gestational weight gain, and birth weight. J Obstet Gynecol Neonatal Nurs. 2002;31(3):263–74.

50. Bodnar LM, Wisner KL, Moses-Kolko E, Sit DK, Hanusa BH. Prepregnancy body mass index, gestational weight gain, and the likelihood of major depressive disorder during pregnancy. J Clin Psychiatry. 2009;70(9):1290–6. Research Support, N.I.H., Extramural.
51. Milgrom J, Skouteris H, Worotniuk T, Henwood A, Bruce L. The association between ante- and postnatal depressive symptoms and obesity in both mother and child: a systematic review of the literature. Womens Health Issues. 2012;22(3):e319–28.
52. Jenkin W, Tiggemann M. Psychological effects of weight retained after pregnancy. Women Health. 1997;25(1):89–98.
53. Vernon MM, Young-Hyman D, Looney SW. Maternal stress, physical activity, and body mass index during new mothers' first year postpartum. Women Health. 2010;50(6):544–62.
54. Lacoursiere DY, Baksh L, Bloebaum L, Varner MW. Maternal body mass index and self-reported postpartum depressive symptoms. Matern Child Health J. 2006;10(4):385–90.
55. LaCoursiere DY, Barrett-Connor E, O'Hara MW, Hutton A, Varner MW. The association between prepregnancy obesity and screening positive for postpartum depression. BJOG. 2010;117(8):1011–8.
56. Sundaram S, Harman JS, Peoples-Sheps MD, Hall AG, Simpson SH. Obesity and postpartum depression: does prenatal care utilization make a difference? Matern Child Health J. 2012;16(3):656–67.
57. Lacoursiere DY, Baksh L, Bloebaum L, Varner MW. Maternal body mass index and self-reported postpartum depressive symptoms. Matern Child Health J. 2006 Jul;10(4):385–90. PMID: 16673179 [PubMed – indexed for MEDLINE].
58. LaCoursiere DY, Barrett-Connor E, O'Hara MW, Hutton A, Varner MW. The association between prepregnancy obesity and screening positive for postpartum depression. BJOG. 2010;117(8):1011–8. doi:10.1111/j.1471-0528.2010.02569.x. PMID: 20536433 [PubMed – indexed for MEDLINE].
59. Sundaram S, Harman JS, Peoples-Sheps MD, Hall AG, Simpson SH. Obesity and postpartum depression: does prenatal care utilization make a difference? Matern Child Health J. 2012;16(3):656–67. doi:10.1007/s10995-011-0808-7.
60. Vernon MM, Young-Hyman D, Looney SW. Maternal stress, physical activity, and body mass index during new mothers' first year postpartum. Women Health. 2010;50(6):544–62. doi:10.1080/03630242.2010.516692.
61. Boury JM, Larkin KT, Krummel DA. Factors related to postpartum depressive symptoms in low-income women. Women Health. 2004;39(3):19–34.
62. Claesson IM, Josefsson A, Sydsjö G. Prevalence of anxiety and depressive symptoms among obese pregnant and postpartum women: an intervention study. BMC Public Health. 2010;10:766. doi:10.1186/1471-2458-10-766.
63. Krause KM, Ostbye T, Swamy GK. Occurrence and correlates of postpartum depression in overweight and obese women: results

from the active mothers postpartum (AMP) study. Matern Child Health J. 2009;13(6):832–8. doi:10.1007/s10995-008-0418-1. Epub 2008 Oct 4.
64. Harris HE, Ellison GT, Clement S. Do the psychosocial and behavioral changes that accompany motherhood influence the impact of pregnancy on long-term weight gain? J Psychosom Obstet Gynaecol. 1999;20(2):65–79. PMID: 10422038 [PubMed – indexed for MEDLINE].
65. Huang TT, Wang HS, Dai FT. Effect of pre-pregnancy body size on postpartum weight retention. Midwifery. 2010;26(2):222–31. doi:10.1016/j.midw.2008.05.001. Epub 2008 Jul 26.
66. Pedersen P, Baker JL, Henriksen TB, Lissner L, Heitmann BL, Sørensen TI, Nohr EA. Influence of psychosocial factors on postpartum weight retention. Obesity (Silver Spring). 2011;19(3):639–46. doi:10.1038/oby.2010.175. Epub 2010 Aug 12.
67. Siega-Riz AM, Herring AH, Carrier K, Evenson KR, Dole N, Deierlein A. Sociodemographic, perinatal, behavioral, and psychosocial predictors of weight retention at 3 and 12 months postpartum. Obesity (Silver Spring). 2010;18(10):1996–2003. doi:10.1038/oby.2009.458. Epub 2009 Dec 24. PMID: 20035283 [PubMed – indexed for MEDLINE].
68. Walker LO. Weight and weight-related distress after childbirth: relationships to stress, social support, and depressive symptoms. J Holist Nurs. 1997;15(4):389–405.
69. Krause KM, Ostbye T, Swamy GK. Occurrence and correlates of postpartum depression in overweight and obese women: results from the active mothers postpartum (AMP) study. Matern Child Health J. 2009;13(6):832–8.
70. Claesson IM, Sydsjo G, Brynhildsen J, Cedergren M, Jeppsson A, Nystrom F, et al. Weight gain restriction for obese pregnant women: a case–control intervention study. BJOG. 2008;115(1):44–50.
71. Claesson IM, Josefsson A, Sydsjo G. Prevalence of anxiety and depressive symptoms among obese pregnant and postpartum women: an intervention study. BMC Public Health. 2010;10:766.
72. Pedersen P, Baker JL, Henriksen TB, Lissner L, Heitmann BL, Sorensen TI, et al. Influence of psychosocial factors on postpartum weight retention. Obesity (Silver Spring). 2011;19(3):639–46.
73. Huang TT, Wang HS, Dai FT. Effect of pre-pregnancy body size on postpartum weight retention. Midwifery. 2010;26(2):222–31.
74. Siega-Riz AM, Herring AH, Carrier K, Evenson KR, Dole N, Deierlein A. Sociodemographic, perinatal, behavioral, and psychosocial predictors of weight retention at 3 and 12 months postpartum. Obesity (Silver Spring). 2010;18(10):1996–2003.

Chapter 7
Body Image as a Contributor to Weight in Pregnancy and Postpartum: Racial Differences

Tiffany L. Carson, Kesha Baptiste-Roberts, and Tiffany L. Gary-Webb

Abstract The alarming disparities in obesity and related conditions for African-Americans compared to Whites have prompted the investigation of social and cultural influences of the obesogenic environment as potential contributors. One such cultural influence may be body image, which encompasses one's perception of body size and the emotional attitude toward that perception. While studies show that body image is significantly associated with weight, studies during pregnancy have been few, particularly among minority

---

T.L. Carson, PhD, MPH
Division of Preventive Medicine, University of Alabama
at Birmingham School of Medicine, Birmingham, AL, USA

K. Baptiste-Roberts, PhD, MPH
School of Nursing and College of Medicine, Department
of Public Health Sciences, The Pennsylvania State University,
Hershey, PA, USA

T.L. Gary-Webb, PhD, MHS (✉)
Department of Epidemiology, Columbia University Mailman
School of Public Health, New York, NY, USA
e-mail: tlg2124@cumc.columbia.edu

W. Nicholson, K. Baptiste-Roberts (eds.),
Obesity During Pregnancy in Clinical Practice,
DOI 10.1007/978-1-4471-2831-1_7,
© Springer-Verlag London 2014

populations. The concept of body image and its influence on weight control should be considered in various phases of a woman's life, including pregnancy.

Keywords Body image • Racial/ethnic disparities • Cultural influences • Weight control • Prepregnancy • Postpartum

> **Key Points**
> - Body image is an important contributor to weight and significant racial/ethnic disparities exist.
> - Body image changes with different phases of life and should be considered during the very important pregnancy and postpartum phases.
> - Results of studies during pregnancy and postpartum suggest that body image dissatisfaction increases and that there are many factors (i.e., prepregnancy weight and behaviors, psychosocial factors) that influence this association.
> - Health professionals have an opportunity to help pregnant women adapt to their changing bodies in healthy ways. They should implement strategies to improve body image satisfaction during this critical phase.

Understanding How Cultural Influences May Impact Health

African-Americans experience extremely high rates of obesity compared to their White counterparts particularly among women. In fact, over 75 % of African-American women aged 20 and above are overweight or obese [1], and this disparity is only partially explained by differences in socioeconomic status (SES). Given that obesity is also a risk factor for diabetes, heart disease, stroke, and many other chronic problems, studies are urgently needed to identify novel risk factors that may contribute to the disproportionate burden of obesity among African-Americans. It has long been recognized that culturally appropriate methods for ethnic minorities are needed for programs targeting weight loss, diabetes care, and improvement in cardiovascular risk factors; however, little work has been done to identify *specific cultural components* that could be incorporated in these programs. Although the existing medical literature has limited exploration of these cultural components, a few studies bringing in perspectives from anthropology and psychology [2–4] have provided key leads to be further explored including similarities between African and African-American dietary patterns, contrast between African-American values and mainstream values, and cultural perceptions concerning body image and weight, just to name a few. This chapter explores in detail the construct of body image.

Conceptual Framework

The conceptual framework guiding this chapter (see Fig. 7.1) was developed by Ard and analyzes the obesogenic environment from the unique perspective of African-American women [5]. It proposes that, unlike mainstream US culture which promotes thinness, cultural influences for African-American women may be permissive for weight gain. It has been suggested that many of the cultural norms of African-Americans don't identify being "skinny" as critical to one's health, happiness, and personal sense of well-being [5]. Body image is a unique, multidimensional concept that is influenced by the cultural frameworks that help to shape individuals and groups. Thus, examining the broader social/cultural context above and beyond individual goals is crucial to understanding facilitators and barriers. Careful examination of body image, as well as other social/cultural constructs, will move us closer to identifying solutions for achieving healthy weight in African-American communities.

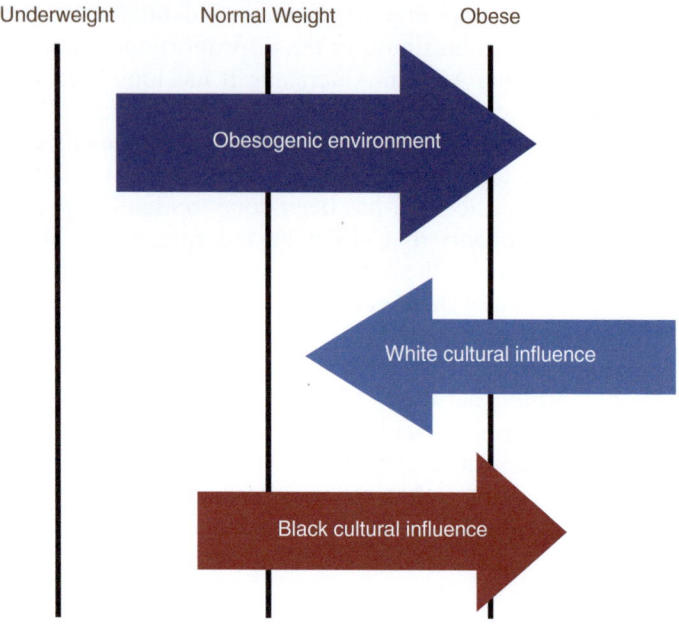

Figure 7.1 Confluence of obesogenic environment and cultural influence. Black cultural influence has an additive interaction with the overall obesogenic environment further promoting obesity among Black women. Conversely, White cultural influence acts as a counterweight to the prevailing obesogenic environment by influencing White women to strive for thinness (Reproduced with permission from: Ard [5])

Body Image as a Construct

Body image, an important factor in weight control, encompasses one's perception of body size and the emotional response or attitude toward that perception [6–8]. Body image is often assessed using attitudinal questionnaires such as the Body Cathexis Scale [9], the Body Shape Questionnaire [10] or by exploring percept evaluations using figure rating exercises. For the figure rating exercises, participants are shown a series of numbered silhouettes ranging from very thin to extremely obese. Participants are asked to select which figure they currently most resemble. This is known as body image$_{current}$. To further explore dimensions of body image, participants are often asked to select which figure they would like to resemble. This is known as body image$_{ideal}$. The calculated difference between body image$_{current}$ and body image$_{ideal}$ is called body image discrepancy or body image dissatisfaction (BID = body image$_{current}$ − body image$_{ideal}$). Several instruments have been developed to facilitate this line of study. The most widely used instrument is the Stunkard Figure Rating Scale, which consists of 9 silhouettes (see Fig. 7.2a) [11]. The Stunkard scale was introduced in the early 1980s as an easy-to-administer self-assessment of body image and has been strengthened by subsequent work, which established BMI norms for adults and children [12]. Several additional figure rating scales have been developed and adapted

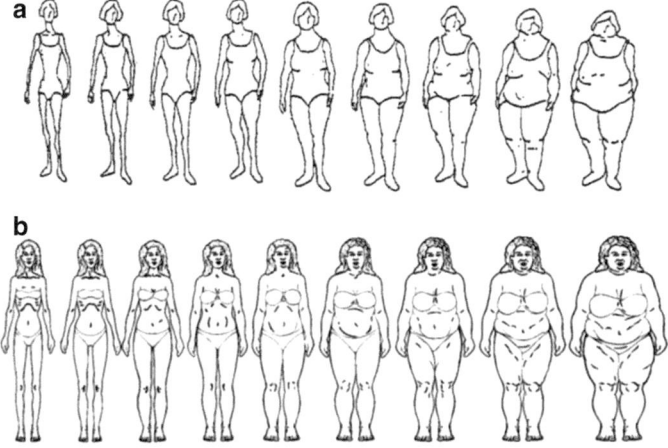

FIGURE 7.2 Selected figure rating scales. (**a**) Stunkard Figure Rating Scale: most widely used instrument developed as an easy-to-administer self-assessment of body image (Reproduced with permission from: Stunkard et al. [11]). (**b**) Pulvers Figure Rating Scale: instrument adapted to be appropriate for diverse populations [13] (Reproduced with permission of John Wiley & Sons, Inc)

to be appropriate for diverse populations [8, 13, 14]. Highlighted at the bottom of Fig. 7.2b is the scale developed by Pulvers et al., who sought to develop an instrument more relatable to a range of cultures with detailed figures, but not specific to any one culture [13]. Scales are currently being developed that better depict body proportions for African-Americans and allow participants to desire change of specific body parts (i.e., chest, hips) vs. change of the entire body. From these figure rating exercises, many conclusions have been drawn about body image among African-American and White women. Research has shown that both African-American and White women report some body image dissatisfaction [15–18]. However, White women typically report greater body image *dissatisfaction* than African-American women, while African-American women generally report body image ideals larger than that of White women [19, 20]. There are a range of proposed factors that may influence body image differences across race/ethnic groups.

Historical Influence

Body image ideals in the United States are thought to have roots in historical conditions where different body sizes were promoted for African-American and White women. The environmental and economic conditions in colonial times made women who were physically strong and able preferable because they were seen as fertile and able to contribute to the land and household chores [21]. Later, with the introduction of slavery, White women were urged to be thin and frail to make them more attractive candidates for marriage to an upper-class man who could then justify the use of slaves by stating that his wife was too frail to work [22]. However, this pressure to be thin was never imposed upon African-American women. In fact, for African-American women, larger, stronger bodies were preferred by Whites because this body type was seen as more equipped to endure the working conditions. Additionally, African-American men also preferred African-American women with larger body types because that suggested to them the strength, productivity, robustness, and fertility of that woman. From this, we might hypothesize that what was once a survival- and strategy-driven rationale for preference of certain body sizes, over generations, has become an inherent social norm in current society.

Current Social Influence

Media

The current media has also been identified as a contributor to body image perceptions of women [21]. Differential depictions of African-American and White women in the media may drive the differences in body image ideals that have persisted for several decades. For example, a 2004 study by Schooler and colleagues reported that White women were negatively influenced by seeing thin White women in the media, but African-American women were not affected by these images [23]. However, for African-American women, viewing African-American-oriented media actually demonstrated some protective effect on their body image [23], which is believed to be a result of the larger body sizes of African-American women that are often seen in the mainstream media.

Opposite Sex Preferences

Male preference for body size has also been cited as a contributor to body image among women [24]. Currently, male's physical appearance preferences for women largely mirror the body image ideals that seemed to develop during slavery. Specifically, African-American men prefer African-American women with at least a moderate-sized body shape compared to White men who prefer White women with a thin body shape [24]. Both African-American and White women are aware of male preferences for their respective body sizes. However, there is limited empirical data to establish how male preferences influence body image and actual body sizes of African-American and White women.

Maternal Influence

Mothers may also play a role in the development of body image in their daughters. Subsequently, the body image ideals developed during the formative years are continued into adulthood. Among African-American women, there is a cultural belief of valuing character over appearance [25]. The lower emphasis on appearance may protect against body image dissatisfaction in African-American females. In contrast, White mothers were more critical of heavy daughters in a 1995 study by Brown and colleagues [26]. Thus, it may be that some of the differences in body image ideals seen today when comparing African-American and White women are the result of different maternal emphasis in childhood.

Acculturation

Among African-American women only, acculturation may also influence body image ideals. Acculturation is defined as "socialization: the adoption of the behavior patterns of the surrounding culture." So, African-American women with greater acculturation with mainstream America are more likely to adopt the "White" standard of beauty which includes thinness. However, African-American women with lower acculturation are more likely to adopt "African-American" standards of beauty, which is ultimately associated with fuller, more voluptuous figures.

To this point, the main focus of this chapter has been on body image differences between African-American and White women largely due to limited body image research in other race/ethnic groups. However, other race/ethnic groups, such as Hispanics and Asian-Americans are not exempt from this discussion and are increasingly being studied by researchers. Challenges for studying body image in Hispanic Americans come from the diversity of this group in terms of lineage (e.g., Mexican, South American, Caribbean) and immigration stage (first generation, second generation, third generation). It is well known that rates of overweight and obesity are also disproportionately high among most Hispanic women [1].

Though the literature for Hispanic body image is not definitive, it suggests that body image beliefs among Hispanics fall somewhere in between that of African-Americans and Whites. Though reporting more body image dissatisfaction than African-Americans, Hispanics still report less body image dissatisfaction than Whites [19]. It has been suggested that body image among Hispanics is influenced by strong familial ties and focus on character. For Asian Americans, for whom overweight and obesity rates are much lower than other groups, there is even less weight-related body image data. Of the literature that is available for body image of Asian-Americans, the findings are mixed. Some studies have found that Asian-Americans are more satisfied with their bodies than Whites and Hispanics [19, 27], while other studies have indicated that Asian-Americans report similar levels of body image dissatisfaction as Whites [28]. The challenges involved in the study of body image of Asian-Americans are similar to that seen in Hispanic Americans (e.g., lineage, immigration stage).

Body Mass Index (BMI)

Though many of the factors influencing body image are psychological in nature and driven by social relationships and norms, one quantitative measure that has a direct association with body image among African-American and White women is BMI. For example, a 2011 study by Cox and colleagues reported that body image ideals differed by obesity class with class I (BMI 30–34 kg/m^2) obese women having the smallest body image ideal and class III (BMI $\geq$40 kg/m^2) obese women having the largest body image ideal [16]. However, the causal direction of this relationship is unclear. Some suggest that women may select an ideal body size based on what they see as more relatable to their current size which would lead women who are currently class III obese to choose body image ideals that are larger than that of women who are class I obese. Conversely, the body size that a woman chooses to maintain may be driven by what she sees as ideal. Thus, a woman with a larger body image ideal may be more likely to have a larger actual body size. Further research is needed to more fully understand this relationship. Not only does BMI have a direct relationship with body image ideals, it is also positively associated with body image dissatisfaction. Thus, as BMI increases, body image dissatisfaction increases for both African-American and White women [16, 29]. Though relationships between BMI and body image exist for African-American and White women, thresholds for and magnitudes of the relationships differ. Specifically, when comparing African-American and White women of similar BMIs, African-American women consistently report more satisfaction with their bodies and higher weight-related quality of life [30].

Body Image During Pregnancy

Body image is a part of a woman's psyche that begins to develop at a young age and continues through the life course. However, body image is not a static concept and may change with the different phases of life that a woman may experience. One such time to consider is the pregnancy phase, which is a very important phase in a woman's life, with implications for both her own well-being and that of her developing fetus. During pregnancy, women experience substantial and sometimes dramatic changes in their body shape, sensations, muscle tone, and weight, over a relatively short period of time, resulting in significant alterations of body image [31]. It is important to understand women's adaptation to their changing bodies during pregnancy because body image dissatisfaction has been shown to be associated with depression, anxiety [32, 33], and unhealthy dieting and eating behaviors [34], which all have serious implications for the health and well-being of the mother and developing fetus [35, 36]. In addition, body image influences the ability of a woman to develop a positive maternal identity, which has a great impact on her ability to accept the maternal role postpartum. Nevertheless, there is a paucity of evidence in this area with almost all of the studies having been conducted in very small samples containing only nonminority participants or no report of race. A summary of studies evaluating body image during pregnancy is presented in Table 7.1.

TABLE 7.1 Summary of studies evaluating body image during pregnancy

Author (year) country, design	Population	Setting	Body image assessment	Summary of results
Boscaglia (2003) Australia, prospective cohort [47]	$N=71$ 40 high exercisers (HE) 31 low exercisers (LE)	Not described	Body Cathexis Scale [BCS]	Changes in BIS across the 4 time points were different for the higher and low-exercise groups At 15–22 weeks HE were significantly more satisfied with their bodies compared to LE HE were more satisfied with their bodies at 15–22 weeks' gestation compared to 6 months prepregnancy and were also more satisfied at both time points during pregnancy compared to their body image satisfaction expectation postpartum For the LE group, no difference in body image satisfaction across the four time points

(continued)

TABLE 7.1 (continued)

Author (year) country, design	Population	Setting	Body image assessment	Summary of results
Chang (2006) Taiwan, qualitative study [50]	N=18	Clinics at a medical center in Taipei, Taiwan	n/a	Loss of the self/body and expressed concern about regaining the prepregnancy feminine self after the birth of baby
				Approximately 50 % of women emphasized dissatisfaction with their overall appearance
				Negative attitudes toward the changes in their body seemed to be dampened, by awareness that other women shared their experiences
				Partner acceptance of body was an important determinant of body image satisfaction and women expressed fear and anxiety that the changes in their body would negatively affect their relationships with their partners
				Women saw changes in their body as reflective of their child's development
				Women felt that changes in their bodies reflected their role as mothers
				Women were ambivalent about gaining weight, while some considered all changes in her body as signs of her new role as mother

Clark et al. (2009) Australia, prospective cohort [48]	N = 116	Australia	Body Attitude Questionnaire [BAQ]	Women reported feeling least fat at 32–35 weeks when compared to all time points (prepregnancy, 6 weeks postpartum, 6 months postpartum, and 12 months postpartum)
				Women reported feeling most fat at 6 months postpartum
				Significant relationship between depression and body dissatisfaction scores
Davies and Wardle (1994) UK, cross-sectional study [45]	N = 173	London antenatal clinics and community sample at a local GP well-woman clinic	Eating Disorder Inventory (The Body Dissatisfaction and the Drive for Thinness subscales were used)	Pregnant women were all in their third trimester (mean = 33 weeks)
	76 pregnant women (all third trimester)		Figure rating scale	Pregnant women had a lower score on the "Drive for Thinness" and the Body Image Dissatisfaction Scale compared to the nonpregnant group
	97 nonpregnant controls		Body part size perception	In both groups there was a significant positive correlation between BMI and body dissatisfaction
				After adjustment for BMI, the pregnant women evaluated themselves as larger than the nonpregnant group

(continued)

TABLE 7.1 (continued)

Author (year) country, design	Population	Setting	Body image assessment	Summary of results
Duncombe et al. (2008) Australia, prospective cohort [33]	N=158	Melbourne and regional Victoria, Australia	Body Attitudes Questionnaire [BAQ] Contour Drawing Rating Scale Pregnancy Figure Rating Scales	Prepregnancy: 20 % were satisfied, 74 % wanted a smaller body size, and 5.7 % wanted a larger body size. Body image remained relatively stable. Women who felt good about their bodies at the start continued to do so and those that did not maintained that concern during pregnancy
Fairburn et al. (1992) UK, prospective cohort [35]	N=100	Maternity hospital in Oxford	Eating Disorder Examination	The degree of concern about body shape increased between early-to-middle and late pregnancy. Significant decline in concern about weight during the early stages of pregnancy and an increase in the later stages
Fox and Yamaguchi (1997) UK, qualitative study [46]	N=76	Antenatal classes and midwifery centers in 4 London hospital and clinics		18 % of normal-weight women (NW) experience positive change in BI, 62 % negative change, and 19 % no change. Of the overweight women, 62 % experience a positive change, 23 % a negative change, and 15 % no change

Goodwin et al. (2000), Australia, prospective cohort [51]	$N=65$	Community- and hospital-based prenatal classes	Body Cathexis Scale [BCS]	Significant change in attitude toward body image from prepregnancy to early pregnancy in a negative direction
				Exercisers did not have a more positive body image compared to non-exercisers
				Exercise group had more positive ratings compared to the non-exercise group on combined waist, hips, bust, and abdomen subscales of the BCS at 30 weeks' gestation
Harris (1979) UK, prospective cohort [53]	$N=85$ Black: 55 White: 30	Clinic patients	Stomach Focus dimension of the Body Focus Questionnaire	White women were more aware of their stomachs at each of the three time points (3 months, 9 months, and postpartum) compared to Black women
			Body Distortion Questionnaire	At 3 months, both groups had similar body distortion; however, body distortion increased for Black women peaking at 9 months and then decreasing fairly close to the score at 3 months. Body distortion decreased for White women most dramatically during postpartum
Hofmeyr et al. (1990) South Africa, cross-sectional [44]	$N=891$	Antenatal clinic at Johannesburg Hospital	Questionnaire	19 % felt more attractive than usual
				20 % reported increased interest in sex
				53 % felt less attractive than usual
				60 % reported being less interested in sex

(continued)

TABLE 7.1 (continued)

Author (year) country, design	Population	Setting	Body image assessment	Summary of results
Richardson (1990) USA, qualitative study [52]	N=63 AA: 14 % Hisp: 41 % White:45 %	Maternity clinics of a large university-affiliated outpatient facility	n/a	Of 463 experiences reported, 70 % indicated changes in body image Of the 305 changes reported, 80 % were satisfactory and 20 % worrisome
Strang and Sullivan (1985) Canada, prospective cohort [31]	N=96	A large urban hospital in western Canada	Attitude to Body Image Scale	Participants felt more negative about their bodies during the last 3 months of pregnancy than they did before the onset of their pregnancy ($p<0.01$)

BAQ Body Attitudes Scale, *BCS* Body Cathexis Scale, *ABIS* Attitude to Body Image Scale

Chapter 7. Body Image as a Contributor to Weight

The current Institute of Medicine [IOM] guidelines recommend that women with normal prepregnancy weight (body mass index [BMI] <25) gain 25–35 lb whereas overweight (25< BMI <30) or obese (BMI ≥30) women are advised to gain 15–25 lb and 11–20 lb, respectively [37]. However, currently, fewer than one third of pregnant women achieve guideline-recommended gains, with the majority gaining above IOM recommended levels [38]. Excessive gestational weight gain is on the rise, with more than 40 % of normal-weight women and 60 % of overweight women exceeding the gestational weight gain recommendations [38]. There are significant racial differences in gestational weight gain with White women more likely than their African-American counterparts to gain in excess of recommended levels [39–41]. However, African-American women are more likely to enter pregnancy overweight or obese compared to their White peers [42]. As mentioned earlier, a significant amount of research indicates that the idealized image of female beauty in western societies is thin [43]. During the course of pregnancy, with the increase in weight, breast size, and thickening of the waist, women depart from this cultural ideal of beauty. A woman's assessment of her body image when nonpregnant is based on her current perceived body image in comparison to her ideal body image. Thus, it can be expected that if the ideal remains stable during pregnancy, there would be an increase in body image dissatisfaction as pregnancy progresses [31].

The body changes that occur during pregnancy are somewhat expected, but there are some inconsistencies in the literature on whether a woman adapts positively to these changes or becomes dissatisfied or concerned about them [44–51]. In addition, it is evident that women have conflicting feelings about the changes in their bodies. Although for the most part, women have a positive perception of themselves during pregnancy, a considerable proportion report feeling unattractive [44]. A qualitative study by Chang et al. [50] reported that over 50 % of the women interviewed expressed dissatisfaction with their overall appearance. Some women talked about loss of the self/body and expressed concern about regaining their prepregnancy feminine self after the birth of baby. However, some women responded positively to their changed bodies. For others, the response was either negative or conflicted and their reactions to changing breasts covered the spectrum. Almost half of the women expressed concern and most expressed strong negative reactions to striae gravidarum (stretch marks). In this study, the reactions of significant others played a crucial role in a woman's adaptation to her pregnant body. As such, Chang et al. concluded that even during pregnancy, women are relying on ideas of men's standards of attractiveness and media representations to assess the changes they are experiencing during pregnancy. In a cross-sectional study [44] of 891 women, more than half of the study population felt less attractive than usual and 60 % reported being less interested in sex.

In contrast, several studies [35, 45, 52] have suggested that the normal societal pressures in western societies to conform to the ideal body shapes may be reduced during pregnancy [35, 45] since women see changes in their body as temporary and specific to childbearing [52]. As such, pregnancy may be the only reprieve from the pressure to be thin in most western societies since the reproductive role supersedes a woman's physical appearance. Fairburn et al. [35] report that among women interviewed 3 days postdelivery, 6 % reported dieting during pregnancy, 26 % experienced overeating episodes, 50 % expressed no concern about weight gain, and 24 % felt distressed about weight gain or felt less concerned than they would have before pregnancy. Approximately two thirds felt positive about their abdominal shape change, while one third felt negative about this change. Furthermore, the pregnant women in this study were more accepting of their body size and made fewer attempts to control their weight.

Chang et al. [50] reported that pregnant women view the changes in their body as reflective of their child's development and their assumption of the role of "mother." The participants in this study tended to compare their bodies with those of other pregnant women to assess whether or not their child was developing normally and attributed some level of success in this comparison. Davies and Wardle [45] compared pregnant and nonpregnant women and found that pregnant women were more accepting of their body size, had lower body dissatisfaction scores, and made fewer attempts to control their weight. In a diverse US sample ($n=63$) consisting of 45 % non-Hispanic White, 41 % Hispanic, and 14 % African-American women, Richardson also found that women were extremely tolerant of body changes. Of the 63 women studied, 70 % indicated changes in body experience, and of these, 80 % described these changes as satisfactory [52]. In a UK study comparing Black and White women, using the Stomach Focus dimension of the Body Focus and the Body Distortion Questionnaire, Harris [53] reported that over the course of pregnancy, White women were more aware of their stomachs at 9 months and least aware of their stomachs postpartum. However, this decrease in stomach awareness following delivery was not observed among Black women. In addition, the level of body distortion was similar for both groups during the first trimester; however, at 9 months and postpartum, Blacks showed more body distortion than Whites. Body distortion increased during pregnancy among Blacks, peaked at 9 months, and then fell to slightly less than their first trimester scores. On the other hand, body distortion decreased during pregnancy and most dramatically to almost half their 9-month score following delivery among Whites.

Determinants of Body Image During Pregnancy

Prepregnancy Body Image

Women who have had a positive body image prior to pregnancy seem to have a more positive attitude toward their pregnancy bodies, while a negative body image prior to pregnancy seems to persist during pregnancy [49]. The consequences of negative body image may include behaviors such as dieting, starving, and purging, and this is of great concern since these behaviors are linked to adverse obstetric outcomes, such as inadequate weight gain, premature delivery, and low birth weight [36].

Prepregnancy Weight Status

In a study by Fox and Yamaguchi [46], pregnancy weight status influenced body image during pregnancy. A sample of pregnant women ($n=76$) provided qualitative data through open-ended questions on how they felt generally about their current appearance and body shape and if, how, and why these feelings differed from prepregnancy feelings. Among women with a normal weight before pregnancy, 62 % reported more body image dissatisfaction during pregnancy, 19 % experienced less body image dissatisfaction, and 19 % experienced no change in body image. On the other hand, among women who were overweight before pregnancy, 62 % experienced less body image dissatisfaction, 23 % experienced more body image dissatisfaction, and 15 % experienced no change. As such, the thin body ideal may not be completely abandoned during pregnancy.

Prepregnancy Eating Behaviors

Fairburn and Welch [35] explained the differences in response to weight gain and shape on the basis of the woman's prepregnancy experience of being a dieter vs. a non-dieter and her previous attitudes toward her shape. The previous non-dieter group reported no feelings of concern about their weight gain and shape change in pregnancy. However, past dieters either had increased fears of weight gain or reduced concern through a license not to worry. These results contrast with Slade's hypothesis [54] that weight gain and loss history contributes to desensitization of concerns about bodily changes during pregnancy, thus, suggesting that past dieters would be more tolerant of weight gain.

Psychological Factors

Body image satisfaction (BIS) during pregnancy not only reflects a cosmetic assessment of appearance but may affect the woman's psychological and physical well-being. Several studies show a significant correlation between psychological characteristics and BIS during pregnancy [33, 48, 55, 56]. Anderson [55] reported that pregnant women who reported more symptoms of depression had lower BIS than those reporting fewer symptoms. In addition, Di Pietro et al. [56] showed that women who were more satisfied with their bodies during pregnancy showed fewer negative mood symptoms and less anger. In studies conducted by Duncombe et al. [33] and Clark et al. [48], the correlation between depressive symptoms and body image dissatisfaction persisted throughout pregnancy when measured prospectively at three and five time points during pregnancy.

Physical Activity

The link between exercise and body image is well established in the general population [57]. Evidence from previous studies indicates that there is a bidirectional relationship between exercise and body image. Individuals engage in exercise to reduce body image dissatisfaction, and engagement in exercise reduces body image dissatisfaction [57]. However, there is a small body of evidence concerning the relationship between exercise and body image satisfaction in pregnant women [47, 51, 58]. In a small pre-post quasi-experimental study, Marquez-Sterling et al. [58] found improvement in body satisfaction following an intervention consisting of 1 h exercise training sessions for a duration of 15 weeks among previously sedentary pregnant women compared to the control group. In another study, Boscaglia [47] compared high exercisers and low exercisers during pregnancy and assessed BIS prepregnancy retrospectively, at 15–22- weeks' and 23–30 weeks' gestations. High-exercising women were found to be significantly more satisfied with their bodies at 15–22 weeks compared to low-exercising women. Relative to their prepregnancy body image, high-exercising women were significantly more satisfied with their body image at 15–22 weeks' gestation and tended to be more satisfied at 23–30 weeks' gestation. No similar pattern was observed for low-exercising women, whose BIS remained relatively stable from prepregnancy to later pregnancy. As such, there seems to be a benefit of moderate levels of exercise particularly in the early phases of pregnancy.

In contrast, Goodwin et al. [51] compared body image satisfaction of 25 exercisers and 18 non-exercising pregnant women at several time points during pregnancy. For both groups, body image satisfaction ratings prepregnancy were more positive than early pregnancy ratings. There were no differences between groups at any of the time points measured (prepregnancy, 17 weeks, and 30 weeks). However, the exercising group had more positive ratings compared to the non-exercise group on combined waist, hips, bust, and abdomen subscales of the Body Cathexis Scale at 30 weeks' gestation. Several studies have suggested that women who exercise regularly throughout pregnancy retain a positive attitude toward their changing bodies as pregnancy progresses. Moreover, exercise may function as an adaptive strategy such that any potential body dissatisfaction due to weight gain is counteracted by general positive feelings about the body due to exercise. Walker and Freeland-Graves [59] posit that exercise may help avoid excessive weight gain and thus reduce weight distress and body dissatisfaction during pregnancy and postpartum.

Body Image Postpartum

Several studies indicate that one main concern of recent mothers during the postpartum period is the return to her normal/prepregnancy size; a summary of these studies is presented in Table 7.2. Studies of women's postpartum body image have yielded mixed results with some finding that

TABLE 7.2 Summary of studies evaluating body image during postpartum

Author (year) country, design	Population	Setting	Body image assessment	Summary of results
Boyington et al. (2007) US, cross-sectional [67]	N=105 100 % AA	4 inner city clinics in Washington, DC	The Reese Figure Rating Scale	75 % exhibited dissatisfaction with current body size 55 % perceived that they were too large and wanted to lose weight
Carter-Edwards et al. (2010) US, randomized controlled trial [66]	N=162 White: 55 % Black: 45 %	Women residing in the Triangle area of North Carolina	Stunkard Figure Rating Scale	Black women had higher mean body mass index [BMI] and higher mean ideal body image ideal mother body image compared to Whites but their body image dissatisfaction was significantly lower even after adjustment for age, BMI, education, income, and marital status
Gjerdingen et al. (2009) US, prospective cohort [63]	N=506 White: 76 % AA: 17.6 % Asian: 6.7 % Other: 8.7 %	7 Minneapolis/St. Paul metropolitan area clinics	Body Shape Questionnaire	Body image dissatisfaction increased significantly from 0–1 to 9 months postpartum

(continued)

TABLE 7.2 (continued)

Author (year) country, design	Population	Setting	Body image assessment	Summary of results
Jenkin and Tiggemann (1997) Australia, prospective cohort [60]	N = 115			On average, women were heavier 4 weeks after having their baby than they were prior to becoming pregnant and were less satisfied with their postnatal weight and shape
				They were also slightly heavier than they had anticipated, particularly in the case of the younger women
Morin (1995) US, cross-sectional [68]	N = 57 AA: 75 % White: 25 %	Not described	Attitude to Body Image Scale	Women with higher obesity measurement had a more negative view of the body as reflected by a higher ABIS score
Morin et al. (2002) US, cross-sectional [65]	N = 45 African-Americans	Not described	Attitude to Body Image Scale	Women had slight positive attitudes about their bodies immediately postpartum

Rallis et al. (2008) Australia, prospective cohort [62]	$N=79$	Prenatal exercise classes or obstetrician and gynecology practices in various suburbs of Melbourne	BAQ Physical Appearance Comparison Scale	Higher BID during postpartum Women reported feeling most fat at 6 months postpartum, even though they weighed less than they did at 6 weeks postpartum and the discrepancy between the stable ideal body size and their actual body size decreased
Walker (1998) US, cross-sectional survey [64]	$N=207$ White: 73 % Hispanic: 19 % Other: 8 %	Residence in Austin, Texas, with a singleton birth and a published mailing address	BCS	No significant difference in body image dissatisfaction between mothers who bottle-feed and those who breastfeed
Strang and Sullivan (1985) Canada, prospective cohort [31]	$N=96$	A large urban hospital in western Canada	Attitude to Body Image Scale	Participants had a slightly positive feeling toward their body image at 2 and 6 weeks postpartum

BAQ Body Attitudes Scale, *BCS* Body Cathexis Scale, *ABIS* Attitude to Body Image Scale, *BID* Body Image Dissatisfaction women are more dissatisfied during postpartum compared to during pregnancy [60–62] and that body image dissatisfaction increases during postpartum [63], while other studies have observed that women felt more positive about their postpartum body image than their pregnant body image [31]. There are a small number of studies examining body image during postpartum, and most of these included minority women in their study population.

Rallis et al. [62], in a small Australian study, found that women in the first-year postpartum felt fatter and less strong and fit and had greater body image dissatisfaction compared to their reports during pregnancy. Even though women are larger in size in their third trimester of pregnancy than during postpartum, they still reported higher body image dissatisfaction during postpartum. In this study, body image was assessed at three time points during the postpartum period. At 6 weeks postpartum, women seemed to perceive their size in the context of the recent pregnancy and are not yet too concerned about the weight gained during pregnancy and returning to their prepregnancy size. Nonetheless, women reported feeling the heaviest at 6 months postpartum, even though they weighed less than they did at 6 weeks postpartum and the discrepancy between the stable ideal body size and their actual body size decreased. These results suggest that the temporary reprieve of pressure to conform to the ideal during pregnancy is eliminated and returns during the postpartum period. Similarly, one study [63] in a diverse US sample ($n=506$) with 17 % African-American and 67 % White women examined the progression of body image dissatisfaction over time during the postpartum period. On average, women lost 10.1 lb (s.d. 16.3) from 0–1 to 9 months postpartum but remained on average 5.4 lb (s.d. 15.6) heavier at 9 months postpartum compared to prepregnancy. Body image dissatisfaction increased significantly from 0–1 to 9 postpartum. Body image dissatisfaction was significantly associated with overeating, higher current weight, poor mental health, single status, race other than African-American, bottle-feeding, and parity.

Walker et al. [59] examined the association between the method of feeding (bottle vs. breast) and body image dissatisfaction and found no significant difference in a diverse sample ($n=207$ with 73 % White, 19 % Hispanic, and 8 % others). However, in the bottle-feeding group, body image dissatisfaction was significantly associated with weight gain, but this association was not observed in the breastfed group. In another publication [64], text data from this study sample suggests that some women who were breastfeeding may minimize or repress their feelings about their weight and, thus, report lower body image dissatisfaction.

Three studies on body image postpartum were conducted in African-American populations. Morin [65], in small sample of 45 African-American women who were assessed 24–48 h postpartum, found that these women had slightly positive attitudes about their bodies immediately postpartum. Similarly, in the Active Mothers Postpartum (AMP) study [66], the authors, in a sample of 162 participants, compared African-American and White women postpartum. They found that although African-American women had higher mean body mass index [BMI], there was no difference by race in current perception of body image. Although African-American women selected heavier figures as ideal compared to Whites, this difference did not achieve statistical significance. However, for ideal mother image, there was a significant race difference with African-American women selecting heavier figures compared to White women. Both groups experienced some level of body image dissatisfaction when their current body image was compared with the ideal image and the ideal mother image. On average, for both groups, body image dissatisfaction was lower when the current body image was compared with the ideal mother image, suggesting greater satisfaction with a larger size as a mother. However, African-American women had significantly lower mean body dissatisfaction than White women indicating a greater degree of satisfaction with a larger size. This difference persisted even after adjustment for age, BMI, education, income, marital status and interactions terms. In a sample of low-income African-American women interviewed between 0 and 6 months postpartum, Boyington [67] reported that over 75 % exhibited dissatisfaction with current body size and 55 %

perceived that they were too large and wanted to lose weight. Similarly, Morin [68], in a study of predominantly African-American women within the first 48 h postpartum, reported that women with higher BMI had a more negative view of their body as reflected by a higher score on the Attitude to Body Image Scale [ABIS] [31]. These results are not consistent with reports indicating that African-American women have lower body image dissatisfaction when compared to their White counterparts [69].

Strategies to Improve Body Image During Pregnancy and Postpartum

Health professionals working with pregnant women have an opportunity to help them adapt to their changing bodies in positive, healthy ways. To accomplish this, they need to create an environment conducive to sharing of feelings and experiences. It is important that health practitioners do not minimize patient's concerns about their changing bodies. Instead, practitioners should be able to discern when a woman is having a difficult time accepting changes in her body that accompany pregnancy and assist with the development of coping strategies for adapting to a woman's growing body. Several strategies have been noted, for example, support groups for networking with other pregnant women have been successful. Another strategy has been to encourage women to treat themselves periodically to something special. When women take the time to look their best during pregnancy, others respond to them in a positive manner. In this way, the pregnant woman's body image improves. Exercise programs designed especially for pregnant women have been shown not only to reduce stress but also to improve body image. In summary, given the dramatic physical changes during pregnancy and postpartum, and the importance of body image to both maternal and neonatal health, these may be opportune times for interventions to address body image dissatisfaction. However, given the paucity of evidence, limited prospective

Chapter 7. Body Image as a Contributor to Weight

data, and the lack of diversity in study populations, our understanding of body image during pregnancy and postpartum is limited. As such, there is a need for further research in diverse populations so that racial/ethnic differences in body image during pregnancy and postpartum can be better understood.

Moreover, intervention strategies for body image have been investigated primarily among persons with eating disorders. One study [70] found that the importance of appearance typically decreased with age in women, and other studies have indicated that engaging in cognitive reappraisal, an active process to accept aging changes, was associated with lower levels of body dissatisfaction [71, 72]. In addition, studies of cognitive behavioral therapy (CBT)-based interventions for body dissatisfaction and disordered eating in young women have shown clinically significant reductions in body dissatisfaction [73, 74]. Finally, engagement in body management or self-care (relaxation, massage, making time for exercise) was reported to be associated with less concern about shape and weight among midlife women [72]. Perhaps these strategies could be used to inform interventions to promote the acceptance of body changes during pregnancy and improve body image during pregnancy and postpartum.

Weight loss has been associated with improvement in body image in several populations [75–77]. However, the expected improvement in body image as a result of weight loss may be less than expected, since it is not uncommon for participants in weight loss programs after having lost weight to still be dissatisfied with their bodies. Nonetheless, weight loss programs tailored for women during postpartum may improve body image. Although several weight loss intervention studies targeting postpartum women are in progress, body image is not usually assessed [78].

Improved understanding of body image during pregnancy and postpartum in ethnically diverse populations, along with lessons learned from the eating disorder literature, can facilitate the development of culturally tailored interventions which may be effective among specific racial/ethnic groups.

Further research is needed to facilitate the development of evidence-based clinical interventions for promoting a healthy body image during pregnancy and postpartum by health-care professionals working with women during this life stage.

Acknowledgment Dr. Gary-Webb was funded by a grant from NHLBI (K01-HL084700).

References

1. Flegal KM, Carroll MD, Kit BK, Ogden CL. Prevalence of obesity and trends in the distribution of body mass index among US adults, 1999–2010. JAMA. 2012;307(5):491–7. Epub 2012/01/19.
2. Airhihenbuwa CO, Kumanyika S, Agurs TD, Lowe A. Perceptions and beliefs about exercise, rest, and health among African-Americans. Am J Health Promot. 1995;9(6):426–9. Epub 1995/06/07.
3. Airhihenbuwa CO, Kumanyika S, Agurs TD, Lowe A, Saunders D, Morssink CB. Cultural aspects of African American eating patterns. Ethn Health. 1996;1(3):245–60. Epub 1996/09/01.
4. Kumanyika SK, Morssink C, Agurs T. Models for dietary and weight change in African-American women: identifying cultural components. Ethn Dis. 1992;2(2):166–75. Epub 1992/01/01.
5. Ard JD. Unique perspectives on the obesogenic environment. J Gen Intern Med. 2007;22(7):1058–60. Epub 2007/05/24.
6. Anderson LA, Janes GR, Ziemer DC, Phillips LS. Diabetes in urban African Americans. Body image, satisfaction with size, and weight change attempts. Diabetes Educ. 1997;23(3):301–8.
7. Liburd LC, Anderson LA, Edgar T, Jack Jr L. Body size and body shape: perceptions of Black women with diabetes. Diabetes Educ. 1999;25(3):382–8. Epub 1999/10/26.
8. Patt MR, Lane AE, Finney CP, Yanek LR, Becker DM. Body image assessment: comparison of figure rating scales among urban Black women. Ethn Dis. 2002;12(1):54–62. Epub 2002/03/27.
9. Secord PF, Jourard SM. The appraisal of body-cathexis: body-cathexis and the self. J Consult Psychol. 1953;17(5):343–7. Epub 1953/10/01.
10. Cooper PJ, Taylor MJ, Cooper Z, Fairbum CG. The development and validation of the body shape questionnaire. Int J Eat Disord. 1987;6(4):485–94.
11. Stunkard AJ, Sorensen T, Schulsinger F. Use of the Danish Adoption Register for the study of obesity and thinness. Res Publ Assoc Res Nerv Ment Dis. 1983;60:115–20.

12. Bulik CM, Wade TD, Heath AC, Martin NG, Stunkard AJ, Eaves LJ. Relating body mass index to figural stimuli: population-based normative data for Caucasians. Int J Obes Relat Metab Disord. 2001;25(10):1517–24. Epub 2001/10/24.
13. Pulvers KM, Lee RE, Kaur H, Mayo MS, Fitzgibbon ML, Jeffries SK, et al. Development of a culturally relevant body image instrument among urban African Americans. Obes Res. 2004;12(10):1641–51.
14. Williamson DA, Womble LG, Zucker NL, Reas DL, White MA, Blouin DC, et al. Body image assessment for obesity (BIA-O): development of a new procedure. Int J Obes Relat Metab Disord. 2000;24(10):1326–32. Epub 2000/11/28.
15. Cox TL, Zunker C, Wingo BC, Thomas DM, Ard JD. Body image and quality of life in a group of African American women. Soc Indic Res. 2010;99:531–40.
16. Cox TL, Ard JD, Beasley TM, Fernandez JR, Howard VJ, Affuso O. Body image as a mediator of the relationship between body mass index and weight-related quality of life in Black women. J Womens Health (Larchmt). 2011;20(10):1573–8. Epub 2011/08/06.
17. Cachelin FM. Ethnic differences in body-size preferences: myth or reality? Nutrition. 2001;17(4):353–4. Epub 2001/05/23.
18. Rucker CE, Cash TF. Body images, body-size perceptions, and eating behaviors among African-American and White college women. Int J Eat Disord. 1992;12(3):291–9.
19. Altabe M. Ethnicity and body image: quantitative and qualitative analysis. Int J Eat Disord. 1998;23(2):153–9. Epub 1998/03/21.
20. Becker DM, Yanek LR, Koffman DM, Bronner YC. Body image preferences among urban African Americans and whites from low income communities. Ethn Dis. 1999;9(3):377–86. Epub 1999/12/22.
21. Derenne JL, Beresin EV. Body image, media, and eating disorders. Acad Psychiatry. 2006;30(3):257–61. Epub 2006/05/27.
22. Thesander M. The feminine ideal. London: Reaktion Books; 1997.
23. Schooler D, Ward M, Merriwether A, Caruthers A. Who's that girl: television's role in the body image development of young White and Black women. Psych Women Q. 2004;28:38–47.
24. Kumanyika S, Wilson JF, Guilford-Davenport M. Weight-related attitudes and behaviors of Black women. J Am Diet Assoc. 1993;93(4):416–22. Epub 1993/04/01.
25. Baturka N, Hornsby PP, Schorling JB. Clinical implications of body image among rural African-American women. J Gen Inter Med. 2000;15(4):235–41. Epub 2000/04/12.
26. Brown K, Schreiber G, McMahon R, Crawford P, Ghee K. Maternal influences on body satisfaction in Black and White girls aged 9 and 10: the NHLBI Growth and Health Study (NGHS). Ann Behav Med. 1995;17(3):213–20.

27. Lucero K, Hicks RA, Bramlette J, Brassington GS, Welter MG. Frequency of eating problems among Asian and Caucasian college women. Psychol Rep. 1992;71(1):255–8. Epub 1992/08/01.
28. Shaw H, Ramirez L, Trost A, Randall P, Stice E. Body image and eating disturbances across ethnic groups: more similarities than differences. Psychol Addict Behav. 2004;18(1):12–8. Epub 2004/03/11.
29. Fitzgibbon ML, Blackman LR, Avellone ME. The relationship between body image discrepancy and body mass index across ethnic groups. Obes Res. 2000;8(8):582–9.
30. Cox T, Ard J, Beasley TM, Fernandez J, Howard V, Kolotkin R, et al. Examining the association between body mass index and weight related quality of life in Black and White women. Appl Res Qual Life. 2012;7(3):309–22.
31. Strang VR, Sullivan PL. Body image attitudes during pregnancy and the postpartum period. J Obstet Gynecol Neonatal Nurs. 1985;14(4):332–7. Epub 1985/07/01.
32. Skouteris H, Carr R, Wertheim EH, Paxton SJ, Duncombe D. A prospective study of factors that lead to body dissatisfaction during pregnancy. Body Image. 2005;2(4):347–61. Epub 2007/12/20.
33. Duncombe D, Wertheim EH, Skouteris H, Paxton SJ, Kelly L. How well do women adapt to changes in their body size and shape across the course of pregnancy? J Health Psychol. 2008;13(4):503–15. Epub 2008/04/19.
34. Conti J, Abraham S, Taylor A. Eating behavior and pregnancy outcome. J Psychosom Res. 1998;44(3–4):465–77. Epub 1998/05/20.
35. Fairburn CG, Stein A, Jones R. Eating habits and eating disorders during pregnancy. Psychosom Med. 1992;54(6):665–72. Epub 1992/11/01.
36. Franko DL, Walton BE. Pregnancy and eating disorders: a review and clinical implications. Int J Eat Disord. 1993;13(1):41–7. Epub 1993/01/01.
37. Rasmussen KM, Yaktine AL, Guidelines CtRIPW, Medicine Io, Council NR, editors. Weight gain during pregnancy: reexamining the guidelines. Washington, DC: The National Academies Press; 2009.
38. Chu SY, Callaghan WM, Bish CL, D'Angelo D. Gestational weight gain by body mass index among US women delivering live births, 2004–2005: fueling future obesity. Am J Obstet Gynecol. 2009;200(3):271 e1–7. Epub 2009/01/10.
39. Fontaine PL, Hellerstedt WL, Dayman CE, Wall MM, Sherwood NE. Evaluating body mass index-specific trimester weight gain recommendations: differences between black and White women. J Midwifery Womens Health. 2012;57(4):327–35. Epub 2012/07/05.
40. Schieve LA, Cogswell ME, Scanlon KS. An empiric evaluation of the Institute of Medicine's pregnancy weight gain guidelines by race. Obstet Gynecol. 1998;91(6):878–84. Epub 1998/06/04.

41. Caulfield LE, Witter FR, Stoltzfus RJ. Determinants of gestational weight gain outside the recommended ranges among black and White women. Obstet Gynecol. 1996;87(5 Pt 1):760–6. Epub 1996/05/01.
42. Vahratian A. Prevalence of overweight and obesity among women of childbearing age: results from the 2002 national survey of family growth. Matern Child Health J. 2009;13(2):268–73. Epub 2008/04/17.
43. Thompson JK, Heinberg LJ, Altabe M, Tantleff-Dunn S. Exacting beauty: theory, assessment, and treatment of body image disturbance. Washington, DC: American Psychological Association; 1999.
44. Hofmeyr GJ, Marcos EF, Butchart AM. Pregnant women's perceptions of themselves: a survey. Birth. 1990;17(4):205–6. Epub 1990/12/01.
45. Davies K, Wardle J. Body image and dieting in pregnancy. J Psychosom Res. 1994;38(8):787–99. Epub 1994/11/01.
46. Fox P, Yamaguchi C. Body image change in pregnancy: a comparison of normal weight and overweight primigravidas. Birth. 1997;24(1):35–40. Epub 1997/03/01.
47. Boscaglia N, Skouteris H, Wertheim EH. Changes in body image satisfaction during pregnancy: a comparison of high exercising and low exercising women. Aust N Z J Obstet Gynaecol. 2003;43(1):41–5. Epub 2003/05/21.
48. Clark A, Skouteris H, Wertheim EH, Paxton SJ, Milgrom J. The relationship between depression and body dissatisfaction across pregnancy and the postpartum: a prospective study. J Health Psychol. 2009;14(1):27–35. Epub 2009/01/09.
49. Berk B. Body image and pregnancy: bridging the mind-body connection. A guide for health care professionals. J Perinatol. 1993;13(4):300–4. Epub 1993/07/01.
50. Chang SR, Chao YM, Kenney NJ. I am a woman and i'm pregnant: body image of women in Taiwan during the third trimester of pregnancy. Birth. 2006;33(2):147–53. Epub 2006/05/31.
51. Goodwin A, Astbury J, McMeeken J. Body image and psychological well-being in pregnancy. A comparison of exercisers and non-exercisers. Aust N Z J Obstet Gynaecol. 2000;40(4):442–7. Epub 2001/02/24.
52. Richardson P. Women's experiences of body change during normal pregnancy. Matern Child Nurs J. 1990;19(2):93–111. Epub 1990/01/01.
53. Harris R. Cultural differences in body perception during pregnancy. Br J Med Psychol. 1979;52(4):347–52. Epub 1979/12/01.
54. Slade PD. Awareness of body dimensions during pregnancy: an analogue study. Psychol Med. 1977;7(2):245–52. Epub 1977/05/01.
55. Anderson VN, Fleming AS, Steiner M. Mood and the transition to motherhood. J Reprod Infant Psychol. 1994;12(2):69–77.
56. Dipietro JA, Millet S, Costigan KA, Gurewitsch E, Caulfield LE. Psychosocial influences on weight gain attitudes and behaviors

during pregnancy. J Am Diet Assoc. 2003;103(10):1314–9. Epub 2003/10/02.
57. Campbell A, Hausenblas HA. Effects of exercise interventions on body image: a meta-analysis. J Health Psychol. 2009;14(6):780–93. Epub 2009/08/19.
58. Marquez-Sterling S, Perry AC, Kaplan TA, Halberstein RA, Signorile JF. Physical and psychological changes with vigorous exercise in sedentary primigravidae. Med Sci Sports Exerc. 2000;32(1):58–62. Epub 2000/01/27.
59. Walker LO, Freeland-Graves J. Lifestyle factors related to postpartum weight gain and body image in bottle- and breastfeeding women. J Obstet Gynecol Neonatal Nurs. 1998;27(2):151–60. Epub 1998/04/29.
60. Jenkin W, Tiggemann M. Psychological effects of weight retained after pregnancy. Women Health. 1997;25(1):89–98. Epub 1997/01/01.
61. Leifer M. Psychological changes accompanying pregnancy and motherhood. Genet Psychol Monogr. 1977;95(1):55–96. Epub 1977/02/01.
62. Rallis S, Skouteris H, Wertheim EH, Paxton SJ. Predictors of body image during the first year postpartum: a prospective study. Women Health. 2007;45(1):87–104. Epub 2007/07/07.
63. Gjerdingen D, Fontaine P, Crow S, McGovern P, Center B, Miner M. Predictors of mothers' postpartum body dissatisfaction. Women Health. 2009;49(6):491–504. Epub 2009/12/17.
64. Walker LO. Weight-related distress in the early months after childbirth. West J Nurs Res. 1998;20(1):30–44. Epub 1998/02/25.
65. Morin KH, Brogan S, Flavin SK. Attitudes and perceptions of body image in postpartum African American women. Does weight make a difference? MCN Am J Matern Child Nurs. 2002;27(1):20–5.
66. Carter-Edwards L, Bastian LA, Revels J, Durham H, Lokhnygina Y, Amamoo MA, et al. Body image and body satisfaction differ by race in overweight postpartum mothers. J Womens Health (Larchmt). 2010;19(2):305–11. Epub 2010/02/02.
67. Boyington J, Johnson A, Carter-Edwards L. Dissatisfaction with body size among low-income, postpartum Black women. J Obstet Gynecol Neonatal Nurs. 2007;36(2):144–51. Epub 2007/03/21.
68. Morin KH. Obese and nonobese postpartum women: complications, body image, and perceptions of the intrapartal experience. Appl Nurs Res. 1995;8(2):81–7. Epub 1995/05/01.
69. Baptiste-Roberts K, Gary TL, Bone LR, Hill MN, Brancati FL. Perceived body image among African Americans with type 2 diabetes. Patient Educ Couns. 2006;60(2):194–200. Epub 2006/01/31.
70. Pliner P, Chaiken S, Flett GL. Gender differences in concern with weight and physical appearance over the lifespan. Pers Soc Psychol Bull. 1990;16:10.

Chapter 7. Body Image as a Contributor to Weight 155

71. Webster J, Tiggemann M. The relationship between women's body satisfaction and self-image across the life span: the role of cognitive control. J Genet Psychol. 2003;164(2):241–52. Epub 2003/07/15.
72. McLean SA, Paxton SJ, Wertheim EH. Factors associated with body dissatisfaction and disordered eating in women in midlife. Int J Eat Disord. 2010;43(6):527–36. Epub 2009/09/01.
73. Paxton SJ, McLean SA, Gollings EK, Faulkner C, Wertheim EH. Comparison of face-to-face and internet interventions for body image and eating problems in adult women: an RCT. Int J Eat Disord. 2007;40(8):692–704. Epub 2007/08/19.
74. Gollings EK, Paxton SJ. Comparison of internet and face-to-face delivery of a group body image and disordered eating intervention for women: a pilot study. Eat Disord. 2006;14(1):1–15. Epub 2006/06/08.
75. Stewart TM, Bachand AR, Han H, Ryan DH, Bray GA, Williamson DA. Body image changes associated with participation in an intensive lifestyle weight loss intervention. Obesity (Silver Spring). 2011;19(6):1290–5. Epub 2010/12/15.
76. Dalle Grave R, Cuzzolaro M, Calugi S, Tomasi F, Temperilli F, Marchesini G. The effect of obesity management on body image in patients seeking treatment at medical centers. Obesity (Silver Spring). 2007;15(9):2320–7. Epub 2007/09/25.
77. Ramirez EM, Rosen JC. A comparison of weight control and weight control plus body image therapy for obese men and women. J Consult Clin Psychol. 2001;69(3):440–6. Epub 2001/08/10.
78. Kuhlmann AK, Dietz PM, Galavotti C, England LJ. Weight-management interventions for pregnant or postpartum women. Am J Prev Med. 2008;34(6):523–8. Epub 2008/05/13.

Part III
The Early Postpartum Period

Chapter 8
Promoting a Healthy Weight After Delivery

Alexander Berger and Wanda Nicholson

"If I don't lose weight, that puts me at high risk for heart disease, heart attacks and stroke," FIRST WIND Trial participant, 2008. [1]

Abstract There are over 1.4 million overweight or obese women who become pregnant each year in the United States. The postpartum period may be a critical period for postpartum weight retention, long-term weight gain, and chronic obesity for young women. Achieving a healthy weight after delivery in women who were overweight or obese prior to pregnancy should be possible, but will require the use of relevant, evidence-based lifestyle interventions. There is a lack of consensus from medical and public health policy organizations about how lifestyle interventions should be implemented

---

A. Berger, MD, MPH
Department of Obstetrics and Gynecology,
Thomas Jefferson University Hospital,
Philadelphia, PA, USA

W. Nicholson, MD, MPH, MBA (✉)
Department of Obstetrics and Gynecology,
Diabetes and Obesity Core, Center for Women's Health Research,
University of North Carolina School
of Medicine, Chapel Hill, NC, USA
e-mail: wanda_nicholson@med.unc.edu

W. Nicholson, K. Baptiste-Roberts (eds.),
Obesity During Pregnancy in Clinical Practice,
DOI 10.1007/978-1-4471-2831-1_8,
© Springer-Verlag London 2014

in the postpartum period. Differences in recommendations may be due in part to limited and inconsistent evidence of the effectiveness of postpartum interventions on weight loss. Larger-scale trials with rigorous methodology, diverse study samples, and consistent outcome measures are needed to confirm intervention effectiveness in the postpartum period. The translation and dissemination of evidence-based interventions to high-risk populations deserves further attention.

Keywords Postpartum care • Lifestyle modification • RE-AIM framework • Lifestyle interventions

> **Key Points**
> - Few women return for their postpartum visit at 6–8 weeks after delivery, limiting the ability of their providers to communicate about weight loss after delivery.
> - There are few published trials comparing weight loss interventions in the postpartum period; few trials use evidence-based lifestyle components.
> - The RE-AIM framework is an established model for assessing the sustainability of community-based lifestyle interventions.
> - The Chronic Care Model may be a reasonable framework to translate lifestyle interventions into routine postpartum care.

Introduction

Based on current estimates, there are over 1.4 million overweight or obese women who become pregnant each year in the United States [2–4]. Helping women to prepare for the postpartum [5–8] and to achieve a healthy weight after delivery [9] continues to be an important challenge for clinicians within the current US model of care. The *postpartum period* is generally defined as the 6- to 8-week period after delivery. The *interconception period* refers to the time between pregnancies, including, but not restricted to, the postpartum period [10]. In many clinical trials and public health reports, the interconception period is referred to as the time frame from delivery to 12–18 months after the birth of an infant. Throughout this chapter, we use the term postpartum broadly to include the standard 6- to 8-week postpartum period and the interconception period.

Using established frameworks, such as RE-AIM or the Chronic Care Model, may help to facilitate the integration of a standard postpartum care model for overweight or obese parturients into the current health system.

Importance of the Postpartum Period

The postpartum period may be a critical period for postpartum weight retention, long-term weight gain, and chronic obesity for young women [3, 4]. Physiological changes of childbirth and sedentary behaviors related to parenting contribute to weight retention and weight gain [11, 12]. Compared with weight gain during other life intervals, excess weight retained after childbirth appears to be particularly harmful, as postpartum weight accumulates centrally rather than peripherally, increasing the risk of developing the chronic disease [13, 14]. Although it is well recognized that the time period after delivery represents a unique opportunity [15] to initiate weight management interventions or to continue interventions that began during pregnancy (Chap. 4), there are relatively few opportunities for ongoing patient-clinician communication after delivery. Insurance coverage for postpartum or interconception care, including third-party payers and Medicaid, ends at 6–12 weeks after delivery. The postpartum visit, which often occurs within a busy clinical practice, focuses primarily on contraception and lactation. Recent estimates show that only 50 % of women, independent of socioeconomic status or insurance, return for the postpartum visit [16], therefore missing an important opportunity to communicate with their providers about important lifestyle modifications after delivery.

Achieving a healthy weight after delivery in women who were overweight or obese prior to pregnancy should be possible, but will require the use of relevant, evidence-based lifestyle interventions [5, 6]. Also, given the one brief postpartum visit, interventions will need to be widely disseminable in order to be deemed successful. In this chapter, we summarize current global recommendations for postpartum weight management and review the findings of seven fair-to-good published studies on the effectiveness of diet and physical activity interventions to prevent postpartum weight retention, highlighting current gaps in our knowledge of the best practices for postpartum weight management. Finally, we propose an agenda for future research to improve the development and testing of evidence-based models of care.

Recommendations for Postpartum Weight Management

Global recommendations for postpartum care for overweight and obese women vary widely. The American Congress of Obstetricians and Gynecologists [17] provides general recommendations for postpartum physical activity, but there are no current evidence-based guidelines for dietary or exercise interventions and no recommendations in the United States that specifically target women who were overweight or obese prior to pregnancy (Table 8.1). The most recent recommendation supports the gradual resumption of prepregnancy exercise activities in those women with uncomplicated pregnancies and provides reassurance that moderate physical activity does not interfere with the quality of milk production or neonatal weight. ACOG does not make specific guidelines for nutritional intake, but clinicians are encouraged to provide their patients with information about healthy eating, and a list of resources is available through the ACOG Resource Guide – Nutrition and Physical Activity to Address Overweight and Obesity (http://www.acog.org) [18]. The Canadian Society for Exercise Physiologists [19] recommends the generally healthy women to return to their normal exercise program after receiving medical clearance at the 6–8-week postnatal visit.

TABLE 8.1 Comparison of NICE and ACOG recommendations

	All postpartum women	Postpartum women with BMI ≥30
NICE	6–8-week postnatal check:	6–8-week postnatal check:
	Ask those who are overweight and obese or who have concerns about their weight if they would like any further advice and support now – or later	Explain the increased risks that being obese poses to them and, if they become pregnant again, their unborn child
	Provide clear, tailored, consistent, up-to-date, and timely advice about how to lose weight safely after childbirth	Encourage them to lose weight
	Ensure women have a realistic expectation of the time it will take to lose weight gained during pregnancy	Offer a structured weight loss program or a referral to a dietitian or an appropriately trained health professional
	Discuss benefits of a healthy diet and regular physical activity	Provide women who are not yet ready to lose weight with information about where they can get support when they are ready
	Advice on healthy eating and physical activity should be tailored to her circumstances	Use evidence-based behavior change techniques to motivate and support women to lose weight

(continued)

TABLE 8.1 (continued)

All postpartum women	Postpartum women with BMI ≥30
Advise women, their partners, and family to seek information and advice from a reputable source	Encourage breastfeeding
Provide details of appropriate community-based services	
Encourage women to breastfeed	
Provide advice on recreational exercise:	
1. A mild exercise program consisting of walking, pelvic floor exercises, and stretching may begin immediately	
2. After complicated deliveries, or lower segment caesareans, a medical caregiver should be consulted before resuming prepregnancy levels of physical activity, usually after the first checkup at 6–8 weeks after giving birth	
Emphasize the importance of participating in physical activities, such as walking, which can be built into daily life	

ACOG	Rapid return to prepregnancy activities is acceptable after an uncomplicated pregnancy and delivery	No recommendations based on BMI
	Moderate weight reduction after delivery does not interfere with lactation or neonatal weight	
	Postpartum exercise may help to reduce postpartum depression symptoms	
	Refer to consultation with a weight specialist before the next pregnancy	
	Discuss healthy lifestyle behaviors at each visit	

NICE National Institute of Health and Clinical Excellence, *ACOG* American Congress of Obstetricians and Gynecologists

Current recommendations for postpartum dietary interventions and physical activity interventions in the United Kingdom were developed by the National Institute for Health and Clinical Excellence (NICE) [20]. NICE recommendations are developed based on available evidence of effectiveness (including cost-effectiveness), fieldwork data, and incorporating the perspectives of multiple stakeholders (e.g., patients, clinicians) and experts. The recommendations include components of effective aspects of care for obesity in general and identify key dietary, exercise, and behavioral principles, such as eating a low-fat diet, encouraging regular physical activity, and identifying and addressing barriers to behavioral change. In slight contrast to ACOG, NICE provides specific recommendations for postpartum counseling and support to prevent weight retention in overweight or obese women (Table 8.1). NICE recommends that clinicians discuss the need for weight loss with all postpartum women and expand the discussion to include the adverse effects of maternal obesity on pregnancy outcomes for any future pregnancy. Clinicians are encouraged to provide ongoing counseling with their practice or to refer the patient to a dietary expert for further behavioral modification. If patients have not yet committed to making lifestyle modifications, it is recommended that clinicians provide a 6-month follow-up visit to reevaluate the patient's readiness for weight loss. Of particular relevance are the NICE community-based service guidelines. These guidelines encourage communities to create and sustain affordable recreational exercise facilities and to increase the availability of cost-efficient healthy foods. Also, the NICE provides guidelines for health professionals to improve their ability to talk with their patients about weight loss and to provide dietary and exercise counseling. The NICE recommendations are continually updated based on available evidence for effectiveness and expert review.

Evidence for Postpartum Interventions to Promote Weight Loss

Interventions that integrate exercise and dietary changes have been shown to achieve weight loss in middle- and older-aged adults [PREMIER [6], Well-Integrated Screening and

Evaluation for Women Across the Nation (WISEWOMAN) [21], Diabetes Prevention Program (DPP) [22]], though evidence for their efficacy in postpartum women is limited. The paucity of recommendations for postpartum care in the United States may be due, in part, to the small number of clinical trials that compare the effectiveness and safety of dietary and exercise interventions, small sample size, limitations in study design, and a lack of participants that are generalizable to diverse populations of US women. Reducing postpartum weight retention can decrease the proportion of women that develop pregnancy-related hypertension or gestational diabetes in a subsequent pregnancy. Alternatively, if women have completed childbearing, reducing postpartum weight retention can lower the risk of long-term metabolic abnormalities or cardiovascular disease. The PREMIER trial was a National Heart Lung and Blood (NHLBI)-funded intervention designed for adults with Stage 1 hypertension. The intervention was successful in lowering blood pressure and was also found to lower weight. The Diabetes Prevention Program [5] was a clinical study sponsored by the Centers for Disease Control and Prevention (CDC). Subsequent trials have focused on translating these interventions into various settings [23]. Administered through the CDC's Division for Heart Disease and Stroke Prevention, the WISEWOMAN program [21] provides low-income, underinsured, or uninsured women, age 40–64, with lifestyle intervention and referral services in an effort to prevent cardiovascular disease.

We conducted a review of clinical trials comparing diet and exercise interventions for the reduction in postpartum weight retention. Our goal was to identify fair-to-good quality RCTs based on the United States Preventive Services Task Force quality criteria [24] and to assess studies for the use of evidence-based intervention components proven effective in general populations. Twelve trials [25–35] published between 1998 and 2011 met the quality criteria (Table 8.2). Eight trials were conducted in the United States, one in Taiwan [31] and one in Honduras [26] and one in Greece [23] and the United Kingdom [32]. The trials also compared different types of interventions using different modes of delivery. Seven trials compared an in-person diet

Table 8.2 Results from 12 randomized controlled trials of diet and exercise interventions

Author, year, country (reference)	Intervention arms	Intervention enrollment/duration	Study sample, N	Race/ethnicity	Weight change, kg (standard deviation)
Diet plus exercise interventions					
Leermakers and Wing 1998, USA [34]	Intervention (I): Correspondence lessons, group sessions, and telephone follow-up	8 mos	Non-lactating postpartum women	3 % nonwhite	I: −7.8 ± 4.5
	Control (C): usual care, brochure	6 mos	N = 90		C: −4.9 ± 5.4 ($P = 0.03$)[a]
O'Toole et al., 2003, USA [33]	I: Structured diet + exercise with weekly in-person sessions × 12 wks, biweekly sessions × 8 wks, and monthly sessions up to 1 year	6 wks to 6 mos	Postpartum women who were overweight or obese prior to pregnancy	1 AA	I: −4.8 ± 1.7
	C: One session, self-directed	6–10 mos	N = 40		C: −0.8 ± 2.3 ($P < 0.001$)

Craigie et al. 2011, UK [32]	I: Two face-to-face counseling sessions, with telephone follow-up for reinforcement and resources for pamphlet	6–18 mos	Low-income, overweight, and obese postpartum women	3 nonwhite participants	I: −7.3
	C: Information pamphlet	3 mos	$N=52$		C: −1.3 ($P<0.05$) SD-NR
Huang and Tsai 2011, Taiwan [31]	I: Individualized dietary and physical activity plans, including 6 in-person pregnancy sessions and 3 postpartum sessions	1 day	Pregnant and postpartum Taiwanese women; 1 day postpartum	Taiwanese	I: −0.9 ± 5.1
	C: Usual care	6 mos	$N=189$		C: −0.36 ± 4.9 ($P=0.25$)

(continued)

TABLE 8.2 (continued)

Author, year, country (reference)	Intervention arms	Intervention enrollment/duration	Study sample, N	Race/ethnicity	Weight change, kg (standard deviation)
Lovelady et al. 2000, USA [30]	I: Caloric restriction and exercise intervention, including 4 exercise sessions, lasting 43 min with goal of 65–80 % heart rate	5 wks	Overweight postpartum women with BMI 25–30 kg/m2, exclusively breastfeeding	3.5 % AA	I: -1.6 ± 2.0
	C: Usual care	2.5 mos	$N=40$		C: 0.2 ± 2.2 ($P=0.018$)
Ostbye et al. 2009, USA [29]	I: 8 healthy eating classes, 10 physical activity classes, and 6 telephone counseling sessions over 9 mos	2 mos	Overweight or obese postpartum women	I: 45 % AA	I: -11.21
	C: Usual care	9 mos	$N=450$	C: 45 % AA	C: -11.04 (P-value NR) SD-NR

Davenport et al. 2011, USA [35]	I: Diet + low-intensity exercise	8 wks	Overweight or obese women who retained >5 kg after delivery	Intervention groups: 85–90 % white	I: −5.0 ± 2.9 moderate intensity
	I: Diet + moderate-intensity exercise	4 mos	N = 60	No AA	I: −4.2 ± 4.0 low intensity
	C: No intervention			Other race: NR	C: −0.1 ± 3.3
					($P < 0.01$)
Exercise-only interventions					
Zourladani et al. 2011, Greece [23]	I: Instructor led 1-h exercise class with aerobic activity and strength training 3 times per wk for 12 wks	4–6 wks	Primiparous postpartum women	Greek	I: −3.3
	C: No intervention	3 mos	N = 40		C: −1.3
					($P = 0.667$)

(continued)

TABLE 8.2 (continued)

Author, year, country (reference)	Intervention arms	Intervention enrollment/duration	Study sample, N	Race/ethnicity	Weight change, kg (standard deviation)
Maturi and Abedi, 2011, Iran [28]	I: Tailored pedometer-based walking program with baseline counseling session, cell phone and text reminders, and telephone feedback	6 wks to 6 mos	Lactating, normal, or overweight postpartum women	Iranian	I: −2.1
	C: Routine care	3 mos	N=66		C: 0 ($P<0.001$)
Dewey et al., 1994, USA [26]	I: Individually tailored and supervised aerobic activity to achieve 60–70 % heart rate reserve. 45 min–5 times a wk	6–8 wks	Exclusively breastfeeding postpartum women	No AA	I: −1.6
	C: No intervention	3 mos	N=33		C: −1.6 ($p>0.05$)

Diet-only intervention

Krummel et al. 2010, USA [25]	Counseling with dietitian and 10 facilitated discussion groups, monthly personalized feedback on self-monitoring records	30 wks	Postpartum women enrolled in WIC	10 % nonwhite	I: −2.1
	C: Self-directed	12 mos	$N=151$		C: 0 ($P<0.001$) SD-NR

Breastfeeding Intervention

Dewey et al., 2001, Honduras [26]	I: Received counseling on exclusive breastfeeding	4 mos	Two studies: postpartum, primiparous, low-income women	NR	Cohort 1:
	C: Usual care	2 mos	141		I: −0.7 ± 1.5 C: −0.1 ± 1.7 ($P<0.05$)

NR not reported, *AA* African American, *mos* months, *wks* weeks, *WIC* Women, Infant, and Children's program
[a]P-values less than or equal to 0.05 represents a statistically significant difference between outcome in the intervention and control groups

and exercise intervention to standard postpartum care. Three trials compared the effects of exercise interventions to standard postpartum care; two were supervised while one was self-directed. One trial compared the effect of individual dietetic counseling and facilitated group sessions with standard postpartum care. The mode of delivery of the interventions varied from mail correspondence to in-person individual and group sessions to telephone follow-up.

The enrollment period for the 12 trials ranged from 1 day to 6 months after delivery. The duration of the interventions was 3–9 months. No trials included evidence-based intervention components. Only three trials reported the percentage of African American participants [29, 33, 36]. Ostbye and colleagues [29] reported that African American women comprised 45 and 44 % of the intervention and standard care groups, respectively. One trial reported 3.5 % of the 40 participants as African American women [30]; another trial reported one African American woman among 40 enrollees [33]; two studies [32, 34] included a small number of nonwhite participants, but the specific racial/ethnic groups for participants were not reported.

There were inconsistent results among the seven trials [29–35] comparing the effect of a postpartum diet and exercise intervention to standard postpartum care on weight (Table 8.2). Five trials [30, 32–35] reported greater postpartum weight loss among women in the intervention group compared to those in the usual care group. One study reported no statistically significant differences in weight. In the largest trial by Ostbye and colleagues [29] ($N=450$), there were no statistically significant differences in mean weight loss between the intervention and usual care groups. Leermakers and colleagues [34] found a statistically significantly higher percentage weight loss (10 % versus 5.8 %; $p<0.04$) among women in the intervention group compared to those in the control group. Also, there were a higher proportion of women returning to their prepregnancy weight (33 % versus 11.5 %, $p<0.05$) in the intervention group versus the standard care group. There were no statistically significant differences in abdominal circumference between women in a diet and exercise intervention and those in usual care. In a small trial, Davenport and colleagues [35] reported statistically significantly lower waist-to-hip ratios in women receiving a diet and exercise intervention compared to usual care.

Further research is needed to determine the effectiveness of postpartum intervention on weight and measures of adiposity (e.g., waist circumference, skinfold thickness) and to increase our understanding of which single or combinations of components are most effective in postpartum women. Large-scale studies that include a diverse sample of participants, improved adherence to intervention protocol, and consistency in outcome measures can provide better insight into the effectiveness of intervention. Further, studies should include an examination of harms including effects on both the mother and infant child. Such studies can inform the development of postpartum care guidelines tailored to overweight or obese women. The LIFE-Moms Consortium [37], sponsored by NIH, consists of six ongoing large studies of pregnancy and postpartum interventions. Findings from these ongoing studies should address some of the existing gaps in our knowledge and inform postpartum care guidelines.

Proposing an Agenda for Future Research

Future research in postpartum care for the overweight or obese parturient might focus on the integration of existing clinical models of care and the ability to disseminate interventions with proven efficacy. The Chronic Disease Model and the RE-AIM framework represent existing strategies that might be applied to the care of overweight and obese women during the perinatal period.

Applying the RE-AIM Framework to Research on Postpartum Interventions

The four RE-AIM dimensions allow for a standard set of evaluation parameters that can be used to quantitatively evaluate each project. These four dimensions can be used to guide planning, development, and testing of population-based interventions for overweight and obese women. While well established within the public health community, the RE-AIM framework has broad applicability to the 1.4 million overweight or obese women who become pregnant each year. The RE-AIM framework is particularly relevant to the topic of postpartum weight retention and prevention of obesity because it provides flexibility for clinicians and researchers to modify the framework to relate to their specific target population, recruitment and outreach approaches, efficacy, adoption, implementation, and maintenance. Given the multiple settings in which women may receive care after delivery (private medical office, health department, hospital-based clinic), a general framework that can be modified for specific populations and settings can be useful in designing dissemination studies. The Weight Loss After Delivery (Fig. 8.1) project was a feasibility study conducted among African American women in West Baltimore to promote postpartum weight loss. The intervention adapted evidence-based components of PREMIER and the Diabetes Prevention Program for use in postpartum African American women who had been overweight or obese at the time of conception. In Phase 1, a pilot trial was planned and conducted in preparation for a larger-scale comparative effectiveness trial. To promote the *reach* of the intervention, the target population for First WIND was postpartum African American women living in West Baltimore City. Statewide data had shown large disparities in overweight and obesity in Baltimore City compared to other areas of Central Maryland and particularly large disparities in obesity and the associated morbidities in African American women in the area. A series of focus groups were conducted with pregnant and postpartum African American women to effectively adapt the components of PREMIER to this specific population. Planning for the feasibility study included multiple meetings with community-based obstetrical practices in the West Baltimore area. Additional discussions were held with the Chief of Obstetrics and Gynecology at the community-based hospitals in which labor and delivery services took place in

Chapter 8. Promoting a Healthy Weight After Delivery

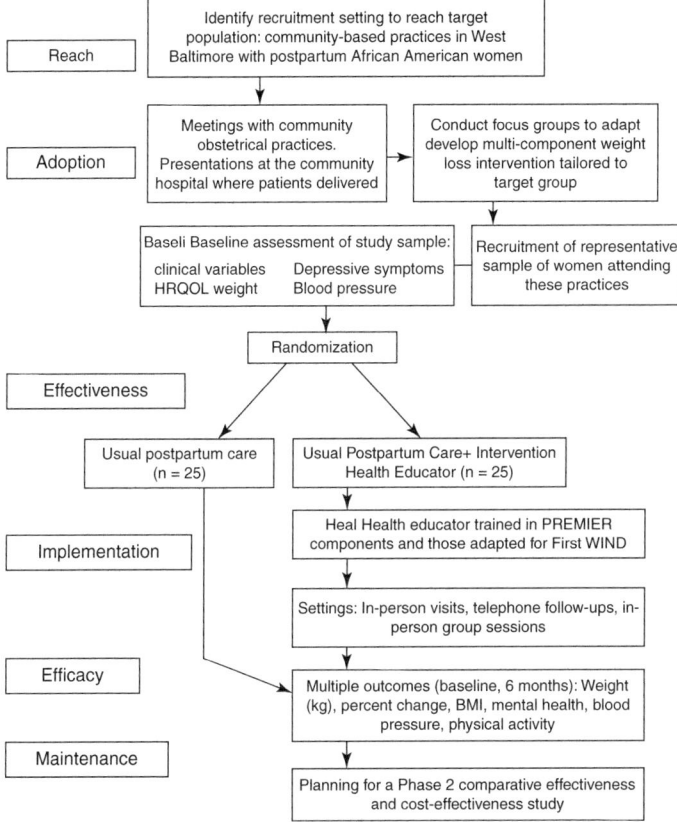

FIGURE 8.1 Using the RE-AIM framework to assess the sustainability of the First WIND intervention (Adapted from Nicholson WK, Ghosh P, Grogan R, Dalcin A, Charleston J, Appel LJ. Translating PREMIER for use in postpartum women (pending publication))

order to promote *adoption* of the intervention by clinicians and the broader health community. The investigative team presented the final plans for the study at the community hospital's monthly grand rounds, where clinicians were able to make additional suggestions and modifications to the research plan. To test the preliminary effectiveness of the intervention,

30 postpartum women were randomized to the adapted intervention (First WIND) or usual care. Women randomized to the usual care + intervention received a 6-month postpartum intervention, consisting of 5 individual sessions with a health educator and 10 group sessions facilitated by the health educator in a community setting. Women randomized to usual care received a series of informational brochures. A key phase of *implementation* will be the training of health educators, the interventionists who have previously undergone training in participatory methods and received additional sessions on implementing the adapted components to postpartum women. Several outcomes were planned at 6 months, including weight, systolic and diastolic blood pressure, mental health, and weekly minutes of physical activity to determine preliminary *efficacy*. Analysis included comparison of outcomes between the usual care and intervention groups. Planned process outcomes included logistical barriers to intervention implementation, participant adherence to study protocol, and staff and participant behaviors. Assessment of clinical and process outcomes is the next step in planning for a larger comparative effectiveness study to set the stage for sustainability or *maintenance* of the intervention within the study community.

A potential theoretical approach to creating effective postpartum care in the overweight or obese parturient is the Chronic Care Model. This model acknowledges the importance of multiple community, health system, and individual level factors (Fig. 8.2) [37–39]. Building from this model, clinicians and public health officials can rigorously engage other community-based providers, including behavioral interventionists, dieticians, exercise physiologists, and lifestyle coaches to assist patients with the important lifestyle modifications necessary to reach their weight loss goals. The Chronic Care Model is particularly relevant to reducing postpartum weight retention because it includes condition-specific decision support and general skill building around prevention. Interventions that share success similar to other interventions based on this model have the potential to provide significant improvements in overall health in preparation for a future pregnancy and for long-term health.

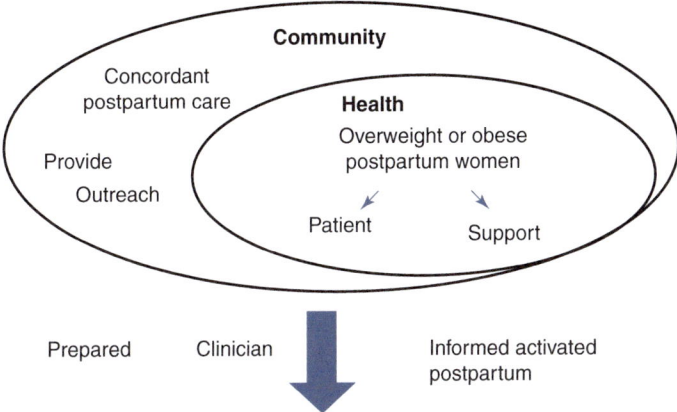

FIGURE 8.2 The Chronic Care Model applied to postpartum care for women at risk for long-term obesity and development of chronic disease

Postpartum weight retention or weight gain is major problem that has received scant attention. Additional efforts are needed to design and test interventions that are readily scalable, able to be implemented in a variety of institutional settings (e.g., perinatal programs, large clinics, HMOs), and applicable to overweight or obesity postpartum women and easily accessible.

References

1. Setse R, Grogan R, Cooper LA, Strobino D, Powe NR, Nicholson W. Weight loss programs for urban-based, postpartum African-American women: perceived barriers and preferred components. Matern Child Health J. 2008;12(1):119–27.
2. Flegal KM, Carroll MD, Kit BK, Ogden CL. Prevalence of obesity and trends in the distribution of body mass index among US adults, 1999–2010. JAMA. 2012;307(5):491–7.
3. Gunderson EP, Abrams B, Selvin S. The relative importance of gestational gain and maternal characteristics associated with the risk of becoming overweight after pregnancy. Int J Obes Relat Metab Disord. 2000;24(12):1660–8.
4. Gore SA, Brown DM, West DS. The role of postpartum weight retention in obesity among women: a review of the evidence. Ann Behav Med. 2003;26(2):149–59.

5. Ratner RE, Christophi CA, Metzger BE, Dabelea D, Bennett PH, Pi-Sunyer X, Fowler S, Kahn SE. Prevention of diabetes in women with a history of gestational diabetes: effects of metformin and lifestyle interventions. J Clin Endocrinol Metab. 2008;93(12):4774–9.
6. Appel LJ, Champagne CM, Harsha DW, Cooper LS, Obarzanek E, Elmer PJ, Stevens VJ, Vollmer WM, Lin PH, Svetkey LP, Stedman SW, Young DR. Effect of comprehensive lifestyle modification on blood pressure control: main results of the PREMIER clinical trial. JAMA. 2003;289:2083–93.
7. Howell EA. Lack of patient preparation for the postpartum period and patients' satisfaction with their obstetric clinicians. Obstet Gynecol. 2010;115(2 Pt 1):284–9.
8. Martin A, Horowitz C, Balbierz A, Howell EA. Views of women and clinicians on postpartum preparation and recovery. Matern Child Health J. 2013. [Epub ahead of print].
9. Ostbye T, Krause KM, Brouwer RJ, Lovelady CA, Morey MC, Bastian LA, Peterson BL, Swamy GK, Chowdhary J, McBride CM. Active Mothers Postpartum (AMP): rationale, design, and baseline characteristics. J Womens Health (Larchmt). 2008;17(10):1567–75.
10. Information for health professionals on preconception and interconception care, Center for Disease Control and Prevention. http://www.cdc.gov/preconception/hcp/recommendations.html. Accessed on 24 Sep 2013.
11. Rooney BL, Schauberger CW, Mathiason MA. Impact of perinatal weight change on long-term obesity and obesity-related illnesses. Obstet Gynecol. 2005;106(6):1349–56.
12. Kral JG. Preventing and treating obesity in girls and young women to curb the epidemic. Obes Res. 2004;12(10):1539–46.
13. Gunderson EP, Murtaugh MA, Lewis CE, Quesenberry CP, West DS, Sidney S. Excess gains in weight and waist circumference associated with childbearing: the Coronary Artery Risk Development in Young Adults Study (CARDIA). Int J Obes Relat Metab Disord. 2004;28(4):525–35.
14. Smith DE, Lewis CE, Caveny JL, Perkins LL, Burke GL, Bild DE. Longitudinal changes in adiposity associated with pregnancy. The CARDIA Study. Coronary Artery Risk Development in Young Adults Study. JAMA. 1994;271(22):1747–51.
15. McBride CM, Emmons KM, Lipkus IM. Understanding the potential of teachable moments: the case of smoking cessation. Health Educ Res. 2003;18(2):156–70.
16. Weir S, Posner HE, Zhang J, Willis G, Baxter JD, Clark RE. Predictors of prenatal and postpartum care adequacy in a medicaid managed care population. Womens Health Issues. 2011;21(4):277–85.
17. Practice ACO. ACOG Committee opinion. Number 267, January 2002: exercise during pregnancy and the postpartum period. Obstet Gynecol. 2002;99(1):171–3.
18. ACOG Resource Guide-Nutrition and Physical Activity to Address Overweight and Obesity. http://www.acog.org/About_ACOG/

ACOG_Departments/Health_Care_for_Underserved_Women/Resource_Guide_-_Nutrition_and_Physical_Activity. Accessed on 24 Sep 2013.
19. Davies GA, Wolfe LA, Mottola MF, MacKinnon C. Joint SOGC/CSEP clinical practice guideline: exercise in pregnancy and the postpartum period. Can J Appl Physiol. 2003;28:330–41.
20. Excellence National Institute for Health and Clinical. Weight management before, during and after pregnancy. London: National Institute for Health and Clinical Excellence; 2010.
21. Nelson TL, Hunt KJ, Rosamond WD, Ammerman AS, Keyserling TC, Mokdad AH, Will JC. Obesity and associated coronary heart disease risk factors in a population of low-income African-American and white women: the North Carolina WISEWOMAN project. Prev Med. 2002;35(1):1–6.
22. Ratner RE, Christophi CA, Metzger BE, Dabelea D, Bennett PH, Pi-Sunyer X, Fowler S, Kahn SE, Diabetes Prevention Program Research G. Prevention of diabetes in women with a history of gestational diabetes: effects of metformin and lifestyle interventions. J Clin Endocrinol Metab. 2008;93(12):4774–9.
23. Zourladani A, Tsaloglidou A, Tzetzis G, Tsorbatzoudis C, Matziari C. The effect of a low impact exercise training programme on the well-being of Greek postpartum women: a randomised controlled trial. Int SportMed J. 2001;12(1):30–8. %O The effect of a low impact exercise training programme on the well-being of Greek postpartum women: A randomised controlled trial %O 1528–3356 %O 2011243572. Language: English. Entry Date: 2020110923. Revision Date: 2020111007. Publication Type: journal article.
24. Atkins D, Best D, Briss PA, Eccles M, Falck-Ytter Y, Flottorp S, Guyatt GH, Harbour RT, Haugh MC, Henry D, Hill S, Jaeschke R, Leng G, Liberati A, Magrini N, Mason J, Middleton P, Mrukowicz J, O'Connell D, Oxman AD, Phillips B, Schünemann HJ, Edejer T, Varonen H, Vist GE, Williams Jr JW, Zaza S. Grading quality of evidence and strength of recommendations. BMJ. 2004;328(7454):1490.
25. Krummel D, Semmens E, MacBride AM, Fisher B. Lessons learned from the mothers' overweight management study in 4 West Virginia WIC offices. Women, Infants, and Children. Journal of Nutrition Education & Behavior. 2010;42(3S):S52–58.
26. Dewey KG, Cohen RJ, Brown KH, Rivera LL. Effects of exclusive breastfeeding for four versus six months on maternal nutritional status and infant motor development: results of two randomized trials in Honduras. J Nutr. 2001;131(2):262–7.
27. Dewey KG, Lovelady CA, Nommsen-Rivers LA, McCory MA, Lonnerdal B. A randomized study of the effects of aerobic exercise by lactating women on breast-milk volume and composition. N Engl J Med. 1994;330:449–53.
28. Maturi SM, Afshary P, Abedi P. Effect of physical activity intervention based on a pedometer on physical activity level and

anthropometric measures after childbirth: a randomized controlled trial. BMC Pregnancy Childbirth. 2011;11(10):103.
29. Ostbye T, Krause KM, Lovelady CA, Morey MC, Bastian LA, Peterson BL, Swamy GK, Brouwer RJN, McBride CM. Active Mothers Postpartum. A randomized controlled weight-loss intervention trial. Am J Prev Med. 2009;37(3):173.
30. Lovelady CA, Garner K, Moreno KL, Williams JP. The effect of weight loss in overweight, lactating women on the growth of their infants. N Engl J Med. 2000;342:449–5.
31. Huang TT, Yeh C, Tsai YC. A diet and physical activity intervention for preventing weight retention among Taiwanese childbearing women: a randomized controlled trial. Midwifery. 2011;27(2):257–64.
32. Craigie AM, Macleod M, Barton KL, Treweek S, Anderson AS. Supporting postpartum weight loss in women living in deprived communities: design implications for a randomized control trial. Eur J Clin Nutr. 2011;65:952–8.
33. O'Toole ML, Sawicki MA, Artal R. Structured diet and physical activity prevent postpartum weight retention. J Womens Health (Larchmt). 2003;12(10):991–8.
34. Leermakers EA, Anglin K, Wing RR. Reducing postpartum weight retention through a correspondence intervention. Int J Obes Relat Metab Disord. 1998;22:1103–9.
35. Davenport MH, Giroux I, Sopper MM, Mottola MF. Postpartum exercise regardless of intensity improves chronic disease risk factors. Med Sci Sports Exerc. 2011;43(6):951–8.
36. Lovelady CA, Nommsen-Rivers LA, McCrory MA, Dewey KG. Effects of exercise on plasma lipids and metabolism of lactating women. Med Sci Sports Exerc. 1995;27(1):22–8.
37. https://portal.bsc.gwu.edu/web/lifemoms.
38. Stuckey HL, Dellasega C, Graber NJ, Mauger DT, Lendel I, Gabbay RA. Diabetes nurse case management and motivational interviewing for change (DYNAMIC): study design and baseline characteristics in the Chronic Care Model for type 2 diabetes. Contemp Clin Trials. 2009;30(4):366–74.
39. Barr VJ, Robinson S, Marin-Link B, Underhill L, Dotts A, Ravensdale D, Salivaras S. The expanded Chronic Care Model: an integration of concepts and strategies from population health promotion and the Chronic Care Model. Hosp Q. 2003;7(1):73–82.

Chapter 9
Obesity and Physical Activity During Pregnancy and Postpartum: Evidence, Guidelines, and Recommendations

Danielle Symons Downs, Kelly R. Evenson, and Lisa Chasan-Taber

> *Those who think they have not time for bodily exercise will sooner or later have to find time for illness.*
> *Edward Stanley, Earl of Derby, 1873*

Abstract This chapter provides clinicians and researchers with an overview of the physical activity and pregnancy/postpartum literature to promote physical activity, understand the

---

D. Symons Downs, PhD (✉)
Departments of Kinesiology and OB/GYN, College of Health and Human Development, The Pennsylvania State University, University Park, PA, USA
e-mail: dsd11@psu.edu

K.R. Evenson, PhD, MS
Department of Epidemiology, Gillings School of Global Public Health, University of North Carolina at Chapel Hill, Chapel Hill, NC, USA

L. Chasan-Taber, ScD
Department of Public Health, School of Public Health and Health Sciences, University of Massachusetts, Amherst, MA, USA

W. Nicholson, K. Baptiste-Roberts (eds.),
Obesity During Pregnancy in Clinical Practice,
DOI 10.1007/978-1-4471-2831-1_9,
© Springer-Verlag London 2014

determinants and outcomes of physical activity participation among pregnant and postpartum women, recognize the scant literature pertaining to overweight and obese women, and inform next steps in practice, prevention, and research. We discuss (a) physical activity guidelines; (b) prevalence rates of physical activity during pregnancy and postpartum; (c) determinants, health outcomes, and critical gaps in the literature of pre- and postnatal physical activity; and (d) recommendations for research and practice to facilitate physical activity initiation, motivation, and maintenance across the transition to motherhood.

Keywords Exercise • Recommendations • Pre- and postnatal periods • Health

> **Key Points**
> - Most pregnant and postpartum women fail to meet national guidelines for physical activity which may elevate their risk for morbidity and contribute to the intergenerational impact of obesity on their offspring.
> - Several key determinants of physical activity behavior in pregnancy and postpartum have been identified (e.g., education, income, social/emotional support, attitude/beliefs, environmental influences); however, these determinants are not well understood among overweight and obese women and therefore warrant future research attention.
> - Prenatal physical activity may reduce negative health outcomes such as gestational diabetes mellitus, preeclampsia, excessive gestational weight gain, and postpartum weight retention; however, currently there is no "gold standard" intervention for effectively promoting pre- and postnatal physical activity to consistently reduce these adverse outcomes across women of diverse socioeconomic and racial backgrounds.
> - Future attention in research and practice is needed to promote and disseminate the physical activity guidelines

> in clinical care, better understand how to motivate overweight/obese pregnant and postpartum women to engage in physical activity, and identify practical, safe, and effective physical activity intervention strategies.

Statement of the Problem

The majority of pregnant and postpartum women do not achieve the minimum physical activity recommendations from either the United States (US) government [1] or the American College of Obstetricians and Gynecologists (ACOG, later "College" became "Congress"); [2] this is of concern, given that physical activity during pregnancy is associated with improved weight control and maintenance of fitness as well as possible reduced risk of gestational diabetes and improved psychological functioning [2–4]. Women who are active in postpartum tend to have less anxiety, depression, lactation-induced bone loss, and urinary stress incontinence, as well as improved cardiovascular fitness and psychological well-being [1, 4–6].

Physical Activity Guidelines

In 1949, the US Children's Bureau issued a standard recommendation for prenatal Physical activity (PA): In the absence of maternal complications, pregnant women can continue housework, gardening, daily walks (up to 1 mile in several short bouts), and even swimming occasionally but should avoid sports participation [7, 8]. Moderate PA formed the basis of prenatal exercise programs of the 1970s and 1980s, which were highly specific and focused mainly on improving maternal fitness and easing labor and delivery.

ACOG issued their first guidelines for prenatal physical activity in 1985 [9]. These guidelines were based on the consensus opinion of a panel of obstetricians and endorsed the safety of most aerobic physical activity but advised caution with high-impact activities, such as running. The guideline included restrictions for exercise duration (not longer than 15 min for strenuous activity), heart rate (not greater than 140 beats/min), and core body temperature (not greater than 100.4 °F/38 °C). These specific parameters for exercise were dropped in later versions of the ACOG guidelines, updated in 1994 [10] and 2002 [2].

The 2002 guidelines recommended at least 30 min of moderate exercise per day on most, if not all, days of the week, provided that there are no medical or obstetric complications. They suggest that participating in a wide range of recreational physical activities is safe and included guidance for absolute and relative contraindications to exercise (Table 9.1) and warning signs to terminate exercise (Table 9.2).

In 2008, the US government [1] released the *"Physical Activity Guidelines for Americans"* which included a section focused on pregnant women. They recommended at least 150 min of moderate-intensity aerobic physical activity per week for pregnant women who were not already highly active or doing vigorous-intensity physical activity and without obstetric/medical complications. This report also put forward, for the first time, guidelines for vigorous-intensity aerobic physical activity, stating that "pregnant women who habitually engage in vigorous-intensity aerobic activity or are highly active can continue physical activity during pregnancy and the postpartum period, provided they remain healthy and discuss with their healthcare provider how and when activity should be adjusted over time" ([1], p. 42). They provided strong scientific evidence for the safety of moderate-intensity physical activity, stating that it does not elevate the risk for low birth weight, preterm delivery, or early pregnancy loss. Moreover, it highlighted the growing but yet inconclusive evidence that physical activity can reduce the risk of pregnancy complications (e.g., preeclampsia, gestational diabetes mellitus) and the length of labor. Both the ACOG and United Status Department of Health and Human Services (USDHHS) guidelines specified specific activities pregnant women should avoid, such as

TABLE 9.1 Absolute and relative contraindications to aerobic exercise from the ACOG (2002) guidelines

Absolute contraindications	Relative contraindications
Hemodynamically significant heart disease	Chronic bronchitis
Incompetent cervix/cerclage	Poorly controlled type 1 diabetes mellitus
Multiple gestation at risk for premature labor	Extreme morbid obesity
Persistent second- or third-trimester bleeding	Extreme underweight
Placenta previa after 26 weeks' gestation	Heavy smoker
Preeclampsia/pregnancy-induced hypertension	History of extremely sedentary lifestyle
Premature labor during the current pregnancy	Orthopedic limitations
Restrictive lung disease	Poorly controlled hypertension
Ruptured membranes	Poorly controlled seizure disorder
	Poorly controlled hyperthyroidism
	Severe anemia
	Unevaluated maternal cardiac arrhythmia
	Intrauterine growth restriction in current pregnancy

See page 172 of the ACOG (2002) guidelines [2]

the supine position during exercise during the second and third trimester. These recommendations are summarized in Table 9.3.

Recent calls have been made for ACOG to update their 2002 prenatal physical activity guidelines in light of the growing body of research on maternal prenatal physical activity over the past decade [11]. Revisions are needed that could provide greater specificity by defining moderate-intensity physical

TABLE 9.2 Warning signs to terminate exercise from the ACOG (2002) guidelines

Warning sign
Vaginal bleeding
Dyspnea prior to exertion
Dizziness
Headache
Chest pain
Muscle weakness
Calf pain or swelling (need to rule out thrombophlebitis)
Preterm labor
Decreased fetal movement
Amniotic fluid leakage

See page 172 of the ACOG (2002) guidelines [2]

TABLE 9.3 Specific physical activities or positions to avoid during pregnancy

Activities or positions to avoid during pregnancy
Supine position (on back face up) during exercise after the first trimester
Motionless standing
Contact sports (i.e., soccer, basketball)
Activities with a high fall risk (i.e., skiing, vigorous racquet sports, horseback riding)
Scuba diving
High altitude exercise (>6,000 ft)

Note: Referenced in ACOG [2] and USDHHS [1]

activity, addressing the specific weekly energy expenditure to be attained, as well as clarifying the impact of incorporating vigorous physical activity on maternal and infant health outcomes. Also, in light of the increasing obesity epidemic worldwide, updated physical activity guidelines are also needed to address the special issues surrounding obesity in pregnancy. In particular, recent findings [12] indicate that fetal exposure in utero to maternal obesity, excessive gestational weight gain, and abnormal glucose tolerance critically influence the risk of subsequent overweight/obesity in the offspring. This evidence highlights the need for physical activity guidelines targeted to overweight/obese pregnant women with the goal of reducing the intergenerational impact of obesity [13].

In terms of postpartum physical activity, the consensus across the guidelines is that prepregnancy physical activity routines should be resumed gradually after giving birth, as soon as it is medically and physically safe to do so [1, 2]. In general, women are able to return to their prepregnancy physical activity levels approximately 6-8 weeks after a normal and healthy vaginal delivery and slightly longer after a cesarean delivery (i.e., following medical approval from one's health-care provider). The 2008 US governmental physical activity guidelines for postpartum women are the same as for the general population (e.g., at least 150 min of moderate-intensity aerobic activity spread throughout the week; [1]). There is no evidence to date that physical activity has a negative impact on postpartum women's health or negatively affects breastfeeding behaviors.

Prevalence of PA During Pregnancy and Postpartum

The US prevalence of physical activity during pregnancy comes from surveillance studies that have relied on self-reported physical activity (see Table 9.4). From the National Health and Nutrition Examination Survey [14], pregnant women reported an average of 0.6 h/week of transportation activity, 1.6 h/week of moderate to vigorous household activity, and 1.8 h of moderate to vigorous leisure activity. A subset of the leisure activities was classified as aerobic (mean 1.5 h/week), accounting for 88.5 % of the proportion of hours/week on aerobic exercise compared to all leisure activities. Pregnant women were classified as meeting the recommendations [1] if

Table 9.4 Summary of US surveillance studies of self-reported physical activity during pregnancy

Acronym	NMIHS	BRFSS	NHANES
Study full name	National Maternal and Infant Health Survey	Behavioral Risk Factor Surveillance System	National Health and Nutrition Examination Survey
Reference	Zhang and Savitz [25]	Evenson et al. [29]; Petersen et al. [139]	Evenson and Wen [14]
Years reported	1988	1994, 1996, 1998, 2000	1999–2006
Method of collection	Telephone survey	Telephone survey	In-person interview
Sample size	9,953	1,979 in the year 2000	1,280
Results	Approximately 35 % reported exercising before and during pregnancy; walking was the most popular exercise, followed by swimming and aerobic exercise	66 % of pregnant women (in 2000) reported any leisure activity in the past month, with walking as the most common activity, followed by gardening, swimming laps, and aerobics	23 % reported any transportation activity (i.e., to/from work/school), 54 % reported any moderate to vigorous household activity, and 57 % reported any moderate to vigorous leisure activity, all in the past month
Limitations	Did not collect gestational age; long period of recall (on average 17 months after delivery); duration and frequency of exercise not collected	Did not collect gestational age	

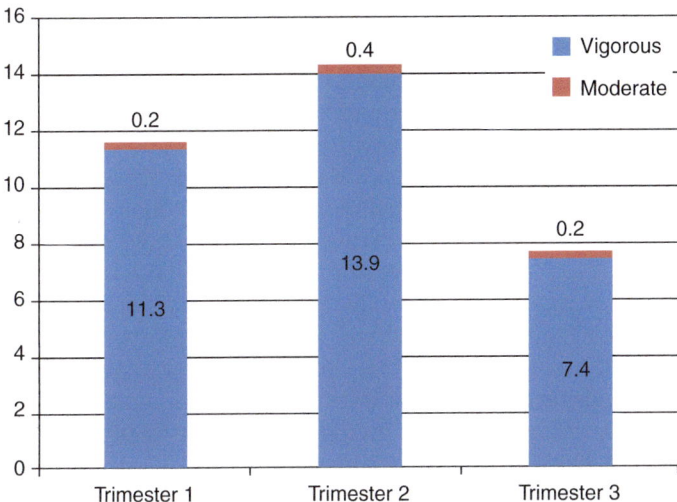

FIGURE 9.1 Weighted mean accelerometer minutes of moderate and vigorous physical activity per day among US pregnant women (From NHANES (2003–2006); Evenson et al. [16]. Open Access Agreement)

they reported at least 150 min/week of moderate-intensity aerobic activity. Overall, 14 % met the recommendation, and when including vigorous activities, almost one-quarter (23 %) met the recommendation for physical activity.

Self-reported physical activity is subject to social desirability bias and misreporting due to the difficulties in recall [15]. In addition, surveillance questions are often limited in number and detail, sometimes missing key components of physical activity behavior. In 2003, accelerometry was added to the NHANES and included a sufficient number of pregnant women who wore the accelerometer to be reported upon [16]. From 2003 to 2006, 359 pregnant women ≥16 years wore an accelerometer for 1 week. Women participated in a mean of 12 min/day of moderate physical activity and 0.3 min/day of vigorous physical activity. Mean moderate to vigorous physical activity varied by trimester: 12 min/day in first trimester, 14 min/day in second trimester, and 8 min/day in third trimester (see Fig. 9.1). On average, women spent 57 % of their monitored time in sedentary behaviors. In multivariable adjusted models, moderate to vigorous physical activity was higher in the first and second trimester compared to the third trimester and among women with higher household income compared to lower household income.

The prevalence of physical activity during postpartum is less well understood, but a number of studies agree that the absolute amounts are below recommendations for most women [17–23]. One observational cohort study found that while pregnant women decreased their physical activity from 17–22 weeks' gestation to 27–30 weeks' gestation, they did increase their physical activity at 3 months postpartum [24]. At 12 months postpartum, physical activity was stable, although the differing modes of activity that made up this activity differed from the prenatal period. For example, while indoor household activities that required at least moderate effort declined during the postpartum period, care-giving activities requiring at least moderate effort increased.

Review of Exercise During Pregnancy and Postpartum: Determinants, Outcomes, and Critical Gaps in the Literature

Determinants of Physical Activity in Pregnancy

Identifying determinants of prenatal physical activity is essential to inform future intervention studies designed to increase prenatal physical activity. However, such studies in overweight/obese women are sparse. This is critical as previous studies have found lower levels of physical activity during pregnancy among women who were overweight [25, 26]. In a recent review, Gaston and Cramp [27] found that the relationship between weight or BMI and prenatal physical activity was conflicting. While some studies observed no association between prepregnancy weight or BMI and physical activity level during pregnancy, others found that women of greater weight or BMI were 1.3–1.79 times more likely to discontinue their involvement in physical activity after becoming pregnant. Similarly, recent findings from the Pregnancy, Infection, and Nutrition 3 Study (PIN3) found that women who were overweight or obese prior to pregnancy were less likely to perform any recreational physical activity in late pregnancy as compared to lean women [28].

In general, two important sociodemographic factors known to be positively associated with participation in prenatal physical activity are greater education and income [27, 29–31], whereas physical activity frequency and duration are well documented to decline with advancing maternal and gestational age [32]. Also, women with higher levels of social support (e.g., perceived sense of accountability, support from friends/family), informational support (e.g., how to safely and effectively engage in prenatal physical activity), and emotional support have higher physical activity levels. At the environmental level, perceived community safety, the use of physical activity as a means of transportation, access to childcare, and access to trails, parks, and built environments that are conducive to physical activity are also commonly cited motivating factors [20, 23]. While studies have found that physical activity levels are higher among nulliparous women than among women with children [30, 31, 33], studies which have included household/childcare in the assessment of physical activity have found that women with children were less likely to become inactive throughout pregnancy [34–37].

Determinants of Physical Activity in Postpartum

Studies evaluating the determinants of postpartum physical activity are sparse. The existing studies suggest that women with greater levels of prenatal physical activity and higher family income are more likely to be active during postpartum [30]. Blum et al. [38] administered the Kaiser Physical Activity Survey (KPAS) to 91 postpartum women in Maine and found that women with older infants reported greater increases in household/childcare physical activity and lower occupational physical activity from prepregnancy to postpartum as compared to women with younger infants. In general, women who maintained or increased activity and/or sports participation from prepregnancy to postpartum had better overall maternal well-being and significantly better perception of partner's/husband's participation in childcare and support for maternal role from family and friends, compared to women reporting no or decreased activity participation. In another study, Hinton and Olsen [39] reported that being married and the husband's physical activity frequency were positively associated with the mother's postpartum physical activity frequency.

Other qualitative and quantitative studies indicate a number of barriers to physical activity during postpartum, including physical discomfort, parenting duties, tiredness, lack of time, not prioritizing their health over other competing responsibilities, lack of spousal/partner support, social isolation, lack of childcare, family responsibilities, higher number of children, financial, neighborhood safety, and weather [17–23, 40–45]. These studies also indicate a number of enablers to physical activity including stress relief and increased energy, weight loss, social support, and returning to work (corresponding with childcare) [17–19, 23, 38, 42, 45–47]. Environmental enablers to physical activity have also been described, such as access to safe places to walk and play [40, 45]. While overweight/obese women may experience many of these same barriers and enablers to pregnancy and postpartum physical activity, research about the unique challenges these women experience with engaging in physical activity before, during, and after pregnancy is sparse.

Outcomes of Physical Activity in Pregnancy: Gestational Diabetes Mellitus, Preeclampsia, and Excessive Gestational Weight Gain in Overweight/Obese Women

Gestational Diabetes Mellitus

Gestational diabetes mellitus (GDM) is one of the most common complications of pregnancy with a prevalence rate varying from 1 to 20 % depending on the population studied and diagnostic criteria applied [48, 49]. Obesity increases the risk of GDM [50, 51]. Indeed, there is evidence that the incidence of GDM may be increasing as the prevalence of obesity among women of reproductive age increases [52–54]. GDM, in turn, increases the risk of subsequent development of diabetes later in life, and this risk is even higher in obese women [55]. Within 15 years of delivery, 70 % of obese women with GDM, compared with 30 % of lean women, will go on to develop type 2 diabetes [56]. GDM is also related to other short- as well as long-term adverse health outcomes for both mothers and their offspring such as maternal hypertensive disorders, cesarean delivery, large-for-gestational-age birth, neonatal hypoglycemia, and neonatal death [57]. In the long term, offspring are at increased risk for obesity, glucose intolerance, and type 2 diabetes [58–60].

Prior observational epidemiologic studies have suggested that prepregnancy physical activity may have a protective role in GDM onset. A meta-analysis found a 55 % lower risk of GDM for women in the highest prepregnancy physical activity quartile compared with those in the lowest quartile (pooled odds ratio [OR]=0.45, 95 % confidence interval [CI] 0.28–0.75; $p=0.002$), as well as a 24 % lower risk of GDM for women in the highest physical activity group during pregnancy compared with those in the lowest physical activity group (pooled OR=0.76, 95 % CI 0.70–0.83; $p<0.0001$) [61].

A recent Cochrane Review comparing the impact of physical activity interventions to usual prenatal care [62] found no significant difference in GDM incidence (three trials, 826 women, risk ratio (RR) 1.10, 95 % confidence interval (CI) 0.66–1.84). In addition, none of the five included trials which evaluated insulin sensitivity found significant differences. Of these studies, two were conducted among obese pregnant women; however, both were small studies and only one evaluated risk of GDM [63, 64]. In the first study, Ong et al. [63] investigated the effect of a supervised 10-week home-based exercise program, beginning at week 18 of gestation, on glucose tolerance and aerobic fitness in 12 previously sedentary obese women. The control arm had reduced glucose tolerance (higher blood glucose levels at 1 and 2 h of the post-intervention oral glucose tolerance test) as compared to the exercise arm, although this was not statistically significant. In the second study, Callaway et al. [64] randomized 50 obese women to an individualized exercise program with an energy expenditure goal of 900 kcal per week ($n=25$) or to routine obstetric care ($n=25$). While insulin resistance did not differ between the groups, 73 % of women in the intervention group achieved more than 900 kcal/week of exercise-based physical activity at 28 weeks compared with 42 % of women in the control arm. The review concluded that there is limited randomized controlled trial evidence available on the effect of physical activity during pregnancy for preventing pregnancy glucose intolerance or GDM. Larger, well-designed randomized trials, with standardized behavioral interventions, are needed to assess the effects of physical activity on preventing GDM. Seven trials are currently ongoing (see Appendix 9.1) [62].

Preeclampsia

Hypertensive disorders of pregnancy affect approximately 8 % of pregnancies [65] and include preeclampsia (defined as gestational hypertension with proteinuria) and gestational hypertension (defined as new onset hypertension in pregnancy after 20 weeks' gestation). Obesity increases the risk of hypertensive disorders of pregnancy [54, 66]. For example, in a large prospective cohort study in Washington State (the Omega Study), Frederick et al. found that every unit increase in prepregnancy BMI resulted in an 8 % increased risk of preeclampsia, with overweight women having almost a twofold increased risk and obese women having over a fourfold increased risk [67]. Consistent with this finding, a significant decrease in risk of hypertensive disorders of pregnancy has been observed when BMI decreases [68]. Hypertensive disorders are the second leading cause of maternal mortality, accounting for 19 % of pregnancy-related deaths for women following a live birth and 20 % of pregnancy-related deaths for women following a still birth [69]. Preeclampsia is associated with an increased risk of preterm delivery, neonatal intensive care unit admission, and fetal death [70].

A recent systematic review [71] found a trend toward a protective effect of PA in the prevention of preeclampsia. Specifically, while six case–control studies found that physical activity had a protective effect on the development of preeclampsia (OR = 0.77, 95 % CI 0.64–0.91), the ten prospective cohort studies found no significant difference (OR = 0.99, 95 % CI 0.93–1.05). The only randomized clinical trial found that the incidence of preeclampsia was 14.6 % (95 % CI, 5.6–29.2) among the walking group and 2.6 % (95 % CI 0.07–13.8) among the stretching group [72].

Because overweight is an established risk factor for preeclampsia, several of these studies evaluated whether physical activity might be particularly beneficial for reduction of preeclampsia risk in this group. In a cohort of 2,793 women in Denmark, Hegaard et al. found that protective effect of recreational physical activity on preeclampsia risk was strongest in overweight women (OR = 0.10, 95 % CI 0.02–1.2), although not significantly so [73]. In contrast, in the Norwegian Mother and Child Cohort Study, Magnus et al. found that the protective effect of exercise was absent among obese women (OR = 1.39, 95 % CI 0.83–2.32), although there was the suggestion of a reduction in risk among overweight women (OR = 0.68, 95 % CI 0.44–1.04) [74, 75]. Rudra et al. found the significant trend of decreased preeclampsia risk with increased perceived exertion was apparent in both overweight and normal weight women [76].

Gestational Weight Gain

High gestational weight gain (GWG) is independently associated with postpartum weight retention and the long-term development of obesity [77]. Indeed, GWG is the strongest predictor for weight retention [78]. Overweight and obese women are at particular risk for excessive GWG [79]. Because overweight is characterized by insulin resistance and increased systemic inflammatory response [80], it is also associated with increased risk of GDM and preeclampsia [81, 82]. Recent studies also indicate a relationship between high GWG, an abnormal metabolic environment in utero, and increased risk of large-for-gestational-age infants, neonatal death [57], and subsequent childhood adiposity and morbidity [60]. There is observational evidence that physical activity may be a modifiable risk factor for excessive GWG [77]. In observational studies, vigorous physical activity, total physical activity, and walking have been associated with a lower risk of excessive GWG [83–85]. A recent systematic review of randomized controlled trials comparing supervised prenatal exercise intervention with routine standard prenatal care in women who were overweight/obese during pregnancy found that supervised exercise interventions were associated with lower GWG (five trials, $n=216$ participants, mean difference of –0.36 kg, 95 % confidence interval –0.64 to –0.09 kg) [86].

Furthermore, a systematic review of lifestyle interventions in overweight/obese pregnant women to improve maternal and perinatal outcomes [51] found that prenatal lifestyle interventions in obese pregnant women reduce maternal pregnancy weight gain (10 RCTs; $n=1,228$; –2.21 kg (95 % confidence interval –2.86 kg to –1.59 kg)) although findings were not significant for non-RCTs (six; $n=1,534$). Both the successful and non-successful studies included those which were personalized, individual-based, and combined physical activity with dietary guidance. Degrees of weight gain restriction achieved were modest overall, and all the trials were assessed to be of low to medium quality [51]. Future studies are therefore needed to determine the optimal intensity, duration, and type of exercise intervention to reduce excessive GWG among pregnant women overall as well as specifically among overweight/obese pregnant women.

Outcomes of Physical Activity During Postpartum

Overweight/obese women tend to retain more weight postpartum because the majority of this group gains more weight during pregnancy than is recommended, and therefore, there is more weight to lose in postpartum [55, 78]. Weight loss can be achieved in the immediate postpartum period [87], with studies finding that both caloric restriction as well as physical activity

Chapter 9. Obesity, Physical Activity, Pregnancy/Postpartum

are needed to reduce weight [88, 89] as compared to physical activity interventions alone [90]. However, few intervention studies have been specifically designed to reduce postpartum weight retention in overweight or obese women [88–90].

Lovelady et al. conducted a 10-week supervised exercise and dietary program in overweight, exclusively breastfeeding women. Women in the intervention group lost more weight (4.8 ± 1.7 kg vs. 0.8 ± 2.3 kg, $p < 0.001$) and increased aerobic fitness as compared with the control groups [88]. A second study which randomized overweight women to an exercise program and a structured diet found that the intervention arm successfully lost weight and most maintained weight loss by 1 year after delivery [89]. However, support from professionals and family is crucial for women to engage in physical activity during the postpartum period [38].

Weight loss interventions which begin during pregnancy [90,91] may be more effective than those initiated only in the postpartum period [89,92,93] given the strong association between GWG and postpartum weight retention and the fact that it may be difficult to reduce postpartum weight retention without first preventing excessive GWG during pregnancy [94].

It remains unclear whether clinically relevant postpartum weight loss can be achieved in obese and overweight postpartum women and what form of physical activity intervention would be optimal. The Active Mothers Postpartum (AMP) trial enrolled a total of 450 overweight or obese women at 6 weeks postpartum [93]. Women randomized to the intervention were offered eight healthy-eating classes, ten physical activity classes, and six telephone-counseling sessions over 9 months. There were no significant group differences in mean weight loss, improvement of diet, or increased physical activity. Findings suggest that home-based interventions via mail, telephone, or the Internet/e-mail may be more feasible and successful in this population.

In addition, O'Toole examined the impact of an individualized, structured diet and physical activity intervention on weight loss in 40 overweight women during the first year postpartum [89]. Women were randomized to either a structured intervention which involved individualized diet and physical activity prescriptions or to a self-directed program. At 1 year postpartum, women in the intervention arm had a significant weight loss (7.3 kg, $p<0.01$), a significant decrease in percent body fat (6 %, $p<0.01$), but no change in fat-free mass, while women in the self-directed program had no significant change in these factors. Also recently, Bertz et al. evaluated whether a combined 12-week dietary and physical activity behavior modification intervention compared with stand-alone dietary and physical activity interventions or to usual care led to reduced body weight in 68 lactating Swedish women with a prepregnancy BMI of 25–35 kg/m^2 [95]. The dietary intervention resulted in clinically relevant weight loss, which was sustained 9 months after treatment. However, the combined physical activity and diet treatment did not yield significant weight or body-composition changes beyond those of dietary treatment alone.

Critical Gaps in the Literature

Despite the increasing body of literature aiming to better understand PA prevalence as well as determinants and outcomes of physical activity in pregnancy and postpartum, there are nevertheless critical gaps in the literature. The following section will discuss the following particular gaps: limitations in measuring physical activity during pregnancy, a general lack of understanding about overweight/obese women's beliefs about being active and strategies for overcoming barriers, and a lack of a "best practice" or a "gold standard" intervention to promote physical activity among overweight/obese pregnant and postpartum women.

Measurement of Physical Activity During Pregnancy

To date, assessment of physical activity during pregnancy and postpartum is predominately conducted via self-report, such as with questionnaires or diaries, rather than with objective measurements, such as accelerometers or pedometers [96]. Several advantages of self-report measures include the lower burden it places on the participant and the reduction in equipment cost as compared to objective assessment of physical activity. Questionnaires can be designed to collect mode of physical activity and perception of intensity. A major disadvantage to both questionnaires and diaries is the potential for recall bias. Moreover, keeping a diary may change the woman's physical activity behavior, and consistent with this concern, diaries have been used as motivational tools in prior intervention studies. Questions to consider when selecting a self-reported instrument can be found in Table 9.5.

Objective measurement of physical activity is becoming more common among studies of pregnant and postpartum women. Several advantages to objective measures of pregnancy physical activity include the elimination or reduction of literacy, recall bias, and cultural differences. These objective measures (e.g., activity monitors) can also provide a more precise estimation of total physical activity. Disadvantages include cost and dependency on the participant to wear the monitor. The monitors are often worn for up to 1 week and thus do not reflect longer-term patterns of physical activity. They may be inadvertently worn incorrectly if placed at the hip, due to changes in the pregnant woman's girth [97]. Several studies have noted that compliance to wearing accelerometers declines during pregnancy [98, 99]. This is most likely to occur when participants are instructed to remove the monitor while sleeping, and periods of sleep increase in later pregnancy. Another reason for decline in compliance may be the increasing discomfort associated with wearing the monitor later in pregnancy. To date, the majority of pedometers that have been used in pregnancy only assess locomotion-type activities well (i.e., running, walking) and have not differentiated intensity level. With newer devices, these limitations will likely be overcome.

Overweight/Obese Women's Beliefs About Physical Activity During Pregnancy and Postpartum

To date, there has been a critical lack of understanding about overweight/obese women's beliefs about being active and strategies for overcoming barriers. Several studies not focused

TABLE 9.5 Questions to consider when choosing a physical activity questionnaire or diary assessment for pregnant women

Question	Common options
How will the assessment be delivered?	Paper, electronic, phone, text messaging, e-mail, interactive website
What is the appropriate length of the recall period?	Today, yesterday, past week, past month, since becoming pregnant
Are the major components of physical activity assessed?	The major components of physical activity include mode (type of physical activity), frequency, duration, and intensity
Is it important to know where or with whom the activity occurred?	Consideration could be given to whether the physical and social context is important to collect, assessed by asking where and with whom the physical activity was performed
Can the method assess recommendations for physical activity?	For the US, this would be based on ACOG [2] and US government [1]
Does the assessment evaluate sedentary behavior?	Sedentary behavior is characterized predominately by sitting and associated with low levels of energy expenditure
Was assessment of validity and reliability conducted in a population that is similar to my population?	Assessments may require cultural adaptation
Should objective assessments of physical activity be considered?	Accelerometers, pedometers

Note: Adapted from Evenson and Wen [96]

among overweight/obese women have documented pregnant women's PA beliefs during pregnancy, including that PA contributes to overall well-being [100–102], relieves stress [103], reduces anxiety and depressive symptoms [104], helps to control gestational weight gain [101, 104], and manages gestational diabetes [45]. In postpartum, salient physical activity beliefs are that physical activity assists with postpartum weight loss [101, 105], improves mood, and reduces stress [40]. Common barriers to physical activity in pregnancy are increased size, fatigue, and fear of harming the baby [101] and in postpartum are lack of time, companionship support for physical activity, childcare responsibilities, and health issues (e.g., recovering from labor/delivery) [19, 23, 40, 101, 102].

While overweight/obese women may experience many of these same physical activity beliefs and barriers, there is nevertheless little understanding about the unique challenges these women experience with engaging in physical activity before, during, and after pregnancy. One US study by Chang and colleagues [17] found that obese postpartum mothers' *personal experience of physical discomfort* (e.g., inability to climb stairs, knee and back pain) and their *body size* made engaging in physical activity difficult. Another study conducted in the United Kingdom by Weir and colleagues [106] also identified *feeling uncomfortable engaging in physical activity due to size* (e.g., harder to move when heavier) as well as the *perception that physical activity was less important than eating healthy for the baby* as salient barriers to prenatal physical activity. Of particular concern, the women in this study were generally unconcerned about weight gain in pregnancy despite the adverse effects of high gestational weight gain on maternal and infant health outcomes. Future research is needed to better understand the physical activity beliefs and barriers of overweight/obese women and the extent to which these psychological factors influence their physical activity attitudes and behaviors and perspectives on gestational weight gain. It is possible that for overweight/obese women, the perceived barriers of physical activity greatly overshadow the benefits, and therefore, there is an important need to identify intervention strategies that effectively reduce barriers and improve their physical activity motivation and behavior.

Lack of "Best Practice" Interventions to Promote Physical Activity During Pregnancy and Postpartum

Although the prenatal physical activity guidelines have been revised on several occasions since the 1985 ACOG recommendations and these adaptations have led to greater support for and promotion of physical activity, there is still a considerable gap in the literature. Specifically, there is an absence of a "gold standard" intervention to promote pre- and postnatal physical activity. A recent systematic review [107] examined interventions to promote physical activity during pregnancy in an effort to identify best practices. Ten intervention studies met the inclusion criteria (i.e., randomized controlled trials measuring efficacy of intervention aiming to change physical activity in pregnant women) of which only two focused on physical activity as the primary target (other targets were gestational weight gain, gestational diabetes, and preeclampsia) and only three reported statistically significant differences between the physical activity intervention and control groups (see Table 9.6). The interventions included a variety of behavioral strategies aiming to promote PA (see Table 9.6); however, none were uniquely associated with positive outcomes. The authors concluded that little is known about the efficacy of interventions for physical activity during pregnancy and offered several suggestions for future research such as designing theoretically based studies to better understand factors influencing physical activity participation, expanding interventions beyond pregnant women to include other important social influences (e.g., family members, social networks, medical providers), and increasing generalizability of evidence to special populations such as ethnic minority groups and overweight and obese pregnant women.

There is also a lack of interventions that have effectively promoted postpartum physical activity. While physical activity in postpartum offers a number of benefits, the primary focus for women in early postpartum is recovering from delivery and taking care of the infant. Physical activity is not generally recommended before 6–8 weeks postpartum (depending on vaginal or cesarean delivery), and from that point on, women are largely left to their own to return to their prepregnancy physical activity

TABLE 9.6 Interventions to promote physical activity

Reference	Sample	Strategies	Summary findings
Ferrara et al. [54]	N = 163 pregnant women with gestational diabetes	*Intervention*: in-person and telephone counseling, self-monitoring diaries *Control*: print materials about gestational diabetes and infant safety	No significant differences between intervention and control groups
Gaston and Prapavessis [138]	N = 70 pregnant women	*Intervention*: educational brochure on exercise during pregnancy *Attention control*: brochure about diet *Usual care control*: no intervention	*Significant increase in PA for intervention group compared to both control groups*
Guelinckx et al. [55]	N = 122 obese pregnant women	*Active intervention*: brochure on nutrition and PA to limit gestational weight gain and group counseling with behavioral modification *Passive intervention*: brochure only *Usual care control*: no intervention	No significant differences between intervention and comparison groups

(continued)

TABLE 9.6 (continued)

Reference	Sample	Strategies	Summary findings
Huang et al. [132]	N=189 pregnant women from Taiwan	*Intervention*: PA counseling, brochure, individualized PA plan, self-monitoring PA records, problem solving, goal setting *Usual care control*: leaflet about PA	*Significant increase in PA for intervention group compared to controls*
Jackson et al. [115]	N=287 pregnant women	*Intervention*: Video Doctor counseling session, in-depth behavioral risk assessment, tailored counseling messages, printed output *Usual care control*: no intervention	Significant increase in PA for intervention group but no significant group differences
Kropp et al. [133]	N=152 pregnant women	*Intervention*: motivational enhancement therapy for pregnant substance abuse users including discussion on substance abuse, personalized feedback about PA *Usual care control*: counseling sessions but no personalized messaging	No significant differences between intervention and control groups
Hui et al.[a] [134]	N=190 pregnant women	*Intervention*: community-based group exercise sessions, instructed home exercise/dietary counseling *Usual care control*: no intervention	*Significant increase in PA for intervention group compared to controls*

Luoto et al. [135, 136]	$N=399$ pregnant women at risk for gestational diabetes	*Intervention*: PA counseling with tailored weekly action plans and review of PA logs, booklet on PA, and optional group meetings/exercise *Usual care control*: no intervention	No significant differences between intervention and control groups
Yeo et al. [72, 137]	$N=79$ sedentary pregnant women	*Walking intervention*: 40-min moderate-intensity walking on 5 days a week with training and supervision *Comparison group*: *stretching intervention*: video-guided stretching on 5 days a week with training and supervision	No significant differences between intervention and comparison groups

Note: Usual care control = received standard of prenatal care; Table adapted from Pearce et al. [107]; [a]Hui et al. [134]; Pearce et al. [107]

routine or initiate physical activity altogether. Furthermore, physical activity guidelines do not exist for postpartum which adds to the complexity of defining how to promote physical activity during this time. Mottola [13] suggested that for postpartum physical activity programs to succeed, they must consider the impact of factors such as time management, social support, cultural sensitivity, breastfeeding, childcare, and promoting physical activities that include mother-child interactions (e.g., stroller walking, interactive classes). In addition, postpartum women should get the approval of their health-care provider before starting a physical activity program, and they should start slowly and gradually increase frequency and intensity over time.

Next Steps in Practice, Prevention, and Research

Despite the increase in empirical evidence over the past several decades aiming to promote physical activity during and after pregnancy, women remain generally inactive during this important time in the life cycle, and this low activity is a precursor to later morbidity such as obesity, diabetes, and cardiovascular diseases. While there is no question that physical activity promotion remains an important and necessary focus of research and intervention efforts, it is of even greater importance to identify *how* to effectively motivate women, particularly overweight and obese women, to engage in physical activity during and after pregnancy. Below, we offer some suggestions for the next steps in research and practice to facilitate pre- and postnatal physical activity initiation, motivation, and maintenance.

Emphasis on Physical Activity Recommendations in Clinical Care

Most health-care providers are not specifically trained to counsel pregnant women about physical activity, and guidance on engaging in prenatal physical activity is not a part of the standard of care. For example, [108] found that 75 % of physicians in the 1990s were not aware of physical activity guidelines for pregnancy/postpartum. Unfortunately, almost two decades later, the general consensus is that counseling pregnant women about physical activity is not the "norm" in clinical care. For example, two recent studies [109, 110] found the two main barriers of prenatal care providers for physical activity counseling were a lack of knowledge/formal training and uncertainty or doubt about one's ability to provide effective physical activity counseling. Although the current physical activity guidelines recommend that healthy pregnant women without obstetric complications can engage in 150 min/week of moderate-intensity physical activity (and with a doctor's consent, continue some forms of vigorous physical activity), Evenson and Pompeii [109] found that 74 % of physicians recommended moderate-intensity physical activity and even less (6 %) recommended vigorous-intensity physical activity to their prenatal patients.

Another study [110] examined health-care provider advice to overweight/obese pregnant women and found that 58 % of women received little to no advice on appropriate physical activity during pregnancy. Also, of the 42 % of women who did discuss physical activity with their providers, the focus of the counseling was on being cautious about and/or limiting physical activity. Moreover, the majority of women perceived that their provider lacked knowledge of physical activity recommendations for frequency and intensity. These authors suggested that providers' insufficient knowledge of physical activity guidelines is unlikely to shape positive physical activity expectations for overweight/obese women. Thus, more focused efforts are needed to better educate and train health-care providers about physical activity benefits, guidelines, and safety aspects in an effort to promote physical activity within standard prenatal care.

Furthermore, recent evidence [111, 112] suggests that provider knowledge varies across subgroups of pregnant women. For example, Stotland et al. [112] found that despite having the highest rates of high GWG nationally, White women were the least likely to receive counseling about health behaviors (e.g., nutrition, physical activity) in pregnancy. Also, Symons Downs et al. [113] found that provider recommendations varied across parity. More specifically, 32 % of women felt they received insufficient prenatal health information (e.g., GWG, physical activity, healthy eating) and attributed this lack of information to physicians' assumptions that they already had health knowledge from prior pregnancies.

Thus, as a general recommendation, health-care providers may consider distributing information on the physical activity guidelines to all of their prenatal patients regardless of their prepregnancy weight or activity status. This information can be delivered on multiple occasions at appointments (e.g., handouts, websites) over the course of prenatal care. There is evidence that when primary care providers ask about physical activity, patients show much higher motivation to change their behavior; such change may not be sustained if women are asked only once [114].

Dissemination of Physical Activity Recommendations

In addition to integrating the physical activity guidelines into standard prenatal care, other strategies to disseminate the guidelines include mechanisms such as websites, social media (e.g., Facebook, Twitter), public health messaging (e.g., radio, TV), and mobile phone applications. For example, a recent randomized trial tested the impact of an interactive, computerized Video Doctor counseling tool on health behaviors in pregnancy [115] and found significant increases in self-reported physical activity and diet behaviors from baseline to follow-up. Understanding how to integrate technology into clinical care can help to assist clinicians with effective physical activity and diet counseling. Studies are also needed to examine different dissemination methods to identify which strategies are most effective across subgroups of pregnant and postpartum women (e.g., whether there are differences in effectiveness of mechanisms across women of different weight, parity, and socioeconomic status groups).

Dissemination of Gestational Weight Gain (GWG) Guidelines Identifying Effective Strategies to Promote Physical Activity

While studies have shown that GWG is influenced by healthcare provider recommendations, approximately one-third of women report that they did not receive prenatal counseling on

GWG [116]. Approximately 30–60 % of pregnant women have reported not receiving weight gain advice, and among those patients who received advice, approximately one-third reported receiving advice that was inconsistent with IOM guidelines [117–119]. Barriers to the provision of such advice and related educational materials may include limited time within the constraints of clinical practices, insufficient training, concern about the sensitivity of the topic, the perception that counseling is ineffective, and lack of third-party payer reimbursement [120].

Understanding How to Motivate Overweight/ Obese Pregnant and Postpartum Women to Engage in Physical Activity

Research studies are needed to identify how to help overweight/obese pregnant and postpartum women overcome physical activity barriers and facilitate physical activity motivation. Interventions should be designed that first consider formative research (e.g., focus groups, structured interviews) with overweight/obese women to understand their unique challenges and needs. This research should also be theoretically driven to better understand the complex interactions among the psychological, behavioral, biological, and social/ecological determinants of physical activity during and after pregnancy to inform intervention design and development.

Identifying Effective Strategies to Promote Physical Activity

Research studies are needed to compare the delivery of multiple behavioral strategies to better understand which approaches are most effective at promoting physical activity during and after pregnancy. Understanding which program components and intervention strategies have the strongest impact will inform the development of future interventions in an effort to identify a "gold standard." For example, research is needed that examines model interventions that have been effective in nonpregnant populations (e.g., the Diabetes Prevention Program: http://diabetes.niddk.nih.gov/dm/pubs/

preventionprogram/) to determine which components and strategies may be effectively modified and applied to pregnant/postpartum women. More specifically, the DPP successfully demonstrated that modest weight loss and increased physical activity could reduce the incidence of diabetes in a group of prediabetic (nonpregnant) patients by 58 %. However, both the recruitment methodology and the intervention were too expensive to implement in real-world settings, leading to requests for proposals requiring less expensive methods to be developed and tested [121]. In addition, the DPP recruited an educated and English-literate population. Translating the DPP as well as other effective intervention studies conducted in nonpregnant populations to be used during pregnancy and postpartum could be promising. Such interventions should be tailored to ethnically/racially and socioeconomically diverse population, and they would also need to consider that the time and childcare pressures faced by pregnant and especially postpartum women are barriers to attendance at group meetings at scheduled times and that travel to and from venues would deter many [122, 123]. In fact, studies in nonpregnant populations [47, 124, 125] have found that *individually tailored* lifestyle interventions delivered in person, via telephone, and via mail produce greater or comparable changes in behavior at a more cost-efficient level compared with group-based interventions.

Example: Best Practice, Prevention Approach, or Research Design

As noted above, there is not a single "gold standard" intervention to promote physical activity during or after pregnancy. However, the following section provides an overview of some recent promising approaches for physical activity promotion among pregnant and postpartum women.

Several ongoing interventions are currently investigating the impact of lifestyle changes including physical activity on GDM risk. In one of the only trials to include a significant proportion of Hispanic women, the Behaviors Affecting Baby and You (B.A.B.Y) Study (clinical trial #NCT00728377) is an ongoing exercise trial among an ethnically diverse sample of prenatal care patients in Western Massachusetts at high risk of gestational diabetes mellitus (60 % Latina; [126]). Women are randomized to a 12-week motivationally targeted, individually tailored physical activity intervention involving multimodal contacts (in person, mail, and telephone) or to a comparison health and wellness intervention. The overall goal of the physical activity intervention is to encourage pregnant women to achieve physical activity guidelines during pregnancy through increasing walking and developing a more active lifestyle. The intervention takes into account the specific social, cultural, economic, and physical environmental challenges faced by pregnant women of diverse socioeconomic and ethnic backgrounds. Preliminary findings among the first 110 randomized prenatal care patients (60 % Hispanic) found that the exercise arm ($n=58$) experienced a smaller decrease (−1.0 MET-h/week) in total activity vs. the control arm ($n=52$) (−10.0 MET-h/week; $p=0.03$) and a higher increase in sports/exercise (0.9 MET-h/week) vs. the control arm (−0.01 MET-h/week; $p=0.02$) [127].

Another ongoing trial, Estudia Vida (clinical trial #NCT01141582), is designed to evaluate the feasibility of implementing a lifestyle intervention among pregnant, overweight, and obese Hispanic women at increased risk for GDM [128]. The lifestyle intervention was a 6-month program consisting of 6 monthly in-person educational sessions and 5 biweekly booster telephone calls. Assessments of physical activity, diet, glycemic control, markers of insulin resistance, and blood lipids were conducted at three time points: at baseline, in midpregnancy, and at 6 weeks postpartum. Health outcomes were abstracted from medical records. Among eligible women, 88 (49.4 %) agreed to participate, and a total of 68 women (77.3 %) were successfully randomized into a lifestyle intervention group ($n=33$, 48.5 %) and a standard care group ($n=35$, 51.5 %). Physical activity, diet, and covariate assessment completion rates ranged from 87.9

to 100 % during pregnancy and from 75 to 87.9 % postpartum, with no statistically significant differences between study groups. On average, women in the intervention group attended 4 (1.45 SD) sessions with 93.5 % attending at least three sessions. Clinical outcomes were obtained for 100 % of the participants. This study suggests that a lifestyle intervention delivered primarily via individualized sessions and telephone is feasible for overweight and obese Hispanic women at risk of GDM. However, strategies for helping pregnant Hispanic women to overcome barriers to participation are needed for such studies to be successful.

Another randomized intervention trial, Active MOMS (DK07586702), compared the effects of two theoretically based interventions (semi-intensive, face-to-face, guided exercise, minimal-contact, home-based lifestyle physical activity) to a standard of care control group on the physical activity behaviors and motivational determinants of 105 pregnant women with and without GDM [129, 130]. From baseline (20 weeks' gestation) to follow-up (32 weeks' gestation), women randomized to the semi-intensive physical activity intervention had higher leisure physical activity min/week, accelerometer counts/min, and physical activity attitude, subjective norm, and intention than women in the control group. They also had higher pedometer steps/day, physical activity attitude, and body satisfaction than women in the minimum-contact intervention. More women in the semi-intensive intervention (43 %) met physical activity guidelines than the minimum-contact intervention (23 %) and control (7 %). Also, GDM women had lower physical activity behaviors and motivational determinants than non-GDM women, placing them at even higher risk for low activity and sedentary behaviors both during and after pregnancy.

Specific to overweight/obese women, Mottola et al. [131] examined the effect of a Nutrition and Exercise Lifestyle Intervention Program (NELIP) on weight-related outcomes among 65 overweight/obese pregnant women compared to a matched historical cohort ($n=260$). NELIP included individualized nutrition plans and a walking program using a pedometer to count steps. They found that 80 % of women in NELIP had GWG within the guidelines and postpartum weight retention was minimal (i.e., average 2.2 kg at 8 weeks postpartum) with no significant difference in weight retention between overweight and obese women. Because women in this trial were not randomized to intervention and control groups, future research is needed to test the efficacy of this intervention approach to replicate the study findings and determine the generalizability of this program at a population-based level.

Furthermore, ongoing interventions designed to reduce postpartum weight retention include Estudia Parto. The overall goal of this new randomized controlled trial (clinical trial # NCT01679210) is to test the efficacy of a culturally and linguistically modified, individually tailored lifestyle intervention to reduce risk factors for type 2 diabetes and cardiovascular disease among postpartum Hispanic women with a history of abnormal glucose tolerance during pregnancy. Specific aims are to evaluate the impact of the intervention on postpartum weight loss, biomarkers associated with insulin resistance (i.e., glucose, insulin, HbA_{1c}, leptin, TNF-α, HOMA, AUCgluc, adiponectin), other cardiovascular risk factors (i.e., blood lipids, blood pressure, CRP, fetuin-A, albumin-to-creatinine ratio), and the adoption and maintenance of postpartum behaviors associated with weight loss and prevention of diabetes risk (i.e., physical activity, diet). Eligible Hispanic women will be recruited after routine GDM screening and randomly assigned to a lifestyle intervention ($n=150$) or a comparison health and wellness (control) intervention ($n=150$). Targets of the intervention are to achieve IOM guidelines for postpartum weight loss, ACOG (2002) PA guidelines, and the American Diabetes Association guidelines for diet. The intervention draws from social cognitive theory and the transtheoretical model and addresses the specific social, cultural, economic, and physical environmental challenges faced by underserved Hispanic women. Measures of adherence will include accelerometers and dietary recalls.

Conclusion

Despite the fact that the physical activity and pregnancy/postpartum literature has evolved significantly over the past several decades and prenatal physical activity guidelines have become more relaxed to promote the maternal-fetal health benefits of exercise, most pregnant and postpartum women are not sufficiently active. Even more concerning is the low prevalence rate of physical activity among overweight and obese pregnant and postpartum women. In an effort to understand how to better promote physical activity during pregnancy and postpartum, salient determinants of activity have been identified; however, these have not been well understood among obese pregnant women and warrant future attention. Moreover, prenatal physical activity may reduce negative health outcomes such as gestational diabetes mellitus, preeclampsia, excessive gestational weight gain, and postpartum weight retention; however, greater dissemination of the physical activity guidelines in clinical practice is needed to educate and inform women of these benefits for widespread impact. Important areas for future research and practice include understanding how to motivate pregnant and postpartum women (especially obese women) to be active and identifying practical, safe, and effective physical activity intervention strategies (including a gold standard intervention for dissemination) to improve maternal health and reduce the onset of long-term morbidity.

Appendix 9.1: Additional Reading Material

Another seven trials (Chasan-Taber et al. 2009;Ko 2008; Melo 2008; Newnham et al. 2011; Oostdam et al. 2009; Ramirez-Velez et al. 2009; Shen 2008) are ongoing and will be considered for inclusion in the next update of this review (*see* Characteristics of ongoing studies).

Chasan-Taber L, Marcus BH, Stanek 3rd E, Ciccolo JT, Marquez DX, Solomon CG, et al. A randomized controlled trial of prenatal physical activity to prevent gestational diabetes: design and methods. J Womens Health. 2009;18(6):851–9.

Ko CW. Effect of physical activity on metabolic syndrome in pregnancy and fetal outcome. ClinicalTrials.gov (http://clinicaltrials.gov/) (Accessed 9 Apr 2008).

Melo A. Exercise and pregnancy: randomised clinical trial. Current Controlled Trials (www.controlled-trials.com/) (Accessed 17 Mar 2010).

Newnham J. Fournier P. Guelfi K. Grove R. Wallman K. Doherty D. Preventing gestational diabetes mellitus using a home-based supervised exercise program during pregnancy. Exercise for pregnant women for preventing gestational diabetes mellitus (Review) 17. Copyright © 2012 The Cochrane Collaboration. Published by JohnWiley & Sons, Ltd. ClinicalTrials.gov (http://clinicaltrials.gov/), (Accessed 25 July 2011). (NCT01283854).

Oostdam N, Van Poppel MN, Eekhoff EM, Wouters MG, Van Mechelen W. Design of FitFor2 study: the effects of an exercise program on insulin sensitivity and plasma glucose levels in pregnant women at high risk for gestational diabetes. BMC Pregnancy Childbirth. 2009;9:1.

Ramirez-Velez R, Aguilar AC, Mosquera M, Garcia RG, Reyes LM, Lopez-Jaramillo P. Clinical trial to assess the effect of physical exercise on endothelial function and insulin resistance in pregnant women. Trials. 2009;10:104.

Shen G. Impact of diet and exercise activity on pregnancy outcomes (IDEA). ClinicalTrials.gov (http://clinicaltrials.gov/) (Accessed 20 Feb 2008).

References

1. 2008 Physical Activity Guidelines for Americans. Washington (D.C.): U.S. Department of Health and Human Services; 2008. ODPHP Publication No. U0036
2. ACOG. Exercise during pregnancy and the postpartum period. ACOG Committee Opinion No. 267. Obstet Gynecol. 2002;99(1):171–3.
3. Brown W. The benefits of physical activity during pregnancy. J Sci Med Sport. 2002;5(1):37–45.
4. Pivarnik JM, Chambliss H, Clapp III J, Dugan S, Hatch M, Lovelady C, Mottola MF, Williams M. Impact of physical activity during pregnancy and postpartum on chronic disease risk. Med Sci Sports Exerc. 2006;38(5):989–1006.
5. Larson-Meyer DE. Effect of postpartum exercise on mothers and their offspring: a review of the literature. Obes Res. 2002;10(8):841–53.
6. Sampselle C, Seng J, Yeo S, Killion C, Oakley D. Physical activity and postpartum well-being. J Obstet Gynecol Neonatal Nurs. 1999;28(1): 41–9.
7. Federal Security Agency and Social Security Administration. Prenatal Care. 1949;4:25–26.
8. Sternfeld B. Physical activity and pregnancy outcome: review and recommendations. Sports Med. 1997;23(1):33–47.

9. Exercise during pregnancy and the postnatal period. Washington (D.C.): American College of Obstetricians and Gynecologists; 1985. 1–6 ACOG Home Exercise Programs.
10. ACOG. Exercise during pregnancy and the postpartum period. ACOG Technical Bulletin Number 189. Int J Gynaecol Obstet. 1994;45(1):65–70.
11. Zavorsky GS, Longo LD. Adding strength training, exercise intensity, and caloric expenditure to exercise guidelines in pregnancy. Obstet Gynecol. 2011;117(6):1399–402.
12. Entringer S, Buss C, Swanson JM, Cooper DM, Wing DA, Waffarn F, Wadhwa PD. Fetal programming of body composition, obesity, and metabolic function: the role of intrauterine stress and stress biology. J Nutr Metab. 2012;2012:632548. doi:10.1155/2012/632548
13. Mottola MF. Exercise prescription for overweight and obese women: pregnancy and postpartum. Obstet Gynecol Clin North Am. 2009;36(2):301–16.
14. Evenson K, Wen F. National trends in self-reported physical activity and sedentary behaviors among pregnant women: NHANES 1999–2006. Prev Med. 2010;50:123–8.
15. Welk G, editor. Physical activity assessments for health-related research. Champaign: Human Kinetics; 2002.
16. Evenson K, Wen F. National prevalence and correlates of objectively measured physical activity and sedentary behaviors among pregnant women. Prev Med. 2011;53:39–43.
17. Chang MW, Nitzke S, Guilford E, Adair CH, Hazard DL. Motivators and barriers to healthful eating and physical activity among low-income overweight and obese mothers. J Am Diet Assoc. 2008;108(6):1023–8.
18. Albright C, Maddock JE, Nigg CR. Physical activity before pregnancy and following childbirth in a multiethnic sample of healthy women in Hawaii. Women Health. 2005;42(3):95–110.
19. Groth SW, David T. New mothers' views of weight and exercise. MCN Am J Matern Child Nurs. 2008;33(6):364–70.
20. Kieffer E, Willis S, Arellano N, Guzman R. Perspectives of pregnant and postpartum Latino women on diabetes, physical activity, and health. Health Educ Behav. 2002;29(5):542–56.
21. Carter-Edwards L, Ostbye T, Bastian LA, Yarnall K, Krause KM, Simmons TJ. Barriers to adopting a healthy lifestyle: insight from postpartum women. BMC Res Notes. 2009;2:161.
22. Setse R, Grogan R, Cooper LA, Strobino D, Powe NR, Nicholson W. Weight loss programs for urban-based, postpartum African-American women: perceived barriers and preferred components. Matern Child Health J. 2008;12(1):119–27.
23. Thornton P, Kieffer E, Salabarria-Pena Y, Odoms-Young A, Willis S, Kim H, et al. Weight, diet, and physical activity-related beliefs and practices among pregnant and postpartum Latino women: the role of social support. Matern Child Health J. 2006;10(1):95–104.

24. Borodulin K, Evenson K, Herring A. Physical activity patterns during pregnancy through postpartum. BMC Womens Health. 2009; 9(32):1–7.
25. Zhang J, Savitz DA. Exercise during pregnancy among US women. Ann Epidemiol. 1996;6(1):53–9.
26. Owe KM, Nystad W, Bø K. Correlates of regular exercise during pregnancy: the Norwegian mother and child cohort study. Scand J Med Sci Sports. 2009;19(5):637–45.
27. Gaston A, Cramp A. Exercise during pregnancy: a review of patterns and determinants. J Sci Med Sport. 2011;14(4):299–305.
28. Jukic AMZ, Evenson K, Herring A, Wilcox A, Hartmann K, Daniels J. Correlates of physical activity at two time points during pregnancy. J Phys Act Health. 2012;9(3):325–35.
29. Evenson K, Savitz D, Huston S. Leisure-time physical activity among pregnant U.S. women. Paediatr Perinat Epidemiol. 2004;18: 400–7.
30. Grace SL, Williams A, Stewart DE, Franche RL. Health-promoting behaviors through pregnancy, maternity leave, and return to work: effects of role spillover and other correlates. Women Health. 2006;43: 51–72.
31. Ning Y, Williams MA, Dempsey JC, Sorensen TK, Frederick IO, Luthy DA. Correlates of recreational physical activity in early pregnancy. J Matern Fetal Neonatal Med. 2003;13(6):385–93.
32. Haakstad LA, Voldner N, Henriksen T, Bø K. Why do pregnant women stop exercising in the third trimester? Acta Obstet Gynecol Scand. 2009;88(11):1267–75.
33. Cramp AG, Bray SR. Understanding leisure-time physical activity during pregnancy: a prospective examination of perceived barriers and self-efficacy. Ann Behav Med. 2009;37:325–34.
34. Schmidt MD, Pekow P, Freedson PS, Markenson G, Chasan-Taber L. Physical activity patterns during pregnancy in a diverse population of women. J Womens Health. 2006;5(8):909–18.
35. Chasan-Taber L, Evenson KR, Sternfeld B, Kengeri S. Assessment of recreational physical activity during pregnancy in epidemiologic studies of birthweight and length of gestation: methodologic aspects. Women Health. 2007;45(4):85–107.
36. Liu J, Blair S, Teng Y, Ness A, Lawlor D, Riddoch C. Physical activity during pregnancy in a prospective cohort of British women: results from the Avon longitudinal study of parents and children. Eur J Epidemiol. 2011;26(3):237–47.
37. Lynch K, Landsbaugh J, Whitcomb B, Pekow P, Markenson G, Chasan Taber L. Physical activity of pregnant Hispanic women. Am J Prev Med. 2012;43(4):434–9.
38. Blum JW, Beaudoin CM, Caton-Lemos L. Physical activity patterns and maternal well-being in postpartum women. Matern Child Health J. 2004;8:163–9.

39. Hinton PS, Olson CM. Predictors of pregnancy-associated change in physical activity in a rural white population. Matern Child Health J. 2001;5(1):7–14.
40. Evenson KR, Aytur SA, Borodulin K. Physical activity beliefs, barriers, and enablers among postpartum women. J Womens Health (Larchmt). 2009;18:1925–34.
41. Keller C, Allan J, Tinkle MB. Stages of change, processes of change, and social support for exercise and weight gain in postpartum women. J Obstet Gynecol Neonatal Nurs. 2006;35:232–40.
42. Symons Downs D, Hausenblas H. Women's exercise beliefs and behaviors during their pregnancy and postpartum. J Midwifery Womens Health. 2004;49:138–44.
43. Doran F, Davis K. Factors that influence physical activity for pregnant and postpartum women and implications for primary care. Aust J Prim Health. 2011;17:79–85.
44. Pereira M, Rifas-Shiman S, Kleinman K, Rich-Edwards J, Peterson K, Gillman M. Predictors of change in physical activity during and after pregnancy: Project Viva. Am J Prev Med. 2007;32:312–9.
45. Symons Downs D, Ulbrecht JS. Understanding exercise beliefs and behaviors in women with gestational diabetes mellitus. Diabetes Care. 2006;29:236–40.
46. Price SN, McDonald J, Oken E, Haines J, Gillman MW, Taveras EM. Content analysis of motivational counseling calls targeting obesity-related behaviors among postpartum women. Matern Child Health J. 2012;16:439–47.
47. Smith BJ, Cheung NW, Bauman AE, Zehle K, McLean M. Postpartum physical activity and related psychosocial factors among women with recent gestational diabetes mellitus. Diabetes Care. 2005;28(11):2650–4.
48. American Diabetes Association. Standards of medical care in diabetes – 2010. Diabetes Care. 2010;33:S11–61.
49. International Association of Diabetes and Pregnancy Study Groups Consensus Panel. International Association of Diabetes and Pregnancy Study Groups recommendations on the diagnosis and classification of hyperglycemia in pregnancy. Diabetes Care. 2010;33:676–82.
50. Torloni MR, Betrán AP, Horta BL, Nakamura MU, Atallah AN, Moron AF, Valente O. Prepregnancy BMI and the risk of gestational diabetes: a systematic review of the literature with meta-analysis. Obes Rev. 2009;10(2):194–203.
51. Oteng Ntim E, Varma R, Croker H, Poston L, Doyle P. Lifestyle interventions for overweight and obese pregnant women to improve pregnancy outcome: systematic review and meta-analysis. BMC Med. 2012;10:47.
52. Cheung NW, Byth K. Population health significance of gestational diabetes. Diabetes Care. 2003;26(7):2005–9.

53. Dabelea D, Snell-Bergeon JK, Hartsfield CL, Bischoff KJ, Hamman RF, McDuffie RS. Increasing prevalence of gestational diabetes mellitus (GDM) over time and by birth cohort: Kaiser Permanente of Colorado GDM Screening Program. Diabetes Care. 2005; 28(3):579–84.
54. Ferrara A, Kahn HS, Quesenberry CP, Riley C, Hedderson MM. An increase in the incidence of gestational diabetes mellitus: Northern California, 1991–2000. Obstet Gynecol. 2004;103(3):526–33.
55. Guelinckx I, Devlieger R, Beckers K, Vansant G. Maternal obesity: pregnancy complications, gestational weight gain and nutrition. Obes Rev. 2008;9(2):140–50.
56. O'Sullivan J. Diabetes mellitus after GDM. Diabetes. 1991;40 Suppl 2:131–5.
57. Siega-Riz A, Viswanathan M, Moos M, Deierlein A, Mumford S, Knaack J, Thieda P, Kux LI, Lohr KN. A systematic review of outcomes of maternal weight gain according to the Institute of Medicine recommendations: birthweight, fetal growth, and postpartum weight retention. Obstet Gynecol. 2009;201(4):339.e1–14.
58. American Diabetes Association. Gestational diabetes mellitus. Diabetes Care. 2004;27 Suppl 1:S88–90.
59. Whitaker RC, Pepe MS, Seidel KD, Wright JA, Knopp RH. Gestational diabetes and the risk of offspring obesity. Pediatrics. 1998;101(2):E9.
60. Oken E, Taveras EM, Kleinman KP, Rich-Edwards JW, Gillman MW. Gestational weight gain and child adiposity at age 3 years. Am J Obstet Gynecol. 2007;196(4):322.e1–8.
61. Tobias D, Zhang C, van Dam R, Bowers K, Hu F. Physical activity before and during pregnancy and risk of gestational diabetes mellitus: a meta-analysis. Diabetes Care. 2011;34(1):223–9.
62. Han S, Middleton P, Crowther C. Exercise for pregnant women for preventing gestational diabetes mellitus. Cochrane Database of Systematic Reviews (Internet) 2012 (Cited 17 Jan 2013) Available from: http://onlinelibrary.wiley.com/doi/10.1002/14651858.CD009021.
63. Ong MJ, Guelfi KJ, Hunter T, Wallman KE, Fournier PA, Newnham JP. Supervised home-based exercise may attenuate the decline of glucose tolerance in obese pregnant women. Diabetes Metab. 2009;35(5):418–21.
64. Callaway L, Colditz P, Byrne N, Lingwood B, Rowlands I, Groves A, Sansome X, O'Connor BR, Croaker S, Foxcroft K, McIntyre HD. Prevention of gestational diabetes: feasibility issues for an exercise intervention in obese pregnant women. Diabetes Care. 2010; 33(7):1457.
65. Roberts J, Pearson G, Cutler J, Lindheimer M. Summary of the NHLBI working group on research on hypertension during pregnancy. Hypertens Pregnancy. 2003;22(2):109–27.
66. O'Brien T, Ray J, Chan W. Maternal body mass index and the risk of preeclampsia: a systematic overview. Epidemiology. 2003;14(3):368–74.

67. Frederick I, Rudra C, Miller R, Foster J, Williams M. Adult weight change, weight cycling, and prepregnancy obesity in relation to risk of preeclampsia. Epidemiology. 2006;17(4):428–34.
68. Villamor E, Cnattingius S. Interpregnancy weight change and risk of adverse pregnancy outcomes: a population-based study. Lancet. 2006;368(9542):1164–70.
69. Chang J, Elam-Evans LD, Berg CJ, Herndon J, Flowers L, Seed KA, Syverson CJ. Pregnancy-related mortality surveillance: United States, 1991–1999. MMWR Surveill Summ. 2003;52(SS02):1–8.
70. Berg CJ, MacKay AP, Qin C, Callaghan WM. Overview of maternal morbidity during hospitalization for labour and delivery in the United States. Obstet Gynecol. 2009;113:1075–81.
71. Kasawara K, Nascimento SLD, Costa M, Surita F, e Silva JLP. Exercise and physical activity in the prevention of pre-eclampsia: systematic review. Acta Obstet Gynecol Scand. 2012;91(10):1147–57.
72. Yeo S, Davidge S, Ronis DL, Antonakos CL, Hayashi R, O'Leary S. A comparison of walking versus stretching exercises to reduce the incidence of preeclampsia: a randomized clinical trial. Hypertens Pregnancy. 2008;27(2):113–30.
73. Hegaard H, Pedersen B, Nielsen B, Damm P. Leisure time physical activity during pregnancy and impact on gestational diabetes mellitus, pre-eclampsia, preterm delivery and birth weight: a review. Acta Obstet Gynecol Scand. 2007;86(11):1290.
74. Østerdal ML, Strøm M, Klemmensen AK, Knudsen VK, Juhl M, Halldorsson TI, Nybo Andersen AM, Magnus P, Olsen SF. Does leisure time physical activity in early pregnancy protect against preeclampsia? Prospective cohort in Danish women. BJOG. 2009;116(1): 98–107.
75. Magnus P, Trogstad L, Owe K, Olsen S, Nystad W. Recreational physical activity and the risk of preeclampsia: a prospective cohort of Norwegian women. Am J Epidemiol. 2008;168(8):952–7.
76. Rudra CB, Williams MA, Lee IM, Miller RS, Sorensen TK. Perceived exertion in physical activity and risk of gestational diabetes mellitus. Epidemiology. 2006;17(1):31–7.
77. Weight gain during pregnancy: reexamining the guidelines. Washington (D.C.): Institute of Medicine and National Academy of Sciences; 2009.
78. Gore S, Brown D, West D. The role of postpartum weight retention in obesity among women: a review of the evidence. Ann Behav Med. 2003;26(2):149–59.
79. Influence of pregnancy weight on maternal and child health. Washington (D.C.): National Research Council and Institute of Medicine; 2007. Workshop Report.
80. Bodnar L, Catov J, Klebanoff M, Ness R, Roberts J. Prepregnancy body mass index and the occurrence of severe hypertensive disorders of pregnancy. Epidemiology. 2007;18(2):234–9.

81. Cedergren M. Maternal morbid obesity and the risk of adverse pregnancy outcome. Obstet Gynecol. 2004;103(2):219–24.
82. Crane JMG, White J, Murphy P, Burrage L, Hutchens D. The effect of gestational weight gain by body mass index on maternal and neonatal outcomes. J Obstet Gynaecol Can. 2009;31(1):28–35.
83. Stuebe A, Oken E, Gillman M. Associations of diet and physical activity during pregnancy with risk for excessive gestational weight gain. Obstet Gynecol. 2009;201(1):58.e1–8.
84. Olson CM, Strawderman MS. Modifiable behavioral factors in a biopsychosocial model predict inadequate and excessive gestational weight gain. J Am Diet Assoc. 2003;103(1):48–54.
85. Chasan-Taber L, Schmidt M, Pekow P, Sternfeld B, Solomon C, Markenson G. Predictors of excessive and inadequate gestational weight gain in Hispanic women. Obesity. 2008;16(7):1657–66.
86. Sui Z, Grivell R, Dodd J. Antenatal exercise to improve outcomes in overweight or obese women: a systematic review. Acta Obstet Gynecol Scand. 2012;91(5):538–45.
87. Kim C. Gestational diabetes: risks, management, and treatment options. Int J Womens Health. 2010;2:339–51.
88. Lovelady CA, Garner KE, Moreno KL, Williams JP. The effect of weight loss in overweight, lactating women on the growth of their infants. N Engl J Med. 2000;342(7):449–53.
89. O'Toole ML, Sawicki MA, Artal R. Structured diet and physical activity prevent postpartum weight retention. J Womens Health (Larchmt). 2003;12(10):991–8.
90. Lovelady CA, Nommsen Rivers LA, McCrory MA, Dewey KG. Effects of exercise on plasma lipids and metabolism of lactating women. Med Sci Sports Exerc. 1995;27(1):22–8.
91. Ferrara A, Hedderson MM, Albright C, Ehrlich SF, Quesenberry CP, Peng T, Ching J, Cites Y. A pregnancy and postpartum lifestyle intervention in women with gestational diabetes mellitus reduces diabetes risk factors: a feasibility randomized control trial. Diabetes Care. 2011;34(7):1519–25.
92. Leermakers EA, Anglin K, Wing RR. Reducing postpartum weight retention through a correspondence intervention. Int J Obes. 1998;22(11):1103–9.
93. Ostbye T, Krause K, Lovelady CA, Morey MC, Bastian LA, Peterson BL, Swamy GK, Brouwer RJ, McBride CM. Active mothers postpartum: a randomized controlled weight-loss intervention trial. Am J Prev Med. 2009;37(3):173–80.
94. Kuhlmann AKS, Dietz P, Galavotti C, England L. Weight-management interventions for pregnant or postpartum women. Am J Prev Med. 2008;34(6):523–8.
95. Bertz F, Brekke H, Ellegård L, Rasmussen K, Wennergren M, Winkvist A. Diet and exercise weight-loss trial in lactating overweight and obese women. Am J Clin Nutr. 2012;96(4):698–705.

96. Evenson K, Chasan-Taber L, Symons Downs D, Pearce E. Review of self-reported physical activity assessments for pregnancy: summary of the evidence for validity and reliability. Paediatr Perinat Epidemiol. 2012;26:479–94.
97. Connolly CP, Coe DP, Kendrick JM, Bassett DR, Thompson DL. Accuracy of physical activity monitors in pregnant women. Med Sci Sports Exerc. 2011;43(6):1100–5.
98. Rousham E, Clarke P, Gross H. Significant changes in physical activity among pregnant women in the UK as assessed by accelerometry and self-reported activity. Eur J Clin Nutr. 2005;60(3):393–400.
99. McParlin C, Robson SC, Tennant PW, Besson H, Rankin J, Adamson AJ, Pearce MS, Bell R. Objectively measured physical activity during pregnancy: a study in obese and overweight women. BMC Pregnancy Childbirth. 2010;10:76.
100. Doran F, O'Brien AP. A brief report of attitudes towards physical activity during pregnancy. Health Promot J Austr. 2007;18(2):155–8.
101. Symons Downs D, Hausenblas HA. Exercising during pregnancy and postpartum: an elicitation study using the framework of the theory of planned behavior. J Midwifery Womens Health. 2004;49:138–44.
102. Symons Downs D, Hausenblas HA. Elicitation studies and the theory of planned behavior: a systematic review of exercise beliefs. Psychol Sport Exerc. 2005;6:1–31.
103. Duncombe D, Wertheim EH, Skouteris H, Paxton SJ, Kelly L. How well do women adapt to changes in their body size and shape across the course of pregnancy? J Health Psychol. 2008;13:503–15.
104. Lieferman J, Swibas T, Koiness K, Marshall JA, Dunn AL. My baby, my move: examination of perceived barriers and motivating factors related to antenatal physical activity. J Midwifery Womens Health. 2011;56(1):33–40.
105. Symons Downs D, Ulbrecht J. Exercise and gestational diabetes: an elicitation study based on the theory of planned behavior. Diabetes Care. 2006;29:236–40.
106. Weir Z, Bush J, Robson SC, McParlin C, Rankin J, Bell R. Physical activity in pregnancy: a qualitative study of the beliefs of overweight and obese pregnant women. BMC Pregnancy Childbirth. 2010;10:18. doi:10.1186/1471-2393-10-18.
107. Pearce E, Evenson K, Symons Downs D, Steckler A. Strategies to promote physical activity during pregnancy: a systematic review. Am J Lifestyle Med. 2013;7(1):37–49.
108. Feinstein RA, Francis KT, Lorish C. Physical activity and fitness assessment. Ala Med. 1991;61(2):10–2, 14.
109. Evenson KR, Pompeii LA. Obstetrician practice patterns and recommendations for physical activity during pregnancy. J Womens Health (Larchmt). 2010;19(9):1733–40.

Chapter 9. Obesity, Physical Activity, Pregnancy/Postpartum 225

110. Stotland NE, Gilbert P, Bogetz A, Harper CC, Abrams B, Gerbert B. Preventing excessive weight gain in pregnancy: how do prenatal care providers approach counseling? J Womens Health (Larchmt). 2010;19(4):807–14.
111. Stengel MR, Kraschnewski JL, Hwang SW, Kjerulff KH, Chuang CH. What my doctor didn't tell me: examining health care provider advice to overweight and obese pregnant women on gestational weight gain and physical activity. Womens Health Issues. 2012;22(6):e535–40.
112. Stotland N, Tsoh JY, Gerbert B. Prenatal weight gain: who is counseled? J Womens Health. 2012;21(6):695–701.
113. Symons Downs D, Savage JS, Rauff EL. Falling short of guidelines? Lacking knowledge to achieve gestational weight gain, diet, and physical activity recommendations in pregnancy. In review.
114. Meriwether RA, Lee JA, Lafleur AS, Wiseman P. Physical activity counseling. Am Fam Physician. 2008;77(8):1129–36.
115. Jackson RA, Stotland NE, Caughey AB, Gerbert B. Improving diet and exercise in pregnancy with video doctor counseling: a randomized trial. Patient Educ Couns. 2011;83(2):203–9.
116. Stotland N, Haas J, Brawarsky P, Jackson R, Fuentes Afflick E, Escobar G. Body mass index, provider advice, and target gestational weight gain. Obstet Gynecol. 2005;105(3):633–8.
117. Stotland N, Cheng Y, Hopkins L, Caughey A. Gestational weight gain and adverse neonatal outcome among term infants. Obstet Gynecol. 2006;108(3):635–43.
118. Cogswell ME, Scanlon KS, Fein SB, Schieve LA. Medically advised, mother's personal target, and actual weight gain during pregnancy. Obstet Gynecol. 1999;94(4):616–22.
119. Tovar A, Chasan-Taber L, Bermudez O, Hyatt R, Must A. Knowledge, attitudes, and beliefs regarding weight gain during pregnancy among Hispanic women. Matern Child Health J. 2010;14(6):938–49.
120. Stotland N, Gilbert P, Bogetz A, Harper C, Abrams B, Gerbert B. Preventing excessive weight gain in pregnancy: how do prenatal care providers approach counseling? J Womens Health. 2010;19(4):807–14.
121. Merriam PA, Tellez TL, Rosal MC, Olendzki BC, Ma Y, Pagoto SL, Ockene IS. Methodology of a diabetes prevention translational research project utilizing a community-academic partnership for implementation in an underserved Latino community. BMC Med Res Methodol. 2009;9:20.
122. King AC, Haskell WL, Taylor CB, Kraemer HC, DeBusk RF. Group-vs home-based exercise training in healthy older men and women. A community-based clinical trial. JAMA. 1991;266(11):1535–42.
123. Oldridge NB. Compliance and exercise in primary and secondary prevention of coronary heart disease: a review. Prev Med. 1982;11(1):56–70.

124. Marcus BH, Lewis BA, Williams DM, Dunsiger S, Jakicic JM, Whiteley JA, Albrecht AE, Napolitano MA, Brock BC, Tate DF, Sciamanna CN, Parisi AF. A comparison of internet and print-based physical activity interventions. Arch Intern Med. 2007;167(9):944–9.
125. Cardinal BJ, Sachs ML. Effects of mail-mediated, stage-matched exercise behavior change strategies on female adults' leisure-time exercise behavior. J Sports Med Phys Fitness. 1996;36(2):100–7.
126. Chasan-Taber L, Marcus BH, Stanek E, Ciccolo JT, Marquez DX, Solomon CG, Markenson G. A randomized controlled trial of prenatal physical activity to prevent gestational diabetes: design and methods. J Womens Health (Larchmt). 2009;18(6):851–9.
127. Chasan-Taber L, Silveira M, Marcus B, Braun B, Stanek E, Markenson G. Feasibility and efficacy of a physical activity intervention among pregnant women: the behaviors affecting baby and you (B.A.B.Y.) study. J Phys Act Health. 2011;8 Suppl 2:S228–38.
128. Chasan-Taber L, Hosker M, Marcus BH, Rosal MC, Braun B, Stanek E. Feasibility of a randomized trial to prevent gestational diabetes in overweight and obese hispanic women. BMC Pregnancy Childbirth. In review.
129. Symons Downs D, DiNallo JM, Rauff EL, Ulbrecht JS, Birch LL, Paul IM. Pregnant women's exercise motivation and behavior: preliminary findings from a randomized physical activity intervention. Paper presented at the North American Society for the Psychology of Sport and Physical Activity, Tucson, AZ; 2010.
130. Symons Downs D. Determinants and outcomes of physical activity in pregnancy: findings from Active MOMS, a randomized physical activity intervention for pregnant women. Paper presented at The Society for Behavioral Medicine, Washington, DC; 2011.
131. Mottola MF, Giroux I, Gratton R, Hammond J, Hanley A, Harris S, McManus R, Davenport MH, Sopper MM. Nutrition and exercise prevent excess weight gain in overweight pregnant women. Med Sci Sports Exerc. 2010;42(2):265–72.
132. Huang TT, Yeh CY, Tsai YC. A diet and physical activity intervention for preventing weight retention among Taiwanese childbearing women: a randomised controlled trial. Midwifery. 2011;27(2):257–64. doi:10.1016/j.midw.2009.06.009. Epub 2009 Sep 22.
133. Kropp F, Winhusen T, Lewis D, Hague D, Somoza E. Increasing prenatal care and healthy behaviors in pregnant substance users. J Psychoactive Drugs. 2010;42(1):73–81.
134. Hui A, Back L, Ludwig S, Gardiner P, Sevenhuysen G, Dean H, Sellers E, McGavock J, Morris M, Bruce S, Murray R, Shen GX. Lifestyle intervention on diet and exercise reduced excessive gestational weight gain in pregnant women under a randomised controlled trial. BJOG. 2012;119(1):70–7. doi:10.1111/j.1471-0528.2011.03184.x. Epub 2011 Oct 21.

135. Luoto R, Kinnunen TI, Aittasalo M, Kolu P, Raitanen J, Ojala K, Mansikkamäki K, Lamberg S, Vasankari T, Komulainen T, Tulokas S. Primary prevention of gestational diabetes mellitus and large-for-gestational-age newborns by lifestyle counseling: a cluster-randomized controlled trial. PLoS Med. 2011;8(5):e1001036. doi:10.1371/journal.pmed.1001036. Epub 2011 May 17.
136. Luoto RM, Kinnunen TI, Aittasalo M, Ojala K, Mansikkamäki K, Toropainen E, Kolu P, Vasankari T. Prevention of gestational diabetes: design of a cluster-randomized controlled trial and one-year follow-up. BMC Pregnancy Childbirth. 2010;10:39. doi:10.1186/1471-2393-10-39.
137. Yeo S. Adherence to walking or stretching, and risk of preeclampsia in sedentary pregnant women. Res Nurs Health. 2009;32(4):379–90. doi:10.1002/nur.20328.
138. Gaston A, Prapavessis H. Maternal-fetal disease information as a source of exercise motivation during pregnancy. Health Psychol. 2009;28(6):726–33.
139. Petersen A, Leet T, Brownson R. Correlates of physical activity among pregnant women in the United States. Med Sci Sports Exerc. 2005;37:1748–53.

Chapter 10
Maternal Obesity, Gestational Weight Gain, and Childhood Growth in the First Year of Life

Deborah B. Ehrenthal, Cynthia S. Minkovitz, and Donna M. Strobino

Abstract Obesity has reached epidemic proportions among women of childbearing age. Prepregnancy obesity and inappropriate gestational weight gain (GWG) have detrimental consequences for maternal health, birth outcomes, and infant growth in the first year of life. Dietary interventions during pregnancy have a modest, although significant, impact on GWG, but their long-term impact is unknown. Studies of interventions to reduce obesity prior to pregnancy are limited, but these interventions have the potential to address

---

D.B. Ehrenthal, MD, MPH
Departments of Internal Medicine and OB/GYN,
Christiana Care Health System, Newark, NJ, USA

Departments of Internal Medicine and OB/GYN,
Thomas Jefferson University, Philadelphia, PA, USA

C.S. Minkovitz, MD, MPP • D.M. Strobino, PhD (✉)
Department of Population, Family and Reproductive Health,
Bloomberg School of Public Health, Johns Hopkins University,
615 N Wolfe St., Baltimore, MD 21205, USA
e-mail: dstrobin@jhsph.edu

W. Nicholson, K. Baptiste-Roberts (eds.),
Obesity During Pregnancy in Clinical Practice,
DOI 10.1007/978-1-4471-2831-1_10,
© Springer-Verlag London 2014

modifiable behavioral, social, and environmental factors that may predispose women and their infants to excessive weight gain and to establish healthy trajectories in weight for both.

Keywords Obesity • Overweight • Gestational weight gain • Maternal health • Newborn health • Infant growth • Interventions

---

Key Points
- Obesity and inappropriate weight gain during pregnancy have a detrimental effect on women's health and birth outcomes, and may affect infant growth in the first year of life.
- Interventions that address obesity among women prior to pregnancy are limited, but have the potential to improve women's health, birth outcomes, and predispose children to optimal health, healthy weight and physical activity.
- Dietary interventions during pregnancy have a modest, although significant, impact on gestational weight gain, but their long term impact is unknown.
- Pregnancy provides an important opportunity to instill and reinforce positive lifelong habits for women and their infants.

Introduction

Obesity has reached epidemic proportions among women of childbearing age in recent years [1]. Increases in the percentage of children who are overweight or obese have added to the concern about the epidemic in adults [2]. In particular, current trends suggest that children are becoming heavier at younger ages. Although the most recent data suggest a tapering off of trends among adults [3, 4], the transition from overweight to obese is particularly a problem from adolescence

Chapter 10. Maternal Obesity, Weight Gain, Infant Growth

into early adulthood [5], the prime childbearing years among most US women, especially among racial and ethnic minorities [6]. These latter groups also suffer more overweight or obesity than their more advantaged counterparts [7, 8]. These trends have important implications for the health and well-being of women during pregnancy and the health of their newborns and infants.

In more recent years, the public health and medical communities have recognized important links between prepregnancy obesity, gestational weight gain (GWG), and adverse outcomes for both the mother and child. Prepregnancy obesity increases the likelihood of developing pregnancy complications [9]. Beyond pregnancy, postpartum retention of weight gained during pregnancy appears to play an important role in the development of adult obesity for women during their childbearing years [10–12]. In addition, the vertical transmission of obesity risk from mother to child is now recognized as important in childhood obesity; an understanding of the factors influencing this risk is evolving [13]. As potentially modifiable risks, achievement of optimal prepregnancy weight and GWG is now viewed as a strategy to improve outcomes for both women and their children, especially among obese women and their offspring, both of whom are at greatest risk for important short- and long-term adverse outcomes.

The objective of this chapter is to evaluate the evidence for the relation between prepregnancy weight, with emphasis on overweight and obesity, and maternal and newborn outcomes and growth of children in the first year of life. It also describes the evidence related to gestational weight gain and these same outcomes. Evaluation of interventions before pregnancy to reduce obesity and during pregnancy to promote optimal weight gain also is discussed. The limitations of the scientific evidence are considered along with future research needs. Finally, the implications of the research are discussed within a life course framework, which addresses the complexity of the determinants of obesity and our ability to stay the increasing trend in rates.

The Overweight/Obese Mother

Overweight and obesity at the start of pregnancy have important implications for outcomes for the mother and the newborn, including the risk of developing pregnancy complications as well as adverse neonatal outcomes [9, 14]. In addition to a consistent association of prepregnancy BMI with outcomes related to birth weight and fetal growth, a higher incidence of birth defects and stillbirth has been reported for obese women [15–17]. Some data suggest an increase in the risk of shoulder dystocia, likely related to the higher birth weight, but this relation has not been consistently identified [18]. Finally, children of overweight or obese mothers appear to be more likely to become obese children. Most of these findings come from observational studies. Assessment of outcomes related to effective interventions, as discussed below, is needed to support causality.

Outcomes for the Child

There is strong and consistent evidence that prepregnancy body mass index (BMI) is directly and independently related to birth weight [13, 19]. The 2013 systematic review and meta-analysis by Yu et al. evaluated the findings of 34 observational studies, including those with cohort, case–control, and cross-sectional designs, and examined the relation of prepregnancy BMI with size for gestational age, low birth weight (LBW), and macrosomia [20]. In nearly all studies, obese women were relatively protected from delivery of a small for gestational age (SGA) or LBW baby, but the odds of large for gestational age (LGA), high birth weight, or macrosomia were increased. For example, the authors reported a 67 % greater odds of macrosomia for women who were overweight prior to pregnancy and greater than a 3-fold increase if the mother was obese [20]. Analysis of outcomes of the well-characterized prospective cohort from the Hyperglycemia and Adverse Pregnancy Outcomes (HAPO) study suggests that the association of obesity and birth weight is independent of a diagnosis of gestational diabetes mellitus (GDM), common among obese mothers [21].

Similar findings were reported by Black et al., who conducted a retrospective study of women enrolled in a large prepaid group-practice managed health care plan [22]. They concluded that, in this population, prepregnancy overweight and obesity contributed significantly to the fraction of babies born LGA, independent of GDM [22]. The findings from both studies suggested that the effects of obesity and GDM on outcomes were additive.

Evidence from observational studies supporting a link between maternal obesity and child obesity continues to accumulate [13, 14, 20]. Of the factors identified during infancy, maternal prepregnancy obesity appears to make the greatest contribution to the risk of obesity during childhood [13, 23–25]. Observational studies, however, are unable to distinguish whether or not there is an independent role of maternal adiposity on the child's future obesity risk. Whether the link between maternal obesity and child obesity is the result of a shared susceptibility, the effect of the fetal intrauterine environment, postnatal factors, or a combination of factors is not yet clear. All or a portion of the obesity link may be due to behavioral and environmental factors passed from mother to child or within the context of family and community, especially with regard to cultural preferences in food choices and perceptions of a healthy baby.

Outcomes for the Mother

In their 2012 review, Marshall and Spong described the current literature regarding obesity-related maternal pregnancy complications [9]. Evidence points to an increase in gestational diabetes, gestational hypertensive disorders, and thromboembolic disease among obese women compared to women with normal weight at the start of pregnancy [9, 26, 27]. For example, in the large population-based study of Danish women by Ovesen et al., there was a stepwise increase in gestational diabetes risk with increasing degree of obesity; women with a

BMI of 35 kg/m² or more, had an 11-fold greater odds of gestational diabetes when compared to women of normal weight [18]. At delivery, obese mothers are more likely to experience labor dystocia and deliver by cesarean section [28].

Interventions Among Women of Childbearing Age

An optimal approach to improving obesity-related outcomes in mothers and their newborns is to achieve a more healthy weight prior to pregnancy. This goal should be incorporated into the care of women during their reproductive years, through both primary well women care, which incorporates the notion of reproductive awareness, and a discussion of pregnancy planning. As noted above, obese women present a particularly challenging set of concerns because their weight affects not only their health but that of their future offspring. While interventions to alter lifestyle behaviors focused on diet and physical activity among women of childbearing age may be theoretically ideal [14], research in this area is very limited, often due to questions about which women to study and because most studies include small samples [29], with modest results at best [30]. Most studies of women of childbearing ages have focused on those in the older range of the childbearing population [31, 32] and with children [33, 34] although a few studies involve the inter-pregnancy period. Two major prepregnancy interventions specific to obese women are bariatric surgery and the use of insulin-sensitizing drugs.

Bariatric surgery is not the first line of interventions for weight loss but may be recommended if other attempts at weight loss have failed. It has risen in frequency, however, in recent years among women in the childbearing ages, mirroring in part the rise in obesity in the United States [35]. Its use among adolescent females has plateaued in recent years [36], perhaps in part due to controversies about the appropriateness of surgery for this age group. Bariatric surgery procedures most commonly induce food intake restriction, food malabsorption, or both [37], and in turn promote weight loss, an average of about 30 % in the first year following surgery, although the majority of patients remain overweight [38].

Maggard and colleagues undertook a systematic review of studies of the impact of bariatric surgery on subsequent fertility and pregnancy outcomes [39], followed by more recent reviews by Guelinckx, Devlieger and Vansant, and Kjaer and Nilas [38, 40]. They note that these studies are necessarily observational in nature. The design, sample characteristics, control groups, and type of surgery [41] evaluated are quite heterogeneous across studies [38–40]. Controls among pregnant women may include births to the same women before and after surgery, women who are matched by weight with and without surgery, and in one recent study an additional control group of pregnant women who were the same weight as women with surgery at the time the surgery was performed [42]. Most studies show reduced maternal complications, as measured by GDM and hypertension, and in rates of macrosomic births. Birth weight may be reduced, and there is some suggestion of an increase in SGA births, but this finding is by no means consistent across studies [38–40]. Choice of an appropriate control group remains a challenge in this research.

While the studies of births in women who undergo bariatric surgery generally show that it is safe with some conflicting findings, there may be problems for women with malabsorption and who are at risk for micronutrient deficiencies [40]. Whether or not these deficiencies contribute to birth defects, particularly neural tube defects, is unclear due in part to the difficulty in obtaining adequate samples because of their rare occurrence [40]. Timing of pregnancy is important following surgery especially with regard to potential nutritional deficiencies, and it is recommended that women wait at least 1–2 years following surgery before conception [43]. Nutritional evaluation both before and during pregnancy is recommended to address these risks [38, 39, 43].

A second prepregnancy intervention is the use of insulin-sensitizing drugs for weight loss. Nieuwenhuis-Ruifrok et al. reviewed data from 14 trials of obese or overweight women who were given insulin-sensitizing drugs for weight loss [44].

All but two of the studies included samples of women with polycystic ovary syndrome (PCOS); only data for women completing the trials were included in the analysis. Metformin over 1,500 mg/day was associated with a significant decrease in BMI among overweight and obese women with PCOS; there were no significant findings for lower dosages, but numbers in these studies were small. No additional impact was noted when included with lifestyle interventions. The review had several limitations; only women who completed the trials were included in the analysis, the objectives for the trials were designed with different primary outcomes and clinical questions, the samples across studies were quite heterogeneous, and most studies had small sample size. Moreover, extension of the findings to obese or overweight women prepregnancy without PCOS is unclear.

Studies which address dietary intervention, physical activity, or counseling related to obesity and weight loss are few in young nonpregnant women of childbearing age [29]. The few available studies were conducted among limited populations or women who already have young children and who are unlikely to have subsequent births [33, 34, 45]. The lack of data about potential interventions in young women of childbearing age is a serious gap in the literature. It represents a missed opportunity from a life course perspective and provides clinicians with limited options to prevent obesity or reduce weight gain or high prepregnancy weight among women to whom they provide well woman or preconception care.

Gestational Weight Gain and the Overweight/Obese Woman

Recommendations for GWG have evolved over the past several years as the obesity epidemic has changed the distribution of risk factors for adverse perinatal outcomes and highlighted the importance of balancing the short- and long-term risks for mothers and their children. The link between GWG and birth weight was observed decades ago, and efforts to prevent LBW guided health care and public policy recommendations for GWG [46]. The 1970 Institute of Medicine (IOM) report recommended a 20–27 lb weight gain for all women. Ensuring adequate nutrition for women became a major focus of maternal health interventions.

However, trends in GWG for US populations now show an increasing percentage of women gain in excess of current GWG recommendations [47]. There are important variations in GWG among racial and ethnic groups in the US population [48]. In their review, Headen et al. found excess GWG was most common among. White mothers (>50 %), while inadequate GWG was more common among Asian, Hispanic, and Black mothers [48]. Data from Pregnancy Risk Assessment and Monitoring System (PRAMS) suggest that obese women tend to gain less weight overall than nonobese women, but they are more likely to gain in excess of the current IOM recommendations for their weight [49]. Within the context of the current epidemic of obesity, these differences underscore the importance of understanding the relation of GWG to adverse outcomes.

Components of GWG

Weight gain during pregnancy is a function of a number of factors including maternal weight gain, fetal weight gain, placental weight, and fat mass [47]. The increase in fat mass shows the greatest variability between women and is most reflective of both gestational weight gain and prepregnancy obesity [49]. GWG typically varies by trimester, with a rapid increase in maternal stores during the second trimester preceding the rapid growth of the fetus during the third trimester [49]. Because weight gain in the third trimester is linked closely with the length of pregnancy, it must be taken into account in research on the relation of GWG with preterm birth and low birth weight (LBW).

Determinants of GWG

Weight gain during pregnancy is greatest during the first pregnancy and among pregnancies with multiple gestations (e.g. twins, triplets) [49]. Several maternal factors influence GWG, including prepregnancy BMI, parity, height, smoking, as well as level of education and comorbid conditions [50]. Race and other social and cultural factors also appear to play an important role [50]. Pregnancy-related factors also potentially influence GWG. For example, improvement in diet prompted by a new diagnosis of gestational diabetes may result in weight loss [51]. Conversely, women with a gestational hypertensive disorder may gain more weight as a result of fluid retention and edema related to the syndrome. The influence of bed rest on GWG is unexplored [52].

Current US GWG Guidelines

The medical and public health communities have struggled to define recommendations for GWG. Initially, recommendations focused on the importance of adequate weight gain to prevent LBW. The 1990 IOM revision of recommendations for GWG in the United States reflected the understanding that a mother's adiposity prior to pregnancy influenced fetal growth, and recommendations for GWG were tailored based on prepregnancy BMI, an easily measured value reflecting a proxy for the degree of maternal obesity at the start of gestation. The importance of both short- and long-term outcomes for the mother and child was recognized, but little evidence was available to support recommendations. In addition, there was little evidence that weight gain counseling had an impact on GWG.

Chapter 10. Maternal Obesity, Weight Gain, Infant Growth 239

TABLE 10.1 Current IOM recommendations for GWG [49]

Prepregnancy BMI	Total weight gain		Rates of weight gain, second and third trimester	
	Range in kg	Range in lb	Mean (range) in kg/week	Mean (range) in lb/week
Underweight (<18.5 kg/m^2)	12.5–18	28–40	0.51 (0.44–0.58)	1 (1–1.3)
Normal weight (18.5–24.9 kg/m^2)	11.5–16	25–35	0.42 (0.35–0.50)	1 (0.8–1)
Overweight (25.0–29.9 kg/m^2)	7–11.5	15–25	0.28 (0.23–0.33)	0.6 (0.5–0.7)
Obese (≥30 kg/m^2)	5–9	11–20	0.22 (0.17–0.27)	0.5 (0.4–0.6)

BMI body mass index

The new guidelines for GWG released in 2009 by the IOM were based on a systematic review of the literature (Table 10.1) [47–49]. The recommendations were considered in the context of the recent rise in obesity among women of childbearing age and their children. Evidence of greater GWG among the diverse populations of US mothers was of concern, as was the increasing incidence of obesity-related maternal complications including cesarean delivery, higher rates of fetal macrosomia, and concerns about the impact of GWG on future obesity risk for both the mother and child. To arrive at their recommendations, the committee tried to balance the risks and benefits to the neonate as well as to the mother [47, 49].

The 2009 recommendations changed most significantly for women who are overweight or obese prior to pregnancy. These most recent guidelines recommend gains between 15 and 25 lbs for women who are overweight (BMI 25–29.9 kg/m^2) and 11 and 20 lbs for women with a BMI in the obese range (BMI 30 kg/m^2 or more). Recommendations for teen mothers are not different from those for adult women. It was recommended that short women gain at the lower end of the range. The committee did not have evidence that recommendations should differ based on mother's race or ethnicity, although they do differ for women with multiple gestation pregnancies [47, 49].

With the release of their recommendations, the IOM suggested strategies to help women adhere to GWG recommendations. Pregnancy is now viewed as a teachable moment, a time in women's lives when they may be more motivated to make lifestyle and other changes. Helping women achieve an optimal GWG presents an opportunity to impact short- and long-term outcomes for both the mother and her child. If excess GWG plays an independent role in the development of obesity, focused efforts to avoid excess GWG would be warranted. As discussed below, there is little or no experimental evidence to demonstrate that interventions, which effectively limit GWG, improve long-term outcomes for the mother.

Evidence Linking GWG to Outcomes for Overweight and Obese Mothers and Their Babies

Nearly all evidence supporting the link between GWG and outcomes for mothers and their offspring come from observational studies of women across the BMI spectrum. Although these studies consistently demonstrate several important significant associations between GWG and several short- and long-term outcomes [53], they are constrained by failure in most studies to account for the correlation of weight gain with length of pregnancy and increasing fetal weight as a component of weight gain. Maternal obesity is defined as a BMI of 30 kg/m^2 or more prior to pregnancy; this group is traditionally further divided into three groups: class I (BMI 30–34.9 kg/m^2), class II (35–39.9 kg/m^2), and class III (40+ kg/m^2). The few studies large enough to focus specifically on obese women suggest that the severity of obesity influences the relation of GWG to outcomes [54, 55]. In this section, we summarize the evidence of a relation for short- and long-term outcomes for women who enter pregnancy overweight or obese.

Short-Term Outcomes

Birth Weight

Observational studies show that inadequate GWG increases the odds of SGA, and moderate evidence shows that excess GWG is linked to LGA [53]. These studies may overestimate the effect because most fail to subtract babies' weight from total weight gain; the resulting part-whole correlation between the component of weight gain of the fetus and birth weight necessarily overestimates this relation. Kramer and colleagues showed a similar problem when studying preterm birth, which is further compounded by changes in velocity of weight gain over gestation [56]. Recent studies of large cohorts of women, including obese women suggest these associations are stronger for women of normal weight. Among women who are obese, excess GWG is linked to a greater risk of LGA and macrosomia, whereas inadequate weight gain shows a less strong relation with SGA and LBW [57, 58].

Maternal Outcomes

Overweight and obese women are more likely to develop pregnancy complications including gestational diabetes and hypertensive disorders of pregnancy [9]. Results from the EDEN mother-child cohort suggested that net GWG was directly related to the development of gestational hypertension [59]. Findings from investigations exploring the relation of GWG to the development GDM have been mixed [60, 61]. The relation of GWG to other outcomes may be different for women with pregnancy complications, potentially because the diagnosis may prompt lifestyle changes that may affect overall weight gain [51]. For women entering pregnancy obese, interventions during the prenatal and postpartum periods may also mitigate these risks and improve long- and short-term outcomes for mothers and their children. Key targets for intervention include optimizing GWG, encouraging postpartum weight loss, as well as working to address maternal and infant factors that might play a role in setting children's trajectory towards a healthy weight as they grow.

Prenatal Interventions to Reduce Maternal Weight Gain

Prenatal interventions generally address reduction or restriction in weight gain during pregnancy among samples of pregnant women in general as well as samples of overweight or obese women. The interventions focus primarily on diet, physical activity, and lifestyle alone or in combination. Some studies also evaluated whether additional strategies are needed such as goal setting related to weight loss to enhance the impact of diet and lifestyle interventions. The evidence supporting these interventions is not strong, although it is most consistent for dietary interventions among normal weight women.

Thangaratinam et al. provide the most comprehensive review and meta-analysis of studies of interventions in pregnancy and their impact on maternal weight gain [62, 63]. Their review evaluated 44 randomized controlled trials of interventions related to diet, physical activity, and lifestyle. The results of the meta-analysis show a modest effect of the interventions on reducing weight gain but with considerable heterogeneity across studies. Among the 34 trials evaluating GWG, the impact of any intervention, regardless of the specific intervention, was estimated to result in a reduction of −1.42 kg with 95 % confidence intervals (−0.95; −1.89 kg). The ten trials of dietary interventions alone showed the largest impact with estimates of reduced weight gain of −3.84 kg (−2.45; −5.22 kg) [62]; they also showed the largest effect of all interventions on BMI at delivery, when assessed [63]. The reduction in GWG in the 14 trials of physical activity was modest, −0.72 kg (−1.20; −0.25 kg), as well as in the mixed intervention trials, −1.06 kg (−1.67; −0.46 kg). A small but statistically significant reduction was noted in birth weight in the 28 trials with newborn data. A significantly reduced odds of preeclampsia was shown in 6 trials of dietary interventions and of GDM in 3 trials of dietary interventions. Mixed interventions showed no effect on preeclampsia or GDM, and neither maternal outcome was evaluated in trials of physical activity [62, 63].

The evidence related to weight gain was graded by Thangaratinam et al. as modest, but the overall quality of the evidence for an impact on GDM and gestational hypertension was low [62, 63]. Studies varied by sample characteristics, whether they included overweight or obese women or women of all prepregnancy weight and whether additional components were evaluated such as goal setting. All studies were constrained by selection of women in prenatal care with attendant effects on external validity. Few studies evaluated the impact of the intervention on postpartum weight retention, infant growth, or whether there were real, sustained changes in diet.

The review by Thangaratinam and colleagues included all women regardless of prepregnancy weight [62, 63]. Oteng-Nini et al. reviewed 13 randomized clinical trials and 6 non-randomized studies of prenatal dietary, physical activity, and behavioral and lifestyle interventions among overweight and obese pregnant women [64]. They reported a decrease of −2.21 kg (−2.86; −1.59 kg) in ten trials in which GWG was studied as well as a suggestion of a reduced rate of GDM in studies in which it was evaluated. They found no evidence of a reduction in LGA births. The overall quality of the studies was assessed as low to moderate. The results of a review by Dodd and colleagues also suggested no impact of dietary interventions on LGA births among overweight and obese women [65]. Although they found that women in seven trials gained significantly less weight in the dietary intervention group, adjustment for heterogeneity among studies using random effects models resulted in nonsignificant differences.

Some studies have also evaluated whether interventions may be effective in reducing excessive weight gain during pregnancy [66, 67]. Ronnberg and Nilsson evaluated studies of interventions to reduce excessive GWG and found the evidence to be of insufficient quality to develop recommendations for clinical practice [68]. In an alternative approach, Brown et al. reviewed five studies of goal setting in combination with modifications in diet, physical activity, or both [69]. Although goal setting appeared to be useful to women, the impact of specific aspects of goal setting was unclear.

The results reported by Thangaratinam and colleagues are similar to other reviews conducted on specific interventions [68–72], suggesting some promise for the dietary interventions in particular but limited impact overall of interventions to reduce GWG. There are a number of gaps in the literature, particularly failure to evaluate the long-term impact of the interventions on women or their infants, as noted above. Studies also lack theory or conceptual models to support the interventions from a behavioral modification perspective [70], although some attention was given to goal-setting strategies as a component of the intervention [69]. There is also limited information about specific interventions, making it difficult to replicate studies or to develop clinical practice recommendations. Studies are needed with adequate samples to evaluate the reasons for heterogeneity of findings across studies and to evaluate whether there are subgroups of women who would benefit most from specific interventions. In addition, it is reasonable to postulate that dietary interventions which result in close to a 4 kg reduction in weight gain may also reduce postpartum weight retention, but the magnitude of the impact may be small over the life course of a woman if the intervention does not result in long-term change in diet or alter whether or not a woman becomes overweight or obese.

Maternal Prepregnancy BMI Associated with Decreased Initiation and Shorter Duration of Breastfeeding

High prepregnancy BMI can adversely effect breastfeeding rates. Despite Healthy People 2020 Goals [73], recommendations of the American Academy of Pediatrics [74], and widespread recognition of the benefits of breastfeeding, the percentage of women who breastfeed in the United States did not meet the Healthy People 2010 goals. Among all births in the United States in 2006, 74 % of mothers ever breastfed and

44 % continued through 6 months of age. The corresponding the American Academy of Pediatrics similarly recommends exclusive breastfeeding through 6 months of age and continued breastfeeding for 1 year or longer as complementary foods are introduced and as mutually desired by mother and infant [74].

In a review of the literature, Wojicki reported 12 studies of breastfeeding initiation; the results of 9 studies showed an association between overweight and obesity prior to pregnancy and failure to initiate breastfeeding [75]. Of the 12 studies that considered duration, 10 reported an association between maternal overweight or obesity and decreased duration. Among 2 of the 9 studies of breastfeeding initiation and 2 of the 10 focusing on duration, these relations were observed for selected subgroups, although most studies did not stratify analyses by race and ethnicity. Wojicki suggests that differences by race and ethnicity may reflect underlying sociocultural, environmental, or physiological factors and that these factors are important to address in interventions to promote breastfeeding.

Most studies of breastfeeding have not considered the role of medical complications. Kistantis et al. conducted a study that stratified analyses by presence or absence of medical and delivery complications (e.g., hypertension, fetal distress, gestational diabetes, meconium) [76]. The study results showed that decreased initiation and duration was limited to overweight or obese women with complications. Wojicki noted that possible reasons underlying the association between obesity and breastfeeding may relate to biological changes (delayed prolactin response), mechanical issues (positioning the infant), behavioral factors (choice and intentions), and psychological factors [75].

In a Belgian retrospective cohort study of 200 women, Guelinckx et al. reported decreased initiation and duration of breastfeeding among both obese and underweight women with no association between initiation and hypertensive disorders [77]. More recently, in a sample of 550 women participating in the Pregnancy, Infection, and Nutrition Postpartum

Study, Mehta and colleagues confirmed the link between prepregnancy overweight and obesity and reduced initiation and duration of breastfeeding [78]. Most importantly, they found that these relations were not mediated by depressive symptoms, perceived stress, or anxiety during pregnancy.

Although the association between obesity and decreased initiation and breastfeeding well established in the literature, there is little understanding of the underlying mechanisms. While primary efforts are needed to reduce obesity, further studies also are needed to understand the underlying mechanisms in order to determine whether interventions should address mutable factors that may increase breastfeeding among obese women. These factors may include anatomic barriers that require support of breasts to facilitate appropriate latch-on, reduced willingness to seek support for breastfeeding that requires enhanced and targeted outreach, and concerns over body image which might necessitate strategies to promote comfort of breastfeeding in public [77]. In the absence of studies, it is difficult to understand the barriers to breastfeeding among obese women.

Maternal Prepregnancy BMI and Gestational Weight Gain Influence Infant Growth at 1 Year

In addition, to birth outcomes discussed previously, prepregnancy weight also is associated with infant postnatal growth. Growth in the first year of life is of particular interest given the association between rapid early growth and subsequent childhood obesity [79–81] and cardiovascular disease and diabetes in adulthood [82, 83]. In addition, growth in the first year of life reflects the establishment of early feeding, physical activity, and sleep practices which, when unfavorable, may contribute to the development of obesity in later childhood. Numerous studies have also determined early growth rate to be a strong predictor of childhood obesity [84].

Using data from the Pregnancy, Infection, and Nutrition Study, Deierlein et al. reported that prepregnancy overweight and obesity were associated with greater weight for age and weight for length at 6 months, but not with length for age, after accounting for other infant and maternal characteristics [85]. The relations were attenuated, however, when birth weight was taken into account in the analysis, the effect of prepregnancy overweight and obesity on growth indices at 6 months were largely explained by the relation of prepregnancy weight with prenatal growth.

With regard to body composition, Chandler-Laney et al. observed that prepregnancy BMI was also associated with a child's total lean mass, but not total fat mass or trunk fat mass at 12 months, after adjusting for infant length and rate of weight gain in the first year [86]. The authors speculate that the association may be attributed to genetic susceptibility or the intrauterine environment. Total and trunk fat mass, in their study, was associated with weight gain in the first year of life, particularly in the first 6 months; this association is of particular interest given the role of rapid weight gain in early infancy on future body composition and fat deposition.

Data from the Pregnancy, Infection, and Nutrition Study also inform our understanding of the relation of GWG to infant growth [87]. Infants born to women with GWG up to 199 % of the 2009 Institute of Medicine (IOM) recommendations had higher weight for age and length for age z-scores between birth and 3 years of age than women with appropriate GWG, while infants born to women with GWG of 200 % or more of the recommendations experienced higher weight for age, length for age, and weight for length z-scores. These findings were first observed in early infancy and persisted through 3 years of age. Also, these associations remained after adjusting for prepregnancy BMI, maternal diabetes prior to pregnancy, and demographic characteristics. The authors note that "in utero programming effects beyond fetal growth" may contribute to persistent faster rates of growth as might the postnatal feeding environment (e.g., feeding behaviors, diet quality) and genetic susceptibility to rapid growth.

Multiple studies suggest that increased GWG in pregnancy is associated with higher growth parameters in the first year of life, through adolescence and into adulthood. The extent to which the accompanying adiposity, hypertension, and lipid abnormalities that track into adulthood are related to subsequent obesity, in utero exposures, or genetic susceptibility remains unclear. Moreover, the association of GWG with childhood BMI and adiposity likely varies by prepregnancy BMI status with inconsistent results reported, although generally stronger relations are found among women who are under or normal weight [13, 88]. Gillman argues that prepregnancy BMI, rather than GWG, is a more relevant, modifiable factor and suggests further need to understand the different components of weight gain during pregnancy including maternal tissue, fluid accumulation, the placenta, and the fetus [89]. Chandler-Laney explored the role of GWG in predicting lean mass at 12 months and found no association independent of prepregnancy BMI [86], while others, as reviewed by Poston, have reported associations between GWG and greater fat mass later in childhood and adulthood [90].

Further work is needed to understand the independent effects of prepregnancy BMI and GWG on infant growth and body composition in order to design more effective interventions [91]. A two pronged approach of optimizing the health of women prior to pregnancy and assuring appropriate weight gain during pregnancy may be needed to improve pregnancy outcomes and assure that infants start life on a healthy trajectory with regard to nutritional and metabolic status.

Conclusion

Obesity is widely recognized to be associated with multiple chronic diseases and to adversely affect women's health across the life course, regardless of pregnancy status. As discussed in this chapter, obesity and inappropriate weight gain during pregnancy have detrimental consequences for women's health, birth outcomes, and infant growth in the first year of life. Reducing obesity prior to pregnancy has the potential to address modifiable behavioral, social, and environmental factors that may predispose both women and their infants to excessive weight gain and to establish healthy trajectories that are more likely to achieve healthy weight for both. It also has potential to decrease health care utilization by decreasing the incidence of chronic conditions resulting from obesity-related effects in the mother such as gestational hypertension and diabetes.

Interventions that address obesity among women prior to pregnancy are limited to date but have the potential to improve women's health, improve birth outcomes, and predispose children to optimal health, healthy weight, and physical activity. Interventions that address GWG may have additional positive impacts but may be too little or too late and should be considered as adjunct therapies in addition to addressing maternal obesity. If these interventions, particularly related to diet and physical activity, have long-term impact including behavior change, then they should be part of a life course strategy to maintain healthy weight in women. Long-term evidence, however, is not available.

Pregnancy provides an important opportunity to instill and reinforce positive lifelong habits for women and their infants, particularly among women who have not been receiving routine health care services. The Affordable Care Act, which promotes delivery of preventive services through a yearly well women visit without copayments or other cost sharing mechanisms for women, provides an important opportunity to deliver more regular health care services to women prior to pregnancy. This approach includes an opportunity to recognize and address obesity among women of childbearing age.

References

1. Huffman MD, Capewell S, Ning H, Shay CM, Ford ES, Lloyd-Jones DM. Cardiovascular health behavior and health factor changes (1988–2008) and projections to 2020: results from the National Health and Nutrition Examination Surveys. Circulation. 2012;125(21): 2595–602.
2. Ogden CL, Carroll MD, Kit BK, Flegal KM. Prevalence of obesity and trends in body mass index among US children and adolescents, 1999–2010. JAMA. 2012;307(5):483–90.

3. Flegal KM, Carroll MD, Kit BK, Ogden CL. Prevalence of obesity and trends in the distribution of body mass index among US adults, 1999–2010. JAMA. 2012;307(5):491–7.
4. Flegal KM, Carroll MD, Ogden CL, Curtin LR. Prevalence and trends in obesity among US adults, 1999–2008. JAMA. 2010;303(3):235–41.
5. Gordon-Larsen P, The NS, Adair LS. Longitudinal trends in obesity in the United States from adolescence to the third decade of life. Obesity (Silver Spring). 2010;18(9):1801–4.
6. Lee H, Lee D, Guo G, Harris KM. Trends in body mass index in adolescence and young adulthood in the United States: 1959–2002. J Adolesc Health. 2011;49(6):601–8.
7. Grabner M. BMI trends, socioeconomic status, and the choice of dataset. Obes Facts. 2012;5(1):112–26.
8. Rossen LM, Schoendorf KC. Measuring health disparities: trends in racial-ethnic and socioeconomic disparities in obesity among 2- to 18-year old youth in the United States, 2001–2010. Ann Epidemiol. 2012;22(10):698–704.
9. Marshall NE, Spong CY. Obesity, pregnancy complications, and birth outcomes. Semin Reprod Med. 2012;30(6):465–71.
10. Bobrow KL, Quigley MA, Green J, Reeves GK, Beral V. Persistent effects of women's parity and breastfeeding patterns on their body mass index: results from the Million Women Study. Int J Obes (Lond). 2013;37(5):712–7.
11. Lee SK, Sobal J, Frongillo EA, Olson CM, Wolfe WS. Parity and body weight in the United States: differences by race and size of place of residence. Obes Res. 2005;13(7):1263–9.
12. Wolfe WS, Sobal J, Olson CM, Frongillo Jr EA. Parity-associated body weight: modification by sociodemographic and behavioral factors. Obes Res. 1997;5(2):131–41.
13. Oken E. Maternal and child obesity: the causal link. Obstet Gynecol Clin North Am. 2009;36(2):361–77, ix–x.
14. Poston L, Harthoorn LF, Van Der Beek EM. Obesity in pregnancy: implications for the mother and lifelong health of the child. A consensus statement. Pediatr Res. 2010;69(2):175–80.
15. Stothard KJ, Tennant PW, Bell R, Rankin J. Maternal overweight and obesity and the risk of congenital anomalies: a systematic review and meta-analysis. JAMA. 2009;301(6):636–50.
16. Salihu HM, Dunlop AL, Hedayatzadeh M, Alio AP, Kirby RS, Alexander GR. Extreme obesity and risk of stillbirth among black and white gravidas. Obstet Gynecol. 2007;110(3):552–7.
17. Flenady V, Koopmans L, Middleton P, Froen JF, Smith GC, Gibbons K, et al. Major risk factors for stillbirth in high-income countries: a systematic review and meta-analysis. Lancet. 2011;377(9774):1331–40.
18. Ovesen P, Rasmussen S, Kesmodel U. Effect of prepregnancy maternal overweight and obesity on pregnancy outcome. Obstet Gynecol. 2011;118(2 Pt 1):305–12.

19. Catalano PM, Ehrenberg HM. The short- and long-term implications of maternal obesity on the mother and her offspring. BJOG. 2006;113(10):1126–33.
20. Yu Z, Han S, Zhu J, Sun X, Ji C, Guo X. Pre-pregnancy body mass index in relation to infant birth weight and offspring overweight/obesity: a systematic review and meta-analysis. PLoS One. 2013;8(4): e61627.
21. Catalano PM, McIntyre HD, Cruickshank JK, McCance DR, Dyer AR, Metzger BE, et al. The hyperglycemia and adverse pregnancy outcome study: associations of GDM and obesity with pregnancy outcomes. Diabetes Care. 2012;35(4):780–6.
22. Black MH, Sacks DA, Xiang AH, Lawrence JM. The relative contribution of prepregnancy overweight and obesity, gestational weight gain, and IADPSG-defined gestational diabetes mellitus to fetal overgrowth. Diabetes Care. 2013;36(1):56–62.
23. Weng SF, Redsell SA, Swift JA, Yang M, Glazebrook CP. Systematic review and meta-analyses of risk factors for childhood overweight identifiable during infancy. Arch Dis Child. 2012;97(12):1019–26.
24. Ehrenthal DB, Maiden K, Rao A, West DW, Gidding SS, Bartoshesky L, et al. Independent relation of maternal prenatal factors to early childhood obesity in the offspring. Obstet Gynecol. 2013;121(1):115–21.
25. Rooney BL, Mathiason MA, Schauberger CW. Predictors of obesity in childhood, adolescence, and adulthood in a birth cohort. Matern Child Health J. 2010;15(8):1166–75.
26. Weiss JL, Malone FD, Emig D, Ball RH, Nyberg DA, Comstock CH, et al. Obesity, obstetric complications and cesarean delivery rate–a population-based screening study. Am J Obstet Gynecol. 2004;190(4): 1091–7.
27. Cedergren MI. Maternal morbid obesity and the risk of adverse pregnancy outcome. Obstet Gynecol. 2004;103(2):219–24.
28. Chu SY, Kim SY, Schmid CH, Dietz PM, Callaghan WM, Lau J, et al. Maternal obesity and risk of cesarean delivery: a meta-analysis. Obes Rev. 2007;8(5):385–94.
29. Eiben G, Lissner L. Health hunters–an intervention to prevent overweight and obesity in young high-risk women. Int J Obes (Lond). 2006;30(4):691–6.
30. Poobalan AS, Aucott LS, Precious E, Crombie IK, Smith WC. Weight loss interventions in young people (18 to 25 year olds): a systematic review. Obes Rev. 2010;11(8):580–92.
31. Levine MD, Klem ML, Kalarchian MA, Wing RR, Weissfeld L, Qin L, et al. Weight gain prevention among women. Obesity (Silver Spring). 2007;15(5):1267–77.
32. Lewis BA, Martinson BC, Sherwood NE, Avery MD. A pilot study evaluating a telephone-based exercise intervention for pregnant and postpartum women. J Midwifery Womens Health. 2011;56(2): 127–31.

33. Lombard C, Deeks A, Jolley D, Teede HJ. Preventing weight gain: the baseline weight related behaviors and delivery of a randomized controlled intervention in community based women. BMC Public Health. 2009;9:2.
34. Lombard CB, Deeks AA, Ball K, Jolley D, Teede HJ. Weight, physical activity and dietary behavior change in young mothers: short term results of the HeLP-her cluster randomized controlled trial. Nutr J. 2009;8:17.
35. Pickett-Blakely OE, Huizinga MM, Clark JM. Sociodemographic trends in bariatric surgery utilization in the USA. Obes Surg. 2012;22(5):838–42.
36. Kelleher DC, Merrill CT, Cottrell LT, Nadler EP, Burd RS. Recent national trends in the use of adolescent inpatient bariatric surgery: 2000 through 2009. JAMA Pediatr. 2013;167(2):126–32.
37. Karmon A, Sheiner E. Pregnancy after bariatric surgery: a comprehensive review. Arch Gynecol Obstet. 2008;277(5):381–8.
38. Kjaer MM, Nilas L. Pregnancy after bariatric surgery–a review of benefits and risks. Acta Obstet Gynecol Scand. 2013;92(3):264–71.
39. Maggard MA, Yermilov I, Li Z, Maglione M, Newberry S, Suttorp M, et al. Pregnancy and fertility following bariatric surgery: a systematic review. JAMA. 2008;300(19):2286–96.
40. Guelinckx I, Devlieger R, Vansant G. Reproductive outcome after bariatric surgery: a critical review. Hum Reprod Update. 2009;15(2):189–201.
41. Vrebosch L, Bel S, Vansant G, Guelinckx I, Devlieger R. Maternal and neonatal outcome after laparoscopic adjustable gastric banding: a systematic review. Obes Surg. 2012;22(10):1568–79.
42. Lesko J, Peaceman A. Pregnancy outcomes in women after bariatric surgery compared with obese and morbidly obese controls. Obstet Gynecol. 2012;119(3):547–54.
43. American College of Obstetricians and Gynecologists. ACOG practice bulletin no. 105: bariatric surgery and pregnancy. Obstet Gynecol. 2009;113(6):1405–13.
44. Nieuwenhuis-Ruifrok AE, Kuchenbecker WK, Hoek A, Middleton P, Norman RJ. Insulin sensitizing drugs for weight loss in women of reproductive age who are overweight or obese: systematic review and meta-analysis. Hum Reprod Update. 2009;15(1):57–68.
45. Wilcox S, Sharpe PA, Parra-Medina D, Granner M, Hutto B. A randomized trial of a diet and exercise intervention for overweight and obese women from economically disadvantaged neighborhoods: sisters taking action for real success (STARS). Contemp Clin Trials. 2011;32(6):931–45.
46. Oliveira V, Frazao E. The WIC program: background, trends, and economic issues, 2009 Edition. Economic Research Report No. (ERR-73). April 2009. Available from: http://www.ers.usda.gov/publications/err-economic-research-report/err73.aspx. Cited 3 June 2013.

47. Rasmussen KM, Yaktine AL. Weight gain during pregnancy: reexamining the guidelines. Washington, DC: The National Academies Press; 2009.
48. Headen IE, Davis EM, Mujahid MS, Abrams B. Racial-ethnic differences in pregnancy-related weight. Adv Nutr. 2012;3(1):83–94.
49. Rasmussen KM, Abrams B, Bodnar LM, Butte NF, Catalano PM, Maria Siega-Riz A. Recommendations for weight gain during pregnancy in the context of the obesity epidemic. Obstet Gynecol. 2009;116(5):1191–5.
50. Caulfield LE, Witter FR, Stoltzfus RJ. Determinants of gestational weight gain outside the recommended ranges among black and white women. Obstet Gynecol. 1996;87(5 Pt 1):760–6.
51. Katon J, Reiber G, Williams MA, Yanez D, Miller E. Weight loss after diagnosis with gestational diabetes and birth weight among overweight and obese women. Matern Child Health J. 2013; 17(2):374–83.
52. Maloni JA, Margevicius SP, Damato EG. Multiple gestation: side effects of antepartum bed rest. Biol Res Nurs. 2006;8(2):115–28.
53. Siega-Riz AM, Viswanathan M, Moos MK, Deierlein A, Mumford S, Knaack J, et al. A systematic review of outcomes of maternal weight gain according to the Institute of Medicine recommendations: birth weight, fetal growth, and postpartum weight retention. Am J Obstet Gynecol. 2009;201(4):339 e1–14.
54. Bodnar LM, Siega-Riz AM, Simhan HN, Himes KP, Abrams B. Severe obesity, gestational weight gain, and adverse birth outcomes. Am J Clin Nutr. 2010;91(6):1642–8.
55. Nohr EA, Vaeth M, Baker JL, Sorensen TI, Olsen J, Rasmussen KM. Pregnancy outcomes related to gestational weight gain in women defined by their body mass index, parity, height, and smoking status. Am J Clin Nutr. 2009;90(5):1288–94.
56. Kramer MS, McLean FH, Eason EL, Usher RH. Maternal nutrition and spontaneous preterm birth. Am J Epidemiol. 1992;136(5): 574–83.
57. Ferraro ZM, Barrowman N, Prud'homme D, Walker M, Wen SW, Rodger M, et al. Excessive gestational weight gain predicts large for gestational age neonates independent of maternal body mass index. J Matern Fetal Neonatal Med. 2012;25(5):538–42.
58. Vesco KK, Sharma AJ, Dietz PM, Rizzo JH, Callaghan WM, England L, et al. Newborn size among obese women with weight gain outside the 2009 Institute of Medicine recommendation. Obstet Gynecol. 2011;117(4):812–8.
59. Heude B, Thiebaugeorges O, Goua V, Forhan A, Kaminski M, Foliguet B, et al. Pre-pregnancy body mass index and weight gain during pregnancy: relations with gestational diabetes and hypertension, and birth outcomes. Matern Child Health J. 2012;16(2):355–63.

60. Gibson KS, Waters TP, Catalano PM. Maternal weight gain in women who develop gestational diabetes mellitus. Obstet Gynecol. 2012;119(3):560–5.
61. Herring SJ, Oken E, Rifas-Shiman SL, Rich-Edwards JW, Stuebe AM, Kleinman KP, et al. Weight gain in pregnancy and risk of maternal hyperglycemia. Am J Obstet Gynecol. 2009;201(1):61 e1–7.
62. Thangaratinam S, Rogozinska E, Jolly K, Glinkowski S, Duda W, Borowiack E, et al. Interventions to reduce or prevent obesity in pregnant women: a systematic review. Health Technol Assess. 2012;16(31):iii–iv, 1–191.
63. Thangaratinam S, Rogozinska E, Jolly K, Glinkowski S, Roseboom T, Tomlinson JW, et al. Effects of interventions in pregnancy on maternal weight and obstetric outcomes: meta-analysis of randomised evidence. BMJ. 2012;344:e2088.
64. Oteng-Ntim E, Varma R, Croker H, Poston L, Doyle P. Lifestyle interventions for overweight and obese pregnant women to improve pregnancy outcome: systematic review and meta-analysis. BMC Med. 2012;10:47.
65. Dodd JM, Grivell RM, Crowther CA, Robinson JS. Antenatal interventions for overweight or obese pregnant women: a systematic review of randomised trials. BJOG. 2010;117(11):1316–26.
66. Skouteris H, Hartley-Clark L, McCabe M, Milgrom J, Kent B, Herring SJ, et al. Preventing excessive gestational weight gain: a systematic review of interventions. Obes Rev. 2010;11(11):757–68.
67. Tanentsapf I, Heitmann BL, Adegboye AR. Systematic review of clinical trials on dietary interventions to prevent excessive weight gain during pregnancy among normal weight, overweight and obese women. BMC Pregnancy Childbirth. 2011;11:81.
68. Ronnberg AK, Nilsson K. Interventions during pregnancy to reduce excessive gestational weight gain: a systematic review assessing current clinical evidence using the Grading of Recommendations, Assessment, Development and Evaluation (GRADE) system. BJOG. 2010;117(11):1327–34.
69. Brown MJ, Sinclair M, Liddle D, Hill AJ, Madden E, Stockdale J. A systematic review investigating healthy lifestyle interventions incorporating goal setting strategies for preventing excess gestational weight gain. PLoS One. 2012;7(7):e39503.
70. Gardner B, Wardle J, Poston L, Croker H. Changing diet and physical activity to reduce gestational weight gain: a meta-analysis. Obes Rev. 2011;12(7):e602–20.
71. Streuling I, Beyerlein A, Rosenfeld E, Hofmann H, Schulz T, von Kries R. Physical activity and gestational weight gain: a meta-analysis of intervention trials. BJOG. 2012;118(3):278–84.
72. Sui Z, Grivell RM, Dodd JM. Antenatal exercise to improve outcomes in overweight or obese women: a systematic review. Acta Obstet Gynecol Scand. 2012;91(5):538–45.
73. US Department of Health and Human Services. Office of Disease Prevention and Health Promotion. Healthy people 2020. Washington,

DC. Available from: http://www.healthypeople.gov/2020/topicsobjectives2020/objectiveslist.aspx?topicid=26. Cited 13 Jan 2013.
74. Breastfeeding and the use of human milk. Pediatrics. 2012;129(3): e827–41.
75. Wojcicki JM. Maternal prepregnancy body mass index and initiation and duration of breastfeeding: a review of the literature. J Womens Health (Larchmt). 2011;20(3):341–7.
76. Kitsantas P, Pawloski LR. Maternal obesity, health status during pregnancy, and breastfeeding initiation and duration. J Matern Fetal Neonatal Med. 2010;23(2):135–41.
77. Guelinckx I, Devlieger R, Bogaerts A, Pauwels S, Vansant G. The effect of pre-pregnancy BMI on intention, initiation and duration of breast-feeding. Public Health Nutr. 2012;15(5):840–8.
78. Mehta UJ, Siega-Riz AM, Herring AH, Adair LS, Bentley ME. Pregravid body mass index, psychological factors during pregnancy and breastfeeding duration: is there a link? Matern Child Nutr. 2012;8(4):423–33.
79. Dubois L, Girard M. Early determinants of overweight at 4.5 years in a population-based longitudinal study. Int J Obes (Lond). 2006; 30(4):610–7.
80. Nader PR, O'Brien M, Houts R, Bradley R, Belsky J, Crosnoe R, et al. Identifying risk for obesity in early childhood. Pediatrics. 2006;118(3):e594–601.
81. Taveras EM, Rifas-Shiman SL, Sherry B, Oken E, Haines J, Kleinman K, et al. Crossing growth percentiles in infancy and risk of obesity in childhood. Arch Pediatr Adolesc Med. 2011;165(11):993–8.
82. Dunger DB, Salgin B, Ong KK. Session 7: Early nutrition and later health early developmental pathways of obesity and diabetes risk. Proc Nutr Soc. 2007;66(3):451–7.
83. Leunissen RW, Kerkhof GF, Stijnen T, Hokken-Koelega A. Timing and tempo of first-year rapid growth in relation to cardiovascular and metabolic risk profile in early adulthood. JAMA. 2009;301(21): 2234–42.
84. Monteiro PO, Victora CG. Rapid growth in infancy and childhood and obesity in later life–a systematic review. Obes Rev. 2005;6(2): 143–54.
85. Deierlein AL, Siega-Riz AM, Adair LS, Herring AH. Effects of pre-pregnancy body mass index and gestational weight gain on infant anthropometric outcomes. J Pediatr. 2011;158(2):221–6.
86. Chandler-Laney PC, Gower BA, Fields DA. Gestational and early life influences on infant body composition at 1 year. Obesity (Silver Spring). 2013;21(1):144–8.
87. Deierlein AL, Siega-Riz AM, Herring AH, Adair LS, Daniels JL. Gestational weight gain and predicted changes in offspring anthropometrics between early infancy and 3 years. Pediatr Obes. 2012;7(2):134–42.
88. President's Council of Advisors on Science and Technology. Report to the president realizing the full potential of health information

technology to improve healthcare for Americans: the path forward. 2010. Available from: http://www.whitehouse.gov/sites/default/files/microsites/ostp/pcast-health-it-report.pdf. Cited 9 Sep 2013.
89. Gillman MW. Gestational weight gain: now and the future. Circulation. 2012;125(11):1339–40.
90. Poston L. Gestational weight gain: influences on the long-term health of the child. Curr Opin Clin Nutr Metab Care. 2012;15(3):252–7.
91. Zhang S, Rattanatray L, Morrison JL, Nicholas LM, Lie S, McMillen IC. Maternal obesity and the early origins of childhood obesity: weighing up the benefits and costs of maternal weight loss in the periconceptional period for the offspring. Exp Diabetes Res. 2011;2011:585749.

Part IV
Meeting Future Challenges

Chapter 11
Maternal Obesity and Implications for the Long-Term Health of the Offspring

Kesha Baptiste-Roberts

Abstract The current epidemic of obesity among women of childbearing age has serious implications for both the woman and her potential offspring. The adverse pregnancy outcomes associated with maternal obesity, as well as the long-term implications for the mothers' health, are well established. However, there is increasing evidence indicating that offspring of obese mothers have an increased risk of obesity, cardiometabolic risk, adverse neurodevelopmental outcomes, and respiratory challenges, which follow them all the way to adulthood. This chapter provides clinicians and researchers with an overview of the long-term health implications for offspring exposed to maternal obesity.

Keywords Maternal obesity • Developmental programming • Offspring health • Cardiometabolic risk • Neurodevelopmental outcomes • Asthma

---

K. Baptiste-Roberts, PhD, MPH
School of Nursing and College of Medicine,
Department of Public Health Sciences,
The Pennsylvania State University, Heshey, PA, USA
e-mail: kab50@psu.edu

W. Nicholson, K. Baptiste-Roberts (eds.),
Obesity During Pregnancy in Clinical Practice,
DOI 10.1007/978-1-4471-2831-1_11,
© Springer-Verlag London 2014

Key Points
- There is substantial evidence linking maternal obesity and excessive gestational weight gain to an increased risk for obesity in the offspring.
- Although only a small body of evidence exists, there is a link between maternal obesity and adverse neurodevelopmental outcomes and asthma.
- The evidence available on the long-term health impact of exposure to maternal obesity during pregnancy warrants the development of intervention strategies targeting reduction of obesity in women of reproductive age prior to initiating pregnancy.
- Future research should focus on the conduct of human studies to elucidate the mechanisms underlying the associations between maternal obesity and long-term offspring health.

Introduction

Given the epidemic increase in overweight/obesity in the United States, it is not surprising that national data show that a substantial number of women begin pregnancy either overweight (12.1 %) or obese (22 %) [1]. In a recent study including 75,403 women from 26 states and New York City, the authors report that one in five women who delivered a live birth were obese [2]. Of this group of women, non-Hispanic blacks had approximately a 70 % higher prevalence of obesity when compared to non-Hispanic whites and Hispanics (black: 28.9 %; white: 17.4 %; Hispanic: 17.4 %) [2].

Maternal obesity is of great significance not only because of adverse effects on maternal health and pregnancy outcomes, but also because of the growing evidence of persistent deleterious effects on the offspring. As detailed in Chap. 9, maternal obesity is associated with short-term risk in the offspring, but there is increasing evidence that maternal obesity may have longer-term influences on offspring health, which may be in part attributed to shared genetic and environmental factors in addition to developmental programming. As such, the potential social and economic costs in terms of health of future generations present a significant burden.

Developmental Programming

There is a growing body of evidence suggesting that events in utero have long-term influences on disease risk later in life [3]. In 1977, epidemiologic studies of Anders Forsdahl in Norway demonstrated a causative link between early-life environmental factors and subsequent disease [4]. More recently, David Barker and colleagues in the United Kingdom have expanded this area of research, giving birth to the *fetal origins hypothesis* which proposes that changes in fetal nutrition and endocrine status result in developmental adaptations that can cause permanent structural, physiological, and metabolic changes in a fetus, which predisposes him/her to cardiovascular, metabolic, and endocrine disease in adult life [3]. Recently this idea of developmental programming has been described as the *developmental origins of health and disease* [*DOHaD*] which proposes that the conditions presented during a critical window of development can lead to permanent programmed alterations in physiology [5]. Over the last decade, population-based studies conducted in the United Kingdom, Sweden, Finland, Japan, India, and the United States consistently support the idea of developmental programming of adult disease [6]. These studies have primarily focused on the effect of undernutrition and low offspring birth weight on increased risk of cardiovascular disease, type 2 diabetes, and hypertension, all of which share obesity as a common risk factor. Moreover, these studies provided the basis for the *thrifty phenotype* hypothesis, where the developing fetus adapts to an adverse intrauterine environment and has a survival advantage if the post birth environment is also poor, but these adaptations may be not well suited to an abundant postnatal environment [7].

Maternal obesity and intrauterine overnutrition are not commonly studied programming factors. However, given the rise in maternal obesity, recent studies have focused on the detrimental effects of intrauterine overnutrition. The pregnant obese mother has increased levels of circulating inflammatory cytokines, increased insulin resistance, glucose levels and lipids, and an elevated supply of nutrients to the developing fetus. A developmental overnutrition hypothesis has been developed which proposes that increased fuel supply to the developing fetus leads to permanent changes in offspring metabolism, behavior, appetite regulation with increased risk of obesity, metabolic, and behavioral problems in adult life [5, 8, 9]. Most of the studies designed to test the overnutrition hypothesis have been primarily conducted using animal models which allows for in depth investigation of the complex pathways involved. These pathways are quite complex and multifactorial. There is the complex maternal-fetal relationship during pregnancy and the potential influence of the postnatal environment. As such, it is difficult to disentangle these effects in human studies. In this developing area, most of the research thus far report phenotypic outcomes, but the underlying mechanisms are yet to be understood.

Consequences of Maternal Obesity on Offspring Outcomes

We have only recently begun to investigate the influence of maternal obesity on long-term offspring outcomes. This is due in part to the lack of suitable data sets with good records on maternal obesity prior to and during pregnancy and offspring of a suitable age to manifest outcomes of interest. However, there is accumulating evidence of the influence of maternal obesity on childhood and adolescent obesity, as well as metabolic outcomes including insulin resistance, hypertension dyslipidemia, adverse neurodevelopmental outcomes, and asthma.

Obesity

Offspring obesity risk is the most studied long-term effect of maternal obesity. There is consistent evidence, which suggests that maternal obesity has long-term detrimental effects on offspring obesity risk [8]. Several studies have demonstrated a relationship between increased pre-pregnancy body mass index [BMI] and maternal BMI during pregnancy with increased BMI in the offspring [8, 10–15]. One large cohort study with 8,400 children, reported that children born to obese mothers (using BMI in the first trimester) were twice as likely to be obese by 2 years of age [10]. This risk of obesity persisted with increasing age, such that for women with BMI ≥30, the prevalence of childhood obesity in their offspring at ages 2, 3, and 4 years was 15.1, 20.6, and 24.2 %, respectively. Offspring of obese mothers had between 2.4 and 2.7 times the obesity prevalence of offspring of mothers with normal BMI (18.5–24.9 kg/m^2) at the different ages assessed. In addition, there is also evidence of alterations in body composition of offspring of obese mothers, specifically fat mass [16–18]. In several studies, the influence of maternal obesity on offspring obesity persists into adulthood even after adjustment for current lifestyle factors up until the age of 31 [8].

Gestational Weight Gain

In humans, there are no studies addressing overnutrition specifically during pregnancy; however, gestational weight gain may closely reflect this exposure in utero for the developing fetus. A number of studies have demonstrated an association between maternal gestational weight gain and later obesity in childhood [19–21], adolescence [12, 22, 23], and early adulthood [15, 24, 25], while some have not shown this association [26, 27]. The effects in these studies are less than that observed with maternal obesity, but given the high prevalence of excessive gestational weight gain, these associations are important. Nevertheless, there is some evidence that the effect of excessive gestational weight gain is stronger among underweight/normal weight women [24]. In contrast, there is evidence showing modest association between excessive gestational weight gain among normal weight women and a stronger association among mothers with higher pre-pregnancy BMI [15]. Interestingly, Stuebe et al. [15] also reported an increased risk of offspring obesity for obese mothers who gained less than 15 lb, thus suggesting the importance of adequate nutrition during fetal development.

Interpregnancy weight gain is another important contributor to offspring obesity. Maternal weight gain and increased BMI between pregnancies has also been found to be associated with increased risk of overweight in offspring compared with their siblings [28]. In addition, interventional strategies to reduce the weight of obese women via bariatric surgery also reduce the risk of obesity in subsequent offspring compared to those born before the weight loss intervention [29, 30]. These data show a disproportionate risk in offspring from the same mother under different in utero conditions. One 21 year prospective study [24] reported that the offspring of mothers who became overweight or remained overweight or obese over 21 years were more likely to be overweight at age 21. These results persisted even after adjustment for age, education, tobacco consumption during pregnancy, offspring birth weight, breastfeeding, TV watching, sports participation, and family meals. These findings suggest that if mothers maintain a healthy weight over a long postpartum period, their offspring may have a reduced risk of obesity.

Although there is consistent evidence of an association between maternal obesity and offspring obesity risk, the mechanisms underpinning this association are not well understood. However, the use of animal models has highlighted the possible role of altered leptin production and regulation, changes in hypothalamic regulation of key genes involving appetite control and energy balance, alterations in skeletal muscle metabolism, and altered placental structure and function [8].

Metabolic Outcomes

Human studies assessing the relationship between maternal obesity and offspring cardiometabolic risk are limited. A small number of studies have explored other cardiometabolic outcomes such as insulin sensitivity, glucose levels, lipids, and even type 2 diabetes. These studies are summarized in Table 11.1.

There have only been a few studies to examine the relationship between maternal obesity and blood pressure [31–35]. Most of these have examined blood pressure during childhood only [31–33], and just one study has examined offspring blood pressure during adolescence [34] and in adulthood, respectively [35]. These studies consistently report a significantly positive association between maternal obesity and blood pressure as shown in Table 11.1. To our knowledge, to date, only two studies have examined the association between maternal obesity and metabolic markers such as insulin and glucose in offspring beyond 1 year. Mingrone et al. [37] compared insulin sensitivity, insulin secretion, and body composition in offspring of obese mothers with those born to mothers with normal weight. They found that offspring of obese mothers were significantly more insulin resistant (410 ± 91 vs. 500 ± 60 ml^{-1} · min^{-1}) and had higher prevalence of hyperinsulinemia than offspring of normal weight mothers, but found no difference in β-cell glucose sensitivity impairment. Similarly, in the Jewish Perinatal Family Follow-Up Study birth cohort, Hochner and colleagues investigated the association between maternal obesity and cardiometabolic risk factors in offspring at age 32 [35]. In this study, maternal obesity was independently associated with insulin, triglycerides levels, and lower HDL as shown in Table 11.1. These findings concur with the findings of Catalano et al. who reported that at birth, offspring of obese mothers had higher insulin resistance, leptin, and IL-6, suggesting that maternal obesity results in a high cardiometabolic risk phenotype, with increased cardiometabolic risk beginning at birth [38]. One study [11] examined the association between maternal obesity and metabolic syndrome in offspring. Boney et al. [11] reported an independent effect of maternal obesity on risk of metabolic syndrome in a study of 179 children at ages 6–11 years.

TABLE 11.1 Obesity during pregnancy and offspring cardiometabolic disease risk

Series (year) [reference]	Design	Sample/setting	Maternal obesity measure	Cardiometabolic outcome	Age at follow-up	Key findings
Blood pressure						
Filler et al. (2008) [31]	Cohort	Children's Hospital, London Health Science Centre, UK $N=1,915$ children	Pre-pregnancy BMI reported retrospectively by mother at 24–28 weeks GA	Systolic blood pressure [SBP] and diastolic blood pressure [DBP]	Mean age = 8.3 ± 5.2 years	BMI z-score correlated significantly with SBP (Spearman $r=0.214, p<0.0001$), and DBP z-scores (Spearman $r=0.143, p<0.0001$)
Lawlor et al. (2004) [32]	Cohort	Mater-University study of pregnancy and its outcomes (MUSP) $N=3,864$	Maternal pre-pregnancy BMI	Systolic blood pressure [SBP]	5	For every standard deviation unit increase in maternal pre-pregnancy BMI, there was a 0.38 increase in SBP, respectively ($p<0.05$), after adjustment for potential confounders
Wen et al. (2011) [33]	Cohort	Collaborative Perinatal Project $N=30,461$	Maternal pre-pregnancy BMI	Systolic blood pressure [SBP]	7	Compared to normal weight, pre-pregnancy overweight obesity was associated with a higher offspring SBP (0.89 mmHg 95 % CI: 0.52, 1.26)

Laor et al. (1997) [34]	Cohort	Jerusalem $N=10{,}883$	Maternal pre-pregnancy BMI	Systolic blood pressure [SBP] and diastolic blood pressure [DBP] from military draft records	17	*Women*: Pearson correlation 0.053 and 0.049 for SBP and DBP, respectively *Men*: Pearson correlation 0.053 and 0.060 for SBP and DBP, respectively
Hochner et al. (2012) [35]	Cohort	Jerusalem Perinatal Study [JPS] $N=1{,}400$	Maternal pre-pregnancy BMI	Systolic blood pressure [SBP] and diastolic blood pressure [DBP]	32	For every unit increase in maternal pre-pregnancy BMI, there was a 0.441 and a 0.287 increase in SBP and DBP, respectively ($p<0.05$)
Fraser et al. (2010) [36]	Cohort	Avon Longitudinal Study of Parents and Children [ALSPAC] $N=3{,}457$	Maternal pre-pregnancy weight	Systolic blood pressure [SBP] and diastolic blood pressure [DBP]	9	For every unit increase in maternal pre-pregnancy weight, there was a 0.108 increase in SBP (95 % CI: 0.087, 0.130) For every unit increase in maternal pre-pregnancy weight, there was a 0.028 increase in SBP (95 % CI: 0.013, 0.043)

(continued)

TABLE 11.1 (continued)

Metabolic markers

Series (year) [reference]	Design	Sample/setting	Maternal obesity measure	Cardiometabolic outcome	Age at follow-up	Key findings
Mingrone et al. (2008) [37]	Case control	$N=67$ Cases=52 Offspring of mothers with BMI ≥ 30 kg/m^2 Control=15 Offspring of mothers with normal weight, BMI <25 kg/m^2	Maternal pre-pregnancy BMI	Insulin sensitivity calculated from OGTT	23.8 ± 4.5 years	Cases were more insulin resistant than controls *Women:* (398.58 ± 79.32 vs. 513.81 ± 70.70 ml$^{-1} \cdot$ min^{-1}, $p<0.0001$; *Men:* $416.42 \_ 76.17$ vs. 484.242 ± 45.76 ml$^{-1} \cdot$ min^{-1}, $p<0.05$) Insulin secretion after OGTT was higher in cases than control *Men:* (63.94 ± 21.20 vs. 35.71 ± 10.02 nmol $\cdot$ m^{-2}, $p<0.01$) but did not differ significantly in women

| Hochner et al. (2012) [35] | Cohort | Jerusalem Perinatal Study [JPS] $N=1,400$ | Maternal pre-pregnancy BMI | Insulin Glucose LDL HDL Triglycerides | 32 | For every unit increase in maternal pre-pregnancy BMI, there was a 0.008 increase in insulin ($p=0.007$) For every unit increase in maternal pre-pregnancy BMI there was a 0.001 decrease in glucose ($p=0.875$) For every unit increase in maternal pre-pregnancy BMI, there was a 0.010 decrease in HDL ($p=0.033$) For every unit increase in maternal pre-pregnancy BMI, there was a 0.012 ($p=0.240$) and a 0.007 ($p=0.020$) increase in LDL and triglycerides, respectively |

(continued)

TABLE 11.1 (continued)

Series (year) [reference]	Design	Sample/setting	Maternal obesity measure	Cardiometabolic outcome	Age at follow-up	Key findings
Fraser et al. (2010) [36]	Cohort	Avon Longitudinal Study of Parents and Children [ALSPAC] $N=3,457$	Maternal pre-pregnancy weight	Lipids: HDL, triglycerides	9	For every unit increase in maternal pre-pregnancy weight, there was a 0.002 decrease in HDL (95 % CI: −0.003, −0.001) For every unit increase in maternal pre-pregnancy weight, there was a 1.002 increase in triglycerides (95 % CI: 1.000, 1.003)

OGTT: 75 g oral glucose tolerance test

Asthma

Previous studies have found that obesity and asthma occur concurrently in both children and adults. However, the causal direction and mechanisms are not understood [39]. Overweight is associated with increased levels of proinflammatory cytokines. As such, offspring of obese mothers are exposed to increased levels of proinflammatory cytokines during fetal development which may affect the immunological and pulmonary development and result in asthma symptoms after birth. There is a very small body of literature on the association between maternal obesity and asthma and asthma-related symptoms [40–46]. All of these studies consistently show an increased risk of asthma [41, 43–46] or wheezing [40, 42] as shown in Table 11.2 among children between 6 months and 16 years for offspring of mothers who are obese compared to offspring of nonobese mothers. One study even demonstrated a dose response relationship between the degree of maternal overweight status during pregnancy and increased risk of asthma in the offspring [43].

Neurodevelopmental Outcomes

The cardiovascular and endocrine systems may not be the only systems altered by maternal obesity during pregnancy. In fact, a systematic review suggests that infants born to obese mothers are at increased risk of central nervous system (CNS) developmental problems [47]. There is substantial evidence from animal models which suggests that maternal obesity increases the risk of the development of neurological and psychological dysfunction. Results from extant human studies provide additional support that maternal obesity may be linked to mental health disorders in children as summarized in Table 11.3. In a recent systematic review [58] of 12 studies reviewed, five provided clear support for an association between maternal obesity and neurodevelopmental problems including childhood IQ [53], attention-deficit/hyperactivity disorder [ADHD] [55], schizophrenia [49, 51], and eating disorders [59].

TABLE 11.2 Obesity during pregnancy and asthma in the offspring

Series (year) [reference]	Design	Sample/setting	Maternal obesity measure	Asthma measure	Age at follow-up	Findings
Reichman et al. (2008) [45]	Birth cohort study	Fragile Families and Child Wellbeing study, an ongoing longitudinal birth cohort study 1998–2000 75 hospitals in 20 US cities $N=1,971$	Pre-pregnancy weight and height abstracted from medical record	Maternal interview self-report	3 years	Obese mothers had 52 % higher odds than nonobese mothers of having a child diagnosed with asthma (OR = 1.52; 95 % CI: 1.18, 1.93) in the univariate and a 34 % higher odds (OR = 1.34; 95 % CI: 1.03, 1.76) after adjustment for covariates (sociodemographic, medical obstetric, and behavioral factors)

| Harpsoe et al. (2013) [41] | Danish birth cohort study | $N = 38,874$ mother-child pairs from the Danish National Birth Cohort [DNBC] (enrollment 1996–2002) | Self-reported weight and height measures from baseline interview and self-reported gestational weight gain | Self-reported doctor-diagnosed asthma | 7 years | Compared with children of normal weight mothers, children of mothers with high BMI had significantly increased odds of doctor-diagnosed asthma ever ($p < 0.0001$), children of obese mothers (adjusted OR, 1.54; 95 % CI: 1.34, 1.76) or very obese (adjusted OR, 1.52; 95 % CI: 1.21, 1.91). The odds of doctor-diagnosed asthma ever increased significantly with increasing GWG ($p = 0.01$) with the highest odds among mothers gaining ≥25 kg during pregnancy compared with mothers gaining 10–15 kg (adjusted OR, 1.17; 95 % CI: 1.02, 1.33) |

(continued)

TABLE 11.2 (continued)

Series (year) [reference]	Design	Sample/setting	Maternal obesity measure	Asthma measure	Age at follow-up	Findings
Patel et al. (2012) [44]	Prospective cohort study	Northern Finland birth cohort July 1985–June 1986 $N=6,945$	Pre-pregnancy and height were abstracted from medical record and BMI calculated	Self-reported asthma symptoms	15–16 years	High maternal pre-pregnancy weight was significantly associated with ever asthma in adolescents (OR=1.28, 95 % CI: 1.06, 1.54 and for current asthma; OR=1.30, 95 % CI: 1.01, 1.67 for current asthma) Higher maternal pre-pregnancy weight in the top tertile was significantly associated with an increase in the risk of ever wheeze and current wheeze (OR=1.22, 95 % CI: 1.01, 1.47 and OR=1.52, 95 % CI: 1.19, 1.95), respectively

| Lowe et al. (2011) [43] | Retrospective cohort study | Sweden. All children born in Stockholm County, Sweden between 1998 and 2009 $N=129{,}329$ | BMI calculated from initial antenatal visit (8–10 weeks of gestation) BMI ≥ 30 | Asthma in offspring | Higher maternal BMI was consistently associated with an increased risk of asthma in the child both in terms of medicine use and hospitalization Association was linear at all ages. At age 6–8 years, the effect of maternal BMI was somewhat stronger in girls (OR $=1.04$, 95 % CI: 1.02, 1.05) per unit increase in BMI) than in boys (OR $=1.01$, 95 % CI: 1.00, 1.03); p for interaction $=0.01$) and was also weaker in fourth and subsequent children (p for interaction $=.03$) |

(continued)

TABLE 11.2 (continued)

Series (year) [reference]	Design	Sample/setting	Maternal obesity measure	Asthma measure	Age at follow-up	Findings
Haberg et al. (2009) [40]	Cohort study	Norwegian mother and child cohort study (MoBa) N=33,192	Maternal BMI calculated from self-reported pre-pregnancy weight and height obtained via questionnaire	Lower respiratory tract infections [LRTIs], hospitalization for LRTIs and wheeze reported at 6 and 18 months after birth obtained via self-report	6, 18 months	The risk of wheeze increased linearly with maternal BMI in pregnancy and was 3.3 % higher (95 % CI: 1.2, 5.3) for children with mothers who were obese during pregnancy than for children of mothers with normal BMI
Kumar et al. (2010) [42]	Cohort	N=1,191 Boston Birth Cohort (1998-present) followed to a mean age of 3.0±2.4 years	Self-reported pre-pregnancy weight and height	Recurrent wheezing (4 or more episodes of medically attended wheezing illness in the subject's life time using electronic medical record abstraction)	~3 years	Children of obese mothers (BMI≥30) had an increased risk of recurrent wheezing OR=3.51, 95 % CI: 1.68, 7.32

| Scholtens et al. (2010) [46] | Cohort | $N = 3,963$ participants in the prevention and incidence of asthma and mite allergy study | Self-reported pre-pregnancy weight and height | Self-reported wheeze, dyspnea, and use of prescription inhaled corticosteroids | 8 years | Among children predisposed to asthma ($n = 1,058$, i.e., having at least one parent with asthma), pre-pregnancy overweight was associated with increased risk of asthma at 8 years (OR = 1.52, 95 % CI: 1.05, 2.18) |

OR odds ratio

TABLE 11.3 Obesity during pregnancy and long-term neurodevelopment outcomes in offspring

Series (year) [reference]	Design	Sample/setting	Maternal obesity measure	Neurodevelopmental outcome	Age at follow-up	Key findings
Jones et al. (1998) [48]	Cohort study	Finland ($N=10,578$)	Pre-pregnancy BMI reported retrospectively by mother at 24–28 weeks GA	Schizophrenia (psychiatrist diagnosed using DSM III R)	28 years	Odds ratio [OR] = 2.1, 95 % Confidence Interval [CI]: 0.9, 4.6 for children of mothers with BMI > 29 kg/m^2 compared with children of mothers with BMI 19.1–29.0 kg/m^2
Schaefer et al. (2000) [49]	Cohort study	Child Health Development Study [CHDS], USA Births between 1959 and 1967 63 cases of schizophrenia and 6,570 unaffected offspring	BMI measured at study enrolment by healthcare personnel	Schizophrenia and spectrum disorders diagnosed using the DIGS	30–38 years	Relative Risk [RR] = 2.9, 95 % CI: 1.3, 6.6 for children of mothers with BMI > 30 kg/m^2 compared with BMI 20.0–26.9 kg/m^2

Wahlbeck et al. (2001) [50]	Cohort study	Prospective birth cohort, Finland Births between 1924 and 1933 $N = 7,086$	Late pregnancy BMI from birth records	Schizophrenia diagnoses obtained from Hospital Discharge Register		Offspring had a small increased odds of schizophrenia for each unit decrease in maternal late pregnancy BMI (OR = 1.09, 95 % CI 1.02–1.17) Compared to offspring of mothers with a late pregnancy BMI >30, those with mothers with late pregnancy BMI <30 had around a threefold increased odds of schizophrenia
Kawai et al. (2004) [51]	Case–control study	Japan cases: $N = 52$, controls: $N = 6,570$ born on or after 1966	BMI measured at first and last antenatal care visits by clinic personnel	Schizophrenia (psychiatrist diagnosed using DSM IV)	19	For every 1 unit increase in early pregnancy BMI, odds of schizophrenia increased 24 % (OR = 1.24, 95 % CI 1.02–1.50) For every one unit increase in late pregnancy BMI, odds of schizophrenia increased 19 % (OR = 1.19, 95 % CI 1.00, 1.41)

(continued)

TABLE 11.3 (continued)

Series (year) [reference]	Design	Sample/setting	Maternal obesity measure	Neurodevelopmental outcome	Age at follow-up	Key findings
Krakowiak et al. (2012) [52]	Case–control study	California, USA. Data of children enrolled in the CHARGE (Childhood Autism Risks from Genetics and the Environment) study $N=1,004$; ASD(517), DD(172), Control(315)	BMI ≥ 30, with onset before pregnancy	Autism spectrum disorder [ASD], developmental delays [DD]		The risk of having a child with ASD or DD, relative to typical development [TD] was significantly increased among obese women (ASD, OR: 1.67 [95 % CI: 1.10–2.56]; DD, OR: 2.08 [95 % CI: 1.20–3.61]); >20 % of case mothers were obese compared with 14.3 % of controls. The prevalence of any MC was higher in the ASD (28.6 %) and DD (34.9 %) groups compared with controls (19.4 %), with respective adjusted ORs of 1.61 (95 % CI: 1.10–2.37) and 2.35 (95 % CI: 1.43–3.88).

Neggers et al. (2003) [53]	Prospective cohort study	Sample from a prospective cohort (USA). Mother–children pairs (average age <5 years) ($N=355$), born in 1985–1989	Pre-pregnancy BMI self-reported by mother at ~23 weeks after LMP.	Diminished intellectual ability, but not motor skills.	Maternal pre-pregnancy BMI was a significant negative predictor of IQ ($\beta=-0.25$, $P=0.001$) and nonverbal ability ($\beta=-0.29$, $P=0.02$) Each increase of 1 unit in maternal BMI associated with significantly reduced IQ and nonverbal IQ Overall IQ scores of offspring of obese women were 4.7 points lower and nonverbal scores 5.6 points lower than those whose mothers had normal BMI

(continued)

TABLE 11.3 (continued)

Series (year) [reference]	Design	Sample/setting	Maternal obesity measure	Neurodevelopmental outcome	Age at follow-up	Key findings
Heikura et al. (2008) [54]	Cohort	Two Finnish birth cohorts (1966, N=12,058 and 1986, N=9,032) at <11.5 years old	Pre-pregnancy BMI self-reported retrospectively at 25 weeks after LMP	Intellectual disability (ID – IQ<70)		1966 obese: OR=1.3, 95 % CI: 0.5, 3.1 1986 obese: OR=3.6, 95 % CI: 2.0, 6.6 Maternal obesity is a new disadvantageous factor associated with ID, while low socioeconomic status has remained as the major factor associated with ID
Rodriguez et al. (2008) [55]	Prospective birth cohort	3 Prospective birth cohorts (Scandinavia) 7- to 12-year olds (N=12,556). Born 1978–1987	BMI from medical records at <10 weeks after LMP	ADHD		Positive association between high BMI and/or weight gain in moms and core symptoms of ADHD in school-age offspring. For women with high BMI, weight gain further increased odds (OR=1.24, 95 % CI: 1.07, 1.44). Each unit increase in BMI: OR=1.04, 95 % CI: 1.02, 1.07. Overweight (BMI>26): OR=1.43, 95 % CI: 1.12, 1.83

| Rodriguez (2010) [56] | Prospective birth cohort | Prospective birth cohort (Sweden) 5-year olds ($N=1,714$). Born 1999–2000 | Pre-pregnancy BMI from the Swedish Medical Birth Register | ADHD symptom scores (mother and teacher rated) | Parent report: no increased odds for any outcome
Teacher report:
Overweight:
Inattention: OR=2.00, 95 % CI: 1.20, 3.35
Hyperactivity: insignificant
Negative emotionality: OR=1.81, 95 % CI: 1.22, 2.69
Obese:
Inattention: OR=2.09, 95 % CI: 1.19, 4.82
Hyperactivity: insignificant
Negative emotionality: insignificant |

(continued)

Table 11.3 (continued)

Series (year) [reference]	Design	Sample/setting	Maternal obesity measure	Neurodevelopmental outcome	Age at follow-up	Key findings
Fernandes et al. (2012) [57]	Animal case–control study	Lab offspring of obese mice (OO, $N=9$); offspring of control (OC, $N=8$)		Hyperactivity/ADHD		OO were more active and also had enhanced cardiovascular reactivity Results support a direct biological link between in utero exposure to maternal obesity and hyperactivity in the adult offspring

SSD includes schizophrenia, schizoaffective disorder, other non-affective psychosis, and schizotypal personality disorder; DSM III R, DIGS, Diagnostic Interview for Genetic Studies

Schizophrenia

Schizophrenia is fairly common. A review using data from several studies reported the median values per 1,000 persons for the distributions for point and lifetime prevalence as 4.5 and 4.0, respectively [60, 61]. Estimates of the lifetime risk of developing schizophrenia range from 0.3 to 2 % with an average of approximately 0.7 % [60]. As with other neurodevelopmental conditions, schizophrenia risk has genetic and environmental determinants [61, 62]. Accumulating evidence suggests that schizophrenia may have origins in early life like other neurodevelopmental and metabolic conditions. Cohort studies have reported an association between risk of schizophrenia and birth weight, suggesting that adult schizophrenia may be related to alterations in fetal development [63–69]. Several studies have also linked various maternal and obstetric factors with an increased risk of schizophrenia [65, 70–72]. These include gestational diabetes, preeclampsia, emergency cesarean section, and maternal obesity.

There is a paucity of evidence on maternal obesity and schizophrenia risk [48–51, 72]. A recent review included four studies [48–51] with 305 schizophrenia cases and 24,442 controls [72]. All but one study reported an increased risk of schizophrenia among offspring of mothers with high maternal BMI during pregnancy. Two of these studies [48, 49] reported slightly more than a twofold risk of schizophrenia in offspring of mothers with a pre-pregnancy BMI in the highest category (>29 and >30 kg/m^2) compared to offspring of mothers with pre-pregnancy BMI in the lowest category (19.1–29 and 20.0–26.9 kg/m^2). Kawai et al. [51] examined the association between early pregnancy maternal BMI and schizophrenia and found a 24 % increased odds of schizophrenia in the offspring with one unit increase in maternal BMI during early pregnancy. In addition, Kawai et al. [51] also reported a 19 % increase in the odds of schizophrenia with a one unit increase in late pregnancy maternal BMI, while in contrast, Wahlbeck and colleagues reported that offspring of mothers with a late pregnancy BMI <24 kg/m^2 had 3.75 higher odds of schizophrenia compared to offspring of mothers with BMI >30 kg/m^2 [50].

Although there was one discrepant finding, there is evidence of increased risk of schizophrenia in adult offspring of mothers who were obese during pregnancy. Several factors could explain these findings. High pre-pregnancy BMI can increase the risk of obstetric complications, some of which are established risk factors for schizophrenia. As such, the increase in schizophrenia risk observed in offspring of obese mothers may be explained by the increased complication rates in obese mothers. Another possible explanation is the development of gestational diabetes. Maternal obesity is associated with increased risk of gestational diabetes and poor glucose control during pregnancy is also associated with increased risk of neurodevelopmental abnormalities, and there is some evidence of an association with increased risk of schizophrenia [65]. However, Kawai et al. [51] refute this explanation reporting that none of the mothers in their study were diagnosed with diabetes. Khandaker et al. propose maternal infection as a potential mediating factor since there is a strong association between infection and risk of schizophrenia [71] and obese women are more susceptible to infection [72]. In addition, maternal obesity may also contribute to the risk of neurodevelopmental disorders though activation of the innate immune system and/or increasing levels of inflammatory cytokines [72].

There is a great need for further research. Future studies should focus on the untangling of obstetric complications, diabetes, maternal infection, and immune responses that may mediate the association between maternal obesity and schizophrenia.

Attention-Deficit/Hyperactivity Disorder [ADHD]

There is a paucity of literature specifically on the relationship between maternal obesity and attention-deficit/hyperactivity disorder [ADHD]. In the studies reviewed, pre-pregnancy obesity was associated with an increased risk of ADHD [55–57]. One study reported a twofold increase in the risk of emotional intensity regulation [56]. Obesity prior to pregnancy also doubles the risk of the offspring developing ADHD compared to offspring of mothers with a healthy weight status [55]. Although there may be some genetic influences on the development of ADHD, even after adjustment for parental ADHD, the association between maternal obesity and increased risk for ADHD in the offspring persisted [56]. One proposed mechanism is dysfunction in dopaminergic and serotonergic systems that lead to ADHD symptoms [55].

Autism

Recent evidence indicates that fetal exposure to maternal obesity may be associated with an increased risk of developing autism spectrum disorder [ASD] [52]. Leptin, a hormone produced by adipose tissue, when produced in excess is thought to be associated with placental dysfunction that disrupts neurological development in utero [73]. When a group of children with ASD was compared with a group of children without ASD, the group with ASD had higher levels of leptin. However, this possible mechanism is still in the early stages of investigation [74]. Placental dysfunction observed with hyperleptinemia has also been documented with high levels of inflammatory cytokines. Numerous studies have demonstrated that increased exposure of the developing fetus to inflammatory cytokines increases the risk of behavioral abnormalities consistent with ASD [75].

This field is at the budding stages of identifying and understanding the complex mechanisms by which maternal obesity influences the development of neural circuitry that regulates behavior. Despite the fact that few studies have examined the associations between maternal obesity and neurodevelopmental outcomes in the offspring, there is some evidence suggesting an increased risk of cognitive and psychiatric problems across the life span, although there are some inconsistencies. Nevertheless, additional work in this area needs to be done. Certainly there needs to be more evidence before maternal obesity prevention and treatment can be touted as beneficial to offspring neurodevelopment.

Conclusion

This current body of evidence indicates that the current epidemic of maternal obesity will put future generations at greater risk of adverse cardiometabolic, behavioral, and mental health outcomes. There is an opportunity to break the cycle of obesity during pre-pregnancy. The long-term goal must be to reduce the incidence of obesity in pregnancy and increase awareness as to the importance of establishment and maintenance of a healthy weight prior to initiating pregnancy. Patients need to be extensively educated during preconception counseling about the long-term implications of obesity during pregnancy, not only for their own health but that of their offspring which tracks into adulthood. Although this strategy is ideal, the prevalence of unintended pregnancy is fairly high. In the United States almost half (49 %) of pregnancies were unintended in 2006 [76].

Although animal models have been useful in elucidating underlying mechanisms, there is still a lot that remains unknown. Teasing out the relative contributions of the fetal and postnatal periods will be important in the design of effective interventional strategies to ensure optimal long-term health of the offspring. Animal studies have been providing some promising directions in interventional strategies. Some of these strategies include:

- Dietary restriction prior to pregnancy. Results from animal models demonstrated a reduction in the effects of maternal obesity on offspring programming [77, 78].
- Weight loss in obese women prior to pregnancy. There is some evidence of improved offspring metabolic phenotype following weight loss among obese women prior to initiating pregnancy [29, 30].
- Mild dietary restriction during pregnancy. During pregnancy, mild dietary restriction seems to be effective in reversing programming effects [79, 80].

Weight loss strategies and simple dietary changes may improve the metabolic milieu of the mothers and may positively impact the offspring. It is important to increase awareness of healthy dietary behaviors before and during pregnancy in order to reduce maternal obesity with the long-term goal being to reduce health risks for future generations. The current evidence favors actions directed at controlling pre-pregnancy weight and preventing obesity in women of reproductive age. Failure to address maternal obesity may ultimately accelerate the obesity epidemic through successive generations independent of genetic and environmental factors.

References

1. Kim SY, Dietz PM, England L, Morrow B, Callaghan WM. Trends in pre-pregnancy obesity in nine states, 1993–2003. Obesity. 2007;15(4): 986–93. PubMed PMID: 17426334.
2. Chu SY, Kim SY, Bish CL. Prepregnancy obesity prevalence in the United States, 2004–2005. Matern Child Health J. 2009;13(5):614–20. PubMed PMID: 18618231.
3. Barker DJ. Developmental origins of adult health and disease. J Epidemiol Community Health. 2004;58(2):114–5. PubMed PMID: 14729887. Pubmed Central PMCID: 1732687.
4. Forsdahl A. Are poor living conditions in childhood and adolescence an important risk factor for arteriosclerotic heart disease? Br J Prev Soc Med. 1977;31(2):91–5. PubMed PMID: 884401. Pubmed Central PMCID: 479002.
5. Alfaradhi MZ, Ozanne SE. Developmental programming in response to maternal overnutrition. Front Genet. 2011;2:27. PubMed PMID: 22303323. Pubmed Central PMCID: 3268582.
6. Ong KK, Dunger DB. Perinatal growth failure: the road to obesity, insulin resistance and cardiovascular disease in adults. Best Pract Res Clin Endocrinol Metab. 2002;16(2):191–207. PubMed PMID: 12064888.
7. Hales CN, Barker DJ. Type 2 (non-insulin-dependent) diabetes mellitus: the thrifty phenotype hypothesis. Diabetologia. 1992;35(7):595–601. PubMed PMID: 1644236.
8. Drake AJ, Reynolds RM. Impact of maternal obesity on offspring obesity and cardiometabolic disease risk. Reproduction. 2010;140(3): 387–98. PubMed PMID: 20562299.
9. Taylor PD, Poston L. Developmental programming of obesity in mammals. Exp Physiol. 2007;92(2):287–98. PubMed PMID: 17170060.
10. Whitaker RC. Predicting preschooler obesity at birth: the role of maternal obesity in early pregnancy. Pediatrics. 2004;114(1):e29–36. PubMed PMID: 15231970.
11. Boney CM, Verma A, Tucker R, Vohr BR. Metabolic syndrome in childhood: association with birth weight, maternal obesity, and gestational diabetes mellitus. Pediatrics. 2005;115(3):e290–6. PubMed PMID: 15741354.

12. Laitinen J, Jaaskelainen A, Hartikainen AL, Sovio U, Vaarasmaki M, Pouta A, et al. Maternal weight gain during the first half of pregnancy and offspring obesity at 16 years: a prospective cohort study. BJOG. 2012;119(6):716–23. PubMed PMID: 22489762.
13. Lake JK, Power C, Cole TJ. Child to adult body mass index in the 1958 British birth cohort: associations with parental obesity. Arch Dis Child. 1997;77(5):376–81. PubMed PMID: 9487953.
14. Reilly JJ, Armstrong J, Dorosty AR, Emmett PM, Ness A, Rogers I, et al. Early life risk factors for obesity in childhood: cohort study. BMJ. 2005;330(7504):1357. PubMed PMID: 15908441. Pubmed Central PMCID: 558282.
15. Stuebe AM, Forman MR, Michels KB. Maternal-recalled gestational weight gain, pre-pregnancy body mass index, and obesity in the daughter. Int J Obes. 2009;33(7):743–52. PubMed PMID: 19528964. Pubmed Central PMCID: 2710391.
16. Blair NJ, Thompson JM, Black PN, Becroft DM, Clark PM, Han DY, et al. Risk factors for obesity in 7-year-old European children: the Auckland Birthweight Collaborative Study. Arch Dis Child. 2007;92(10):866–71. PubMed PMID: 17855436. Pubmed Central PMCID: 2083229.
17. Burdette HL, Whitaker RC, Hall WC, Daniels SR. Maternal infant-feeding style and children's adiposity at 5 years of age. Arch Pediatr Adolesc Med. 2006;160(5):513–20. PubMed PMID: 16651495.
18. Gale CR, Javaid MK, Robinson SM, Law CM, Godfrey KM, Cooper C. Maternal size in pregnancy and body composition in children. J Clin Endocrinol Metab. 2007;92(10):3904–11. PubMed PMID: 17684051. Pubmed Central PMCID: 2066182.
19. Crozier SR, Inskip HM, Godfrey KM, Cooper C, Harvey NC, Cole ZA, et al. Weight gain in pregnancy and childhood body composition: findings from the Southampton Women's Survey. Am J Clin Nutr. 2010;91(6):1745–51. PubMed PMID: 20375187. Pubmed Central PMCID: 3091013.
20. Oken E, Taveras EM, Kleinman KP, Rich-Edwards JW, Gillman MW. Gestational weight gain and child adiposity at age 3 years. Am J Obstet Gynecol. 2007;196(4):322.e1–8. PubMed PMID: 17403405. Pubmed Central PMCID: 1899090.
21. Olson CM, Strawderman MS, Dennison BA. Maternal weight gain during pregnancy and child weight at age 3 years. Matern Child Health J. 2009;13(6):839–46. PubMed PMID: 18818995.
22. Oken E, Rifas-Shiman SL, Field AE, Frazier AL, Gillman MW. Maternal gestational weight gain and offspring weight in adolescence. Obstet Gynecol. 2008;112(5):999–1006. PubMed PMID: 18978098. Pubmed Central PMCID: 3001295.
23. Reynolds RM. Excess maternal weight gain during pregnancy is associated with overweight/obesity in offspring at age 16 years, but maternal pre-pregnancy obesity has a greater effect. Evid Based Nurs. 2013;16(2):43–4. PubMed PMID: 23100266.

Chapter 11. Maternal Obesity and Implications 291

24. Mamun AA, O'Callaghan MJ, Williams GM, Najman JM. Change in maternal body mass index is associated with offspring body mass index: a 21-year prospective study. Eur J Nutr. 2013;52(6):1597–606. PubMed PMID: 23197072.
25. Reynolds RM, Osmond C, Phillips DI, Godfrey KM. Maternal BMI, parity, and pregnancy weight gain: influences on offspring adiposity in young adulthood. J Clin Endocrinol Metab. 2010;95(12):5365–9. PubMed PMID: 20702520.
26. Catalano PM, Drago NM, Amini SB. Maternal carbohydrate metabolism and its relationship to fetal growth and body composition. Am J Obstet Gynecol. 1995;172(5):1464–70. PubMed PMID: 7755055.
27. Koupil I, Toivanen P. Social and early-life determinants of overweight and obesity in 18-year-old Swedish men. Int J Obes. 2008;32(1):73–81. PubMed PMID: 17667914.
28. Villamor E, Cnattingius S. Interpregnancy weight change and risk of adverse pregnancy outcomes: a population-based study. Lancet. 2006;368(9542):1164–70. PubMed PMID: 17011943.
29. Kral JG, Biron S, Simard S, Hould FS, Lebel S, Marceau S, et al. Large maternal weight loss from obesity surgery prevents transmission of obesity to children who were followed for 2 to 18 years. Pediatrics. 2006;118(6):e1644–9. PubMed PMID: 17142494.
30. Smith J, Cianflone K, Biron S, Hould FS, Lebel S, Marceau S, et al. Effects of maternal surgical weight loss in mothers on intergenerational transmission of obesity. J Clin Endocrinol Metab. 2009;94(11):4275–83. PubMed PMID: 19820018.
31. Filler G, Rayar MS, da Silva O, Buffo I, Pepelassis D, Sharma AP. Should prevention of chronic kidney disease start before pregnancy? Int Urol Nephrol. 2008;40(2):483–8. PubMed PMID: 18246441.
32. Lawlor DA, Najman JM, Sterne J, Williams GM, Ebrahim S, Davey Smith G. Associations of parental, birth, and early life characteristics with systolic blood pressure at 5 years of age: findings from the Mater-University study of pregnancy and its outcomes. Circulation. 2004;110(16):2417–23. PubMed PMID: 15477400.
33. Wen X, Triche EW, Hogan JW, Shenassa ED, Buka SL. Prenatal factors for childhood blood pressure mediated by intrauterine and/or childhood growth? Pediatrics. 2011;127(3):e713–21. PubMed PMID: 21300676. Pubmed Central PMCID: 3065147.
34. Laor A, Stevenson DK, Shemer J, Gale R, Seidman DS. Size at birth, maternal nutritional status in pregnancy, and blood pressure at age 17: population based analysis. BMJ. 1997;315(7106):449–53. PubMed PMID: 9284660. Pubmed Central PMCID: 2127333.
35. Hochner H, Friedlander Y, Calderon-Margalit R, Meiner V, Sagy Y, Avgil-Tsadok M, et al. Associations of maternal prepregnancy body mass index and gestational weight gain with adult offspring cardiometabolic risk factors: the Jerusalem Perinatal Family Follow-up Study. Circulation. 2012;125(11):1381–9. PubMed PMID: 22344037. Pubmed Central PMCID: 3332052.

36. Fraser A, Tilling K, Macdonald-Wallis C, Sattar N, Brion MJ, Benfield L, Ness A, Deanfield J, Hingorani A, Nelson SM, Smith GD, Lawlor DA. Association of maternal weight gain in pregnancy with offspring obesity and metabolic and vascular traits in childhood. Circulation. 2010;121(23):2557–64.
37. Mingrone G, Manco M, Mora ME, Guidone C, Iaconelli A, Gniuli D, et al. Influence of maternal obesity on insulin sensitivity and secretion in offspring. Diabetes Care. 2008;31(9):1872–6. PubMed PMID: 18535193. Pubmed Central PMCID: 2518362.
38. Catalano PM, Presley L, Minium J, Hauguel-de Mouzon S. Fetuses of obese mothers develop insulin resistance in utero. Diabetes Care. 2009;32(6):1076–80. PubMed PMID: 19460915. Pubmed Central PMCID: 2681036.
39. Ali Z, Ulrik CS. Obesity and asthma: a coincidence or a causal relationship? A systematic review. Respir Med. 2013;107(9):1287–300. PubMed PMID: 23642708.
40. Haberg SE, Stigum H, London SJ, Nystad W, Nafstad P. Maternal obesity in pregnancy and respiratory health in early childhood. Paediatr Perinat Epidemiol. 2009;23(4):352–62. PubMed PMID: 19523082. Pubmed Central PMCID: 2827878.
41. Harpsoe MC, Basit S, Bager P, Wohlfahrt J, Benn CS, Nohr EA, et al. Maternal obesity, gestational weight gain, and risk of asthma and atopic disease in offspring: a study within the Danish National Birth Cohort. J Allergy Clin Immunol. 2013;131(4):1033–40. PubMed PMID: 23122630.
42. Kumar R, Story RE, Pongracic JA, Hong X, Arguelles L, Wang G, et al. Maternal pre-pregnancy obesity and recurrent wheezing in early childhood. Pediatr Allergy Immunol Pulmonol. 2010;23(3): 183–90. PubMed PMID: 22375278. Pubmed Central PMCID: 3281288.
43. Lowe A, Braback L, Ekeus C, Hjern A, Forsberg B. Maternal obesity during pregnancy as a risk for early-life asthma. J Allergy Clin Immunol. 2011;128(5):1107–9.e1-2. PubMed PMID: 21958587.
44. Patel SP, Rodriguez A, Little MP, Elliott P, Pekkanen J, Hartikainen AL, et al. Associations between pre-pregnancy obesity and asthma symptoms in adolescents. J Epidemiol Community Health. 2012;66(9):809–14. PubMed PMID: 21844604. Pubmed Central PMCID: 3412048.
45. Reichman NE, Nepomnyaschy L. Maternal pre-pregnancy obesity and diagnosis of asthma in offspring at age 3 years. Matern Child Health J. 2008;12(6):725–33. PubMed PMID: 17987372.
46. Scholtens S, Wijga AH, Brunekreef B, Kerkhof M, Postma DS, Oldenwening M, et al. Maternal overweight before pregnancy and asthma in offspring followed for 8 years. Int J Obes. 2010;34(4): 606–13. PubMed PMID: 19786965.
47. Stothard KJ, Tennant PW, Bell R, Rankin J. Maternal overweight and obesity and the risk of congenital anomalies: a systematic review and meta-analysis. JAMA. 2009;301(6):636–50. PubMed PMID: 19211471.

Chapter 11. Maternal Obesity and Implications 293

48. Jones PB, Rantakallio P, Hartikainen AL, Isohanni M, Sipila P. Schizophrenia as a long-term outcome of pregnancy, delivery, and perinatal complications: a 28-year follow-up of the 1966 north Finland general population birth cohort. Am J Psychiatry. 1998;155(3):355–64. PubMed PMID: 9501745.
49. Schaefer CA, Brown AS, Wyatt RJ, Kline J, Begg MD, Bresnahan MA, et al. Maternal prepregnant body mass and risk of schizophrenia in adult offspring. Schizophr Bull. 2000;26(2):275–86. PubMed PMID: 10885630.
50. Wahlbeck K, Forsen T, Osmond C, Barker DJ, Eriksson JG. Association of schizophrenia with low maternal body mass index, small size at birth, and thinness during childhood. Arch Gen Psychiatry. 2001;58(1):48–52. PubMed PMID: 11146757.
51. Kawai M, Minabe Y, Takagai S, Ogai M, Matsumoto H, Mori N, et al. Poor maternal care and high maternal body mass index in pregnancy as a risk factor for schizophrenia in offspring. Acta Psychiatr Scand. 2004;110(4):257–63. PubMed PMID: 15352926.
52. Krakowiak P, Walker CK, Bremer AA, Baker AS, Ozonoff S, Hansen RL, et al. Maternal metabolic conditions and risk for autism and other neurodevelopmental disorders. Pediatrics. 2012;129(5):e1121–8. PubMed PMID: 22492772. Pubmed Central PMCID: 3340592.
53. Neggers YH, Goldenberg RL, Ramey SL, Cliver SP. Maternal prepregnancy body mass index and psychomotor development in children. Acta Obstet Gynecol Scand. 2003;82(3):235–40. PubMed PMID: 12694119.
54. Heikura U, Taanila A, Hartikainen AL, Olsen P, Linna SL, von Wendt L, Järvelin MR. Variations in prenatal sociodemographic factors associated with intellectual disability: a study of the 20-year interval between two birth cohorts in northern Finland. Am J Epidemiol. 2008;167(2):169–77. Epub 2007 Nov 17.
55. Rodriguez A, Miettunen J, Henriksen TB, Olsen J, Obel C, Taanila A, et al. Maternal adiposity prior to pregnancy is associated with ADHD symptoms in offspring: evidence from three prospective pregnancy cohorts. Int J Obes. 2008;32(3):550–7. PubMed PMID: 17938639.
56. Rodriguez A. Maternal pre-pregnancy obesity and risk for inattention and negative emotionality in children. J Child Psychol Psychiatry. 2010;51(2):134–43. PubMed PMID: 19674195.
57. Fernandes C, Grayton H, Poston L, Samuelsson AM, Taylor PD, Collier DA, et al. Prenatal exposure to maternal obesity leads to hyperactivity in offspring. Mol Psychiatry. 2012;17(12):1159–60. PubMed PMID: 22158015.
58. Van Lieshout RJ, Taylor VH, Boyle MH. Pre-pregnancy and pregnancy obesity and neurodevelopmental outcomes in offspring: a systematic review. Obes Rev. 2011;12(5):e548–59. PubMed PMID: 21414129.

59. Allen KL, Byrne SM, Forbes D, Oddy WH. Risk factors for full- and partial-syndrome early adolescent eating disorders: a population-based pregnancy cohort study. J Am Acad Child Adolesc Psychiatry. 2009;48(8):800–9. PubMed PMID: 19564799.
60. Saha S, Chant D, Welham J, McGrath J. A systematic review of the prevalence of schizophrenia. PLoS Med. 2005;2(5):e141. PubMed PMID: 15916472. Pubmed Central PMCID: 1140952.
61. Messias EL, Chen CY, Eaton WW. Epidemiology of schizophrenia: review of findings and myths. Psychiatr Clin North Am. 2007;30(3):323–38. PubMed PMID: 17720026. Pubmed Central PMCID: 2727721.
62. Mura G, Petretto DR, Bhat KM, Carta MG. Schizophrenia: from epidemiology to rehabilitation. Clin Pract Epidemiol Ment Health. 2012;8:52–66. PubMed PMID: 22962559. Pubmed Central PMCID: 3434422.
63. Rifkin L, Lewis S, Jones P, Toone B, Murray R. Low birth weight and schizophrenia. Br J Psychiatry Suppl. 1994;165(3):357–62. PubMed PMID: 7994506.
64. Abel KM, Wicks S, Susser ES, Dalman C, Pedersen MG, Mortensen PB, et al. Birth weight, schizophrenia, and adult mental disorder: is risk confined to the smallest babies? Arch Gen Psychiatry. 2010;67(9):923–30. PubMed PMID: 20819986.
65. Cannon M, Jones PB, Murray RM. Obstetric complications and schizophrenia: historical and meta-analytic review. Am J Psychiatry. 2002;159(7):1080–92. PubMed PMID: 12091183.
66. Moilanen K, Jokelainen J, Jones PB, Hartikainen AL, Jarvelin MR, Isohanni M. Deviant intrauterine growth and risk of schizophrenia: a 34-year follow-up of the Northern Finland 1966 Birth Cohort. Schizophr Res. 2010;124(1–3):223–30. PubMed PMID: 20933367.
67. Gunnell D, Rasmussen F, Fouskakis D, Tynelius P, Harrison G. Patterns of fetal and childhood growth and the development of psychosis in young males: a cohort study. Am J Epidemiol. 2003;158(4):291–300. PubMed PMID: 12915493.
68. Wegelius A, Tuulio-Henriksson A, Pankakoski M, Haukka J, Lehto U, Paunio T, et al. An association between high birth weight and schizophrenia in a Finnish schizophrenia family study sample. Psychiatry Res. 2011;190(2–3):181–6. PubMed PMID: 21664700.
69. Bersani G, Manuali G, Ramieri L, Taddei I, Bersani I, Conforti F, et al. The potential role of high or low birthweight as risk factor for adult schizophrenia. J Perinat Med. 2007;35(2):159–61. PubMed PMID: 17302511.
70. Hamlyn J, Duhig M, McGrath J, Scott J. Modifiable risk factors for schizophrenia and autism – shared risk factors impacting on brain development. Neurobiol Dis. 2013;53:3–9. PubMed PMID: 23123588.
71. Khandaker GM, Zimbron J, Lewis G, Jones PB. Prenatal maternal infection, neurodevelopment and adult schizophrenia: a systematic review of population-based studies. Psychol Med. 2013;43(2):239–57. PubMed PMID: 22717193. Pubmed Central PMCID: 3479084.

72. Khandaker GM, Dibben CR, Jones PB. Does maternal body mass index during pregnancy influence risk of schizophrenia in the adult offspring? Obes Rev. 2012;13(6):518–27. PubMed PMID: 22188548. Pubmed Central PMCID: 3492912.
73. Hauguel-de Mouzon S, Lepercq J, Catalano P. The known and unknown of leptin in pregnancy. Am J Obstet Gynecol. 2006;194(6): 1537–45. PubMed PMID: 16731069.
74. Ashwood P, Kwong C, Hansen R, Hertz-Picciotto I, Croen L, Krakowiak P, et al. Brief report: plasma leptin levels are elevated in autism: association with early onset phenotype? J Autism Dev Disord. 2008;38(1):169–75. PubMed PMID: 17347881.
75. Onore C, Careaga M, Ashwood P. The role of immune dysfunction in the pathophysiology of autism. Brain Behav Immun. 2012;26(3): 383–92. PubMed PMID: 21906670. Pubmed Central PMCID: 3418145.
76. Finer LB, Zolna MR. Unintended pregnancy in the United States: incidence and disparities, 2006. Contraception. 2011;84(5):478–85. PubMed PMID: 22018121. Pubmed Central PMCID: 3338192.
77. Rattanatray L, MacLaughlin SM, Kleemann DO, Walker SK, Muhlhausler BS, McMillen IC. Impact of maternal periconceptional overnutrition on fat mass and expression of adipogenic and lipogenic genes in visceral and subcutaneous fat depots in the postnatal lamb. Endocrinology. 2010;151(11):5195–205. PubMed PMID: 20861234.
78. Zambrano E, Martinez-Samayoa PM, Rodriguez-Gonzalez GL, Nathanielsz PW. Dietary intervention prior to pregnancy reverses metabolic programming in male offspring of obese rats. J Physiol. 2010;588(Pt 10):1791–9. PubMed PMID: 20351043. Pubmed Central PMCID: 2887995.
79. Gallou-Kabani C, Vige A, Gross MS, Boileau C, Rabes JP, Fruchart-Najib J, et al. Resistance to high-fat diet in the female progeny of obese mice fed a control diet during the periconceptual, gestation, and lactation periods. Am J Physiol Endocrinol Metab. 2007;292(4):E1095–100. PubMed PMID: 17164437.
80. Giraudo SQ, Della-Fera MA, Proctor L, Wickwire K, Ambati S, Baile CA. Maternal high fat feeding and gestational dietary restriction: effects on offspring body weight, food intake and hypothalamic gene expression over three generations in mice. Pharmacol Biochem Behav. 2010;97(1):121–9. PubMed PMID: 20430050.

Chapter 12
Family-Centered Interventions to Reduce Maternal and Child Obesity

Dianne Stanton Ward, Temitope O. Erinosho, Heather M. Wasser, and Paula M. Munoz

> To keep the body in good health is a duty otherwise we shall not be able to keep our mind strong and clear. Buddha
> (c. 563 BC to 483 BC)

Abstract Obesity is associated with multiple health risks for pregnant and postpartum women and can affect their infants, preschoolers, school-aged children, and adolescents. Family-centered intervention strategies may be an important way to prevent or treat maternal and child obesity. This chapter reviews 19 family-centered interventions designed to address excess body weight among mothers and their children. An additional five interventions were classified as "promising."

D.S. Ward, EdD (✉)
Department of Nutrition, UNC School
of Public Health, Chapel Hill, NC, USA

Department of Nutrition, University of North
Carolina at Chapel Hill, Chapel Hill, NC, USA
e-mail: dsward@email.unc.edu

T.O. Erinosho, PhD • H.M. Wasser, PhD, MPH, RD
P.M. Munoz
Department of Nutrition, University of North
Carolina at Chapel Hill, Chapel Hill, NC, USA

W. Nicholson, K. Baptiste-Roberts (eds.),
Obesity During Pregnancy in Clinical Practice,
DOI 10.1007/978-1-4471-2831-1_12,
© Springer-Verlag London 2014

Six of the studies focused on children age 5 and younger including one study targeting infants; half of these studies were prevention based. Thirteen studies addressed school-aged children; all involved overweight or obese children. Only half of these studies targeted and/or measure parent weight. Results suggest that addressing obesity prevention and treatment from a family perspective could be an effective strategy. Clinicians who care for women of childbearing age should stress the importance of family-centered approaches to develop healthy weight in infants, preschoolers, and children, and when necessary address weight management problems using parents as agents of change both for their children's weight and for their own. Promising new studies offer new prevention strategies for maternal and child obesity prevention approaches.

Keywords Families • Obesity prevention • Obesity treatment • Children

Key Points
- Family-centered approaches are useful for preventing unnecessary weight gain in infants, preschoolers, and mothers
- Parents are important "agents of change" for child weight loss
- Targeting family weight loss (rather than child-only) is underutilized strategy
- Multi-country evidence supports family-based approaches to weight management

Background

Maternal and child obesity are major public health problems in the United States (USA), including obesity during pregnancy per se, because national data indicate that about one of five pregnant women in the United States is currently obese

[1]. In addition, about 56 % of women aged 20–39 years old (childbearing age) are overweight or obese, while even more (66 %) women aged 40–59 years old are overweight or obese [2]. Weight problems for US children (aged 2–19 years) also are alarming: approximately 30 % are overweight or obese [3], with higher rates observed in adolescents (34 %) and school-aged children (33 %) than among preschool-aged children (27 %) [3].

Obesity during pregnancy often results in increased use of health-care services, as well as higher risk for such adverse health conditions as gestational diabetes mellitus [1]. Overweight and obesity in childhood are associated with poor health conditions that include greater risks for developing high blood pressure, type 2 diabetes, breathing problems, fatty liver disease, and gallstones [4]. Further, overweight and obesity that develop in childhood are likely to track into adulthood [4–7], increasing the risk for such chronic diseases as type 2 diabetes, hypertension, heart disease, stroke, and several types of cancers in adult life [8].

The prenatal period is a critical stage for the development of childhood obesity [9]. Research shows that pre-pregnancy and early-pregnancy obesity are related to higher risk of obesity in children born to such mothers [9]. For instance, in a study of more than 30,000 pregnant women in the Norwegian Mother and Child Cohort Study, Stamnes and colleagues [10,11] found that higher maternal pre-pregnancy weight gain was associated with higher birth weight in their offspring [10] and increased overweight and obesity at age 3 [11]. Other studies also show that maternal obesity in early pregnancy is associated with overweight and obesity in their offspring in early childhood [12–14] and adolescence [15].

In addition to linking childhood obesity to maternal pre- and early-pregnancy weight, studies indicate that parents, in particular mothers, influence children's weight status through dietary and physical activity practices in the home environment [16, 17]. At home, mothers not only are important role models for children's dietary behaviors; they often are the gatekeepers for foods in the home [18]. Several studies have shown that the types of foods available and accessible at home, child feeding practices (e.g., use of foods as reward or punishment), and dietary role modeling by parents, especially mothers, influence children's dietary behaviors and, ultimately, children's weight [16, 17, 19–28]. In addition, the physical activity of mothers, including their encouragement of children's activity, and their monitoring of children's television viewing and media use (e.g., computer, video game) influence children's physical activity and, consequently, children's weight [17, 27, 29–35]. It is no surprise, therefore, that studies show that children's weight is highly correlated with their mothers' weight [36–38]. Thus, the critical role that mothers play in children's risk for obesity makes it imperative that interventions to promote healthy weight development in children include them.

Defining Family-Centered Interventions for Preventing and Reducing Childhood Obesity

Family-centered interventions (also known as family-based interventions) to reduce childhood obesity are programs that focus on changing weight-related behaviors of multiple family members, and not just those of the child [39]. Such interventions are based on the premises that childhood overweight and obesity develop and are maintained within the context of the family [40, 41]; that parents play a critical role in shaping children's dietary intakes, physical activity behaviors, and body weight [17]; and that involving the family in childhood obesity interventions may provide effective strategies for promoting and sustaining healthy changes in children's diets and physical activity [42].

Since obesity tends to run in families, involving the family in childhood obesity interventions provides an opportunity to simultaneously impact weight-related behaviors of the entire family [42, 43]. Unfortunately, most family-centered interventions focus on obesity *treatment*, particularly in school-aged children and adolescents [44, 45]; family-centered interventions that focus on the *prevention* of childhood obesity are limited [46]. Further, although family-centered interventions that focus on multiple members of a family may be an effective approach, most programs that focus on maternal weight do not include children or other members of the family. However, family-based interventions that focus on children's weight do often include mothers (or fathers). Thus, this chapter will review the evidence base from family-centered interventions for the prevention and treatment of obesity in children and their potential for affecting maternal and/or parent weight as well.

Descriptions of Family-Centered Interventions

Family-Centered Interventions for Infants, Toddlers, and Preschoolers

Six studies were found that used a family-centered intervention approach with infants, toddlers, and/or preschoolers. Details of these interventions are described in Table 12.1.

Family-centered interventions for promoting healthy weight gain in infants and toddlers often target the mother as the primary agent of change. In a home-based, family-centered study, Paul and colleagues [49] examined the independent and combined effects of two behavioral interventions delivered to mothers of newborns. The first intervention, "soothe/sleep," was implemented 2–3 weeks after birth and was designed to increase sleep duration in early infancy by teaching mothers to use alternate soothing and calming strategies instead of feeding as a first response to fussiness. The second intervention, "introduction to solids," was delivered in two parts: the first part taught mothers, at 2–3 weeks after birth, about hunger and satiety cues as well as appropriate timing for introducing solid foods, and the second part, delivered between 4 and 6 months after birth, when mothers reported that their infants were starting to consume solid foods, taught mothers how to use repeated exposure to new foods to overcome infant rejection of healthy foods. One hundred and sixty mother-newborn dyads were recruited from an academic medical center in Hershey, Pennsylvania,

TABLE 12.1 Summary of family-based obesity interventions targeting 0–5-year-olds

Author (year)	Design[a]	Country	Sample size	Age of target child	Focus[b] T	Focus[b] P	Delivery channel	Intervention target Parent only	Intervention target Parent +child	Intervention dose	Length of follow-up	Improved weight outcome[c] Child PI	Child FU	Parent PI	Parent FU
Harvey-Berino (2003) [47]	RCT	United States	43	9–36 months		X	Home visits	X		11 home visits over 16 weeks	None				
Klohe-Lehman (2007) [48]	Pre-post	United States	91	1–3 years	X		Group sessions in community	X		8 (2-h) weekly sessions with mother weigh-in, education, and 30-min of low-to-moderate exercise	4 months	X	X		
Ostybe (2012) [46]	RCT	United States	400	2–6 months		X	Mailed interactive kits + telephone calls + group session	X		8 kits, each followed by 20–30-min telephone coaching plus 1 group session	8 months				

Study	Design	Country	N	Age		Setting		Dose	FU				
Paul (2010) [49]	RCT	United States	160	0–7 days	X	Home visits	X	Up to 2 home visits	1 years	X			
Stark (2011) [50]	RCT	United States	18	2–5 years	X	Group sessions in community + home visits		12 (1.5-h) weekly sessions followed by 6 (1.5-h) biweekly sessions, alternating between clinic and home based	6 months	X	X	X	X
Wen (2012) [51]	RCT	Australia	667	0–2 years		Home visits	X	8 visits over 2 years+telephone support between visits	None	X			

[a]RCT = randomized controlled trial; QE = quasi-experimental
[b]T = treatment; P = prevention
[c]PI = post-intervention; FU = follow-up

and randomized into one of four study arms, using a 2×2 design to receive one, both types, or no intervention. Findings from the 110 participants who completed the intervention showed that at age 1, children whose mothers received both interventions had significantly lower mean weight-for-length percentiles than children whose mothers received only the soothe/sleep intervention, or only the introduction to solids intervention, or were in the control group. Parental weight change was not targeted or reported.

In a study conducted in Australia, Wen and colleagues [51, 52] evaluated the effectiveness of a 24-month, home-based early intervention on children's BMI measured at age 2. Called the "The Healthy Beginnings Trial," it applied theoretical constructs from the Health Belief Model to 667 first-time mothers and their infants in socially and economically disadvantaged areas of Sydney, Australia. Mother-child dyads were randomly allocated to either receive the intervention or to be in a control condition which included usual practice for new mothers supplemented with safety promotion materials. The intervention focused on educational materials promoting breastfeeding, appropriate time to introduce solid foods, tummy time, active play, and proper nutrition and physical activity for the entire family. Participants received eight home visits from specially trained community nurses, timed to coincide with early childhood development milestones. The first visit was during the antenatal period, and seven additional visits were at 1, 3, 5, 9, 12, 18, and 24 months after birth. Child BMI was measured at 24 months and found to be significantly lower in the intervention group than the control group. Mother's weight was not addressed.

In a 16-week, home-based, family-centered intervention, Harvey-Berino and colleagues [47] compared maternal participation in a parenting support intervention with participation in a parenting support *plus obesity prevention* intervention to see whether the latter, *combined* intervention would reduce the prevalence of obesity in high-risk Native American children in the St. Regis Mohawk community in northern New York State and Ontario and Quebec, Canada. Participants were 40 overweight and obese Native American mothers and their children (mean age: 21 months old). Study findings noted that changes in children's weight-for-height z scores showed trends toward statistical significance: children in the parenting support *plus obesity prevention* group had decreased weight-for-height z scores, while children in the parenting support-only group had increased weight-for-height z scores. In addition, children's energy intake declined in the combined group and increased in the parent support-only group, and these changes also approached significance. Mother's weight and BMI decreased more in the combined group than the parenting support-only group, but these changes failed to reach statistical significance.

In an 8-week family-centered intervention conducted in Texas, Klohe-Lehman and colleagues [48] examined the effects of a maternal weight loss program on mothers' BMI, diet, and physical activity as well as the BMI and dietary intake of their 1–3-year-old children. Ninety-one low-income overweight and obese Hispanic, African-American, and White mother-child pairs were recruited from the Special Supplemental Program for Women Infants and Children (WIC) and public health clinics. The intervention was grounded in basic concepts of the social cognitive theory and addressed diet and physical activity. Diet activities included discussion about dietary plans, interactive low-fat cooking demonstrations, recipe modification, and portion size training, while the physical activity component included in-class activities (30 min of walking, stair climbing, and resistance exercises with light weights) and behavioral modification (e.g., self-monitoring, stimulus control, goal setting, and relapse prevention). At the end of the 8-week intervention, children's BMI (or weight-for-length in children under 2 years of age) did not decrease, but the excess energy intake observed in the children at baseline was reduced at the end of the intervention. Mothers in the study lost an average of 2.7 kg in body weight, and their mean BMI reduced significantly from 34.9 to 33.9 kg/m^2. The changes in mothers' weight and BMI were sustained at the 24-week follow-up. It should be noted that this was one of the few interventions that attempted to increase mother's physical activity.

Only two studies were found that used a family-centered approach for either obesity prevention [46] or treatment [50] in preschool-aged children. Obesity prevention was the focus of the Kids and Adults Now – Defeat Obesity (KAN-DO), a family-centered intervention designed to change child BMI [46]. KAN-DO was a 12-month, randomized controlled trial designed to promote healthy lifestyle behaviors in mother-preschooler (2–5 years old) dyads in North Carolina by changing targeting parenting styles and skills, stress management, and healthy eating and activity behaviors. The KAN-DO intervention was based on models of self-regulation and constructs from social cognitive theory. Participants in KAN-DO were 400 postpartum mothers who were overweight or obese prior to pregnancy and their preschool-aged children (no weight-specific inclusion criteria). While KAN-DO did not lead to significant improvement in children's or mother's weight status, an exploratory (completers) analysis showed significant reductions in BMI among mothers who completed at least half of the 16 possible intervention contacts.

Significant improvements in both child and parent weight outcomes were observed in the LAUNCH intervention (Learning about Activity and Understanding Nutrition for Child Health) [50]. LAUNCH was a 6-month, home-based, family-centered intervention conducted at the Cincinnati Children's Hospital Medical Center and was designed to reduce obesity in preschool children (aged 2–5 years) who were at or above the 95th BMI percentile [50]. LAUNCH also was grounded in the social cognitive theory and taught parents to use such child behavior management strategies as praise and attention, ignoring and time-out, modeling, and stimulus control to increase appropriate eating behaviors in their children and themselves. Children received nutrition education through games and art activities, participated in food taste tests, and completed 15 min of moderate to vigorous physical activity during group sessions. Eighteen preschool-aged children with an average BMI percentile of 98 and an overweight parent were randomized to receive either the LAUNCH intervention or an enhanced standard of care through pediatric counseling. Participation in LAUNCH resulted in significant decreases in weight in both children and parents. At 6-month post-intervention, LAUNCH children had a significantly greater decrease in BMI z, BMI percentile, and weight gain compared to children who received pediatric counseling, and these changes were maintained at the 12-month follow-up. In addition, parents in LAUNCH had a significantly greater weight loss at 6-month post-intervention and at the 12-month follow-up than parents who received pediatric counseling.

Family-Centered Interventions for School-Aged Children and Adolescents

Most of the family-centered studies that include school-aged children or adolescents are treatment rather than prevention studies. Family-based approaches to weight control were first developed more than 35 years ago when it was demonstrated that a more structured "lifestyle modification" approach that included family members was more effective for children's weight loss rather than standard weight reduction approaches [53]. For this chapter, 13 studies are reviewed, eight representing shorter-term studies. Most of the existing family-centered obesity treatment interventions for children and adolescents are based on the landmark work of Epstein [39, 54, 55] and Golan [45]. Family-centered studies that produced shorter-term impacts on school-aged children or adolescents are described below and reported in Table 12.2. Following this section is a description of five studies from the United States and abroad that report longer-term results from family-centered studies for school-aged children and/or adolescents.

Shelton and colleagues [68] assessed the impact of a 3-month, parent-based ($n = 43$ families) behavioral intervention on BMI of overweight and obese children in Australia. Although some younger children were included in this study (ages ranged from 3 to 10 years), the average child's age was between 7 and 8 years. In four brief sessions, the intervention promoted healthy family lifestyle changes by addressing nutrition, physical activity, motivation, and behavior management strategies. At the end of the 3 months, children in the intervention group experienced a significant decrease in BMI, but the intervention had no significant effect on parental BMI.

TABLE 12.2 Summary of family-based obesity interventions targeting 5+-year-olds

Author (year)	Design[a]	Country	Sample size	Age of target child (years)	Focus[b] T	Focus[b] P	Delivery channel	Intervention target Parent only	Intervention target Parent +child	Intervention dose	Length of follow-up	Improved weight outcome[c] Child PI	Child FU	Parent PI	Parent FU
Boutelle (2011) [56]	RCT	United States	80	8–12	X		Group sessions in community	X[d]		20 (60-min) weekly sessions conducted separately for parents and/or children	6 months	X	X	X	X
Collins (2012) [57]	RCT	Australia	165	5.5–9.9	X		Group sessions in community + telephone calls		X	10 (2-h) weekly sessions +3 monthly calls	18 months	X	X		
Coppins (2011) [58]	RCT	United Kingdom	65	6–14	X		Groups sessions in community		X	2 (8-h) weekly workshops for parents and children conducted separately +36 biweekly p.a. sessions for children	None				

Study	Design	Country	N	Age		Setting		Intervention	Follow-up				
Edwards (2006) [59]	Pre-post	United Kingdom	33	8–13	X	Group sessions in community	X	8 (1.5-h) weekly sessions + 4 (1.5-h) biweekly sessions conducted separately for parents and children	3 months	X	X		
Epstein (1990) [60]	RCT	United States	28	6–12	X	Clinic-based individualized treatment meetings	X	8 weekly treatment meetings followed by monthly meetings for 6 months	10 years	X	X	X	X
Golan (2006) [61]	Pre-post	Israel	70	4–18	X	Group sessions in community	X	Either a 5-day (40-h) workshop or 12 (3-h) sessions	None	X		X	

(continued)

TABLE 12.2 (continued)

Author (year)	Design[a]	Country	Sample size	Age of target child (years)	Focus[b] T	Focus[b] P	Delivery channel	Intervention target Parent only	Intervention target Parent+child	Intervention dose	Length of follow-up	Improved weight outcome[c] Child PI	Child FU	Parent PI	Parent FU
Gronbaek (2009) [62]		Denmark	100	10–12	X		Group sessions in community + home visit		X	Children's exercise class (1.5-h) twice weekly; ~35 (1-h) child-, parent-, or family-based sessions; 1 (1-h) home visit; 1 (1-h) grocery store tour	1 year	X	X		
Janicke (2008) [63]	RCT	United States	93	8–14	X		Group sessions in community	X	X	8 (90-min) weekly sessions+8 (90-min) biweekly sessions conducted for parents only or separately for parents and children	10 months	X[e] (PO)(B)		X[e]	

Study	Design	Country	N	Age		Setting		Intervention	Follow-up				
Kalarchian (2009) [64]	RCT	United States	192	8–12	X	Group sessions in community	X	20 (1-h) sessions beginning with family weigh-ins and goal setting followed by separate sessions for parents and children+6 booster sessions (3 groups and 3 phone calls during FU[f])	6 and 12 months[f]	X	X[f]	X	X[f]
Margarey (2011) [65]	RCT	Australia	169	5–9.9	X	Group sessions in community		8–12 (1.5- to 2-h) sessions plus 4 telephone sessions over 6 months	1.5 y	X	X		
Robertson (2008) [66] (2011) [67]	Pre-post	United Kingdom	27	7–13	X	Group sessions in community	X	12 weekly (2.5-h) sessions conducted separately for parents and children	2 y	X	X		
Shelton (2007) [68]	RCT	Australia	43	3–10	X	Group sessions in community	X	4 (2-h) weekly sessions	None	X			

(continued)

TABLE 12.2 (continued)

Author (year)	Design[a]	Country	Sample size	Age of target child (years)	Focus[b] T	Focus[b] P	Delivery channel	Intervention target Parent only	Intervention target Parent+child	Intervention dose	Length of follow-up	Improved weight outcome[c] Child PI	Improved weight outcome[c] Child FU	Improved weight outcome[c] Parent PI	Improved weight outcome[c] Parent FU
Williamson (2006) [44]	RCT		57	11–15	X		Face-to-face counseling sessions + secure website	X		4 face-to-face sessions + weekly email counseling for 2 years	None[g]	X[g]			X[g]

[a]RCT = randomized controlled trial; QE = quasi-experimental
[b]T = treatment; P = prevention
[c]PI = post-intervention; FU = follow-up
[d]Tested whether parent-only intervention (PO) as effective as parent+child (PC); testing based on noninferiority of PO group versus PC group
[e]Two intervention groups: parent-only (PO), family-based (FB), waitlist control; both groups decreased BMI z score at FU versus control but no differences between PO and FB
[f]Intervention families received reduced contact between 6 and 12 months and no contact between 12 and 18 months; significant differences between groups only at 12-month FU for children and parents; no significant differences between groups at 18 months
[g]There was no true FU as participants had access to website for full 2 years; however, weight differences between groups were only significant after the 6-month period in which participants also received counseling sessions; there were not significant differences between groups at 2 years

In a randomized controlled trial on child weight loss, Boutelle and colleagues [56] evaluated whether a 5-month standardized, behavioral, parent-only treatment program was inferior to a standardized parent-plus-child program. Eighty parents and their overweight or obese children (aged 8–12 years) were recruited in Minnesota and San Diego and randomly assigned to either a parent-plus-child or a parent-only group. This intervention adapted Epstein's Traffic Light Diet protocol [69] and included strategies for increasing physical activity, behavioral change skills, (viz., self-monitoring of targeted behaviors, positive reinforcement, stimulus control, pre-planning, and modeling), and parenting skills specific for use with children who are overweight. Information presented to children in the parent-plus-child group was similar to that taught to the parents, but was presented in an age-appropriate manner. Weight outcomes of children and parents assessed at baseline, 5-month post-intervention, and at an 11-month follow-up showed that the parent-only group was not inferior to the parent-plus-child group in either child weight loss or parent weight loss. Further exploratory analyses [70] also showed that across both study groups, parent BMI was the only significant predictor of child weight, with a 1 BMI unit reduction in parent weight associated with a 0.255 reduction in child BMI.

In another study using the Epstein Traffic Light Diet protocol, Kalarchian and colleagues [64] evaluated the efficacy of a 6-month, clinic-based, family-centered, behavioral intervention on reducing the weight of 192 severely obese children aged 8–12 years. Families were randomized into either an intervention group that received the family-based intervention, or a control group that received a standard care approach that consisted of two consultation sessions to help them develop individual nutrition plans based on the Traffic Light Diet. Adult and child groups met separately, and each group was presented with similar materials. Overweight adults were encouraged, but not required, to lose weight. At 6 months, the intervention was associated with greater decreases in child percent overweight than the decreases for the children in the control group. Intent-to-treat analyses showed that the intervention was associated with a significant 7.58 % decrease in child percent overweight at 6 months, compared to a 0.66 % decrease for the control group, but differences between the two groups were not significant at 12 or 18 months. In addition, children who attended at least 75 % of the intervention sessions maintained decreases in percent overweight through 18 months, while those who attended less than 75 % of the intervention sessions did not. Parent BMI was reduced significantly in the treatment groups at both the 6- and 12-month measurement periods.

In a family-centered intervention, Janicke and colleagues [63, 71] assessed the effects on the weight of underserved children of Project STORY (Sensible Treatment of Obesity in Rural Youth), a 4-month, family-based, behavioral intervention, and a parent-only behavioral intervention delivered through rural cooperative extension service offices. Participants were 93 overweight or obese children (aged 8–14 years) and their parents recruited from four underserved rural counties in North Central Florida. Participants were randomly assigned to one of three groups: a family-based group in which both children and parents were targeted as active agents of change, a parent-only group that targeted parents as the agents of change, and a waitlist control group that received the intervention following the final follow-up assessments. In general, Project STORY focused on five things: building healthier dietary habits via a modified version of Epstein and colleagues' Traffic Light Diet, increasing moderate intensity physical activity via a pedometer step program, setting goals for reducing sedentary activities, establishing a healthier weight status, and building positive self-worth in participants. Behavioral strategies used in delivering the Project STORY included self-monitoring, goal setting, stimulus control, positive reinforcement, modeling, role playing, and portion size control. At the 4-month assessment, children in the parent-only intervention group showed a greater decrease in BMI z score than children in the waitlist control group. No significant differences, however, were found in BMI z scores between the family-based intervention group and the waitlist control group. At the 10-month follow-up, children in the parent-only and family-based intervention groups showed greater decreases in BMI z score from before treatment (baseline) than the waitlist control group. The intervention did not have any significant effect on parental BMI change score at either month 4 or 10.

In a 2-year randomized controlled trial, Coppins and colleagues [58] evaluated whether a family-based intervention, "The Family Project," was more effective in reducing BMI z score in overweight children aged 6–14 years than just monitoring body composition alone. The intervention focused on healthy eating, physical activity, reducing sedentary behavior, behavior change, and psychological well-being. Sixty-five overweight and obese children were randomly assigned to receive the family-based intervention in either the first or second year and to be in the control group that received body composition monitoring alone during the year when they are not in the family-based intervention group. Siblings and parents or guardians were also encouraged to participate. After year 1, the intervention and control group crossed over, with the control group receiving the family-based intervention program and the intervention group receiving body composition monitoring alone for year 2 of the project. Children who received the intervention in year 1 reduced their BMI z score significantly in the first 12 months, and that score continued to be reduced over the next 12 months, so that by the end of the 2-year study, their BMI z score was 0.44 lower than at the beginning of the study. Children assigned to the body composition monitoring-alone group in year 1 also reduced their BMI z score in the first 12 months, although not significantly, and when they were put in the active family intervention, their BMI z score continued to fall, but only marginally. At the end of the 2-year study, fewer children in the group that received the active family intervention in year 1 were classified as grossly overweight than children who received only body composition monitoring in year 1. At baseline, about 60 % of all the children in the study were above the 99.6th BMI percentile.

By the end of the 24 months, only 19 % of children in the active family intervention group in year 1 were still above the 99.6th BMI percentile, compared with 48 % of children in the group that received only body composition monitoring in year 1. Parent weight was not targeted.

In a one group, pre-post design study conducted in the United Kingdom, Edwards and colleagues [59] assessed the impact of a clinic-based, family behavioral treatment on the weight of obese children aged 8–13 years. Thirty-three families received the 4-month intervention that included two components: advice on whole-family lifestyle change to modify the microenvironment of the home and a behavioral weight control program for the overweight children. The behavioral weight control program was based on learning theory and used such behavior modification techniques as self-monitoring, goal setting, positive reinforcement, and stimulus control to modify the children's eating and exercise behaviors. At the end of the 4-month intervention, children lost 8.4 % BMI and maintained that reduction at 3-month follow-up. Although the focus was "whole-family" lifestyle change, parental weight was not targeted.

In a study conducted in Copenhagen, Gronbaek and colleagues [62] evaluated the impact of an 18-month community and family-based childhood obesity treatment intervention on weight outcomes of 100 obese school-aged children and their families. The intervention consisted of a 6-month intensive phase and a less intensive 1-year follow-up. The intensive phase of the intervention consisted of physical exercises to reduce sedentary practices and nutrition sessions focused on healthy food choices and portion size regulation. The less intensive follow-up phase consisted of group meetings with all families. The meetings focused on families' development of healthy lifestyles and well-being, along with healthy weight development in their children. The 81 (of 100) children who completed the full program significantly decreased their BMI z score from 2.9 to 2.6 during the intensive phase of the intervention, and their BMI z score further decreased from 2.6 to 2.4 during the less intensive follow-up phase. Children who completed the full program also showed a significant decrease in percent body fat from 32.2 to 30.1 during the intensive phase, and this decreased further to 29.5 during the less intensive follow-up phase, although that decrease was nonsignificant. In addition to a 20 % loss to follow-up, this study had no comparison group and parent weight was not monitored.

In a study involving preschool and school-aged children in Australia, Magarey and colleagues [65] assessed the effectiveness of Parenting Eating and Activity for Child Health (PEACH), a 6-month hospital-based intervention for overweight children aged 5–9 years. PEACH targeted parents as the agents of change. One hundred and sixty-nine families were randomized into one of two groups: parenting skills plus healthy lifestyle group or a healthy lifestyle-only group. The parenting skills plus healthy lifestyle sessions encouraged parents to anticipate and manage high-risk situations to achieve a positive energy balance using a problem solving approach, while the healthy lifestyle-only sessions focused only on information that was consistent with traditional nutrition education and clinical advice. Overall, between the baseline and 6-month post-intervention, children's BMI z score decreased by 10 % in both study groups, and this decrease was maintained at the 24-month follow-up assessment. Similar to several studies above, parental weight was not monitored.

Long-Term Effects of Family-Centered Interventions

Researchers in the United States, Australia, United Kingdom, and Israel have demonstrated the long-term effects (up to 2 years) of family-centered obesity interventions on children's and parents' weight. Although some of those reported below are smaller studies, they include long-term follow-up data. Their interesting approaches and promising findings merited inclusion in the chapter.

As noted earlier, much of this research has been guided by the seminal work of Epstein and colleagues [39, 54, 55, 72] who pioneered the family-based treatment model for pediatric obesity. In a follow-up study of 10 years, Epstein et al. [60] evaluated the effect of a family-based behavioral treatment on percent overweight and growth in obese 6- to 12-year-olds, with repeated measurements at the 5- and 10-year periods. The study followed 76 obese children and their parents who were randomized into one of three groups: child and parent target group (group 1), child target group (group 2), or nonspecific target control group (group 3). All families received eight weekly treatment meetings and six additional meetings over a 6-month period. The families were then seen at 21-, 60-, and 120-month follow-up meetings. The three study groups were provided similar information about diet, exercise, and behavioral principles (this included the use of contracting, such as having parents deposit $65 at the beginning of the program and returning $5 at each session, contingent on either parent or child weight loss in groups 1 and 2 or attendance in group 3 along with goal setting, self-monitoring, and social reinforcement and modeling). Children in the child and parent target group (group 1) showed significantly greater decreases in percent overweight after 5 and 10 years, respectively, compared to children in the nonspecific target control group that increased in percent overweight. In contrast, children in the child target group (group 2) showed increases in percent overweight after 5 and 10 years that were midway between those for the child and parent target group and the nonspecific target group, but not significantly different from either. Parent weight decreased in all three groups, with effects lasting until the 21-month follow-up period. However, by the 5-year point, parents had returned to their baseline percent of overweight.

The stability of this approach with children was further demonstrated in a recent paper by Epstein and colleagues [73]. Results from contemporary studies using the Epstein model were compared to those conducted 25 years earlier that had similar results (observed over the 2-year follow-up period) [73]. In the more recent studies, the children and adolescents were, as a rule, heavier than in years past, making the task of obesity reduction even more challenging.

In a pilot study, Robertson and colleagues [66, 67] tested "Families for Health," a 12-week, community-based family intervention for treating obesity in children 7–13 years old in Coventry, England. Twenty-one families (27 children) received the Families for Health intervention that focused on parenting, relationship skills, emotional and social development, and healthy eating strategies in the home environment. Weight outcomes were measured at the end of the 3-month program and at a 9-month follow-up. For the 22 children on whom there is follow-up data, BMI z scores were reduced significantly between baseline and the end of the 3-month intervention, and this reduction was maintained at the 9-month follow-up. In a 2-year follow-up of 19 of the children (13 families), Robertson and colleagues (71 found that the BMI z score observed at 9 months was sustained at 2 years. Although these are promising results, lack of a control group and loss to follow-up prevent further interpretation. Also, parent weight change was neither targeted nor measured.

Most of the family-centered obesity interventions have employed face-to-face counseling. However, compliance (e.g., attendance at group sessions, coming to a university-based program) appears to be difficult for certain populations. Williamson and colleagues [44] evaluated the efficacy of an Internet-based, lifestyle behavior modification program for adolescent African-American girls in a randomized controlled trial and reported their results at the 2-year point. Fifty-seven overweight African-American girls aged 11–15 years and an overweight or obese parent were randomized to receive either an interactive behavioral Internet program or a standard Internet health education program (control condition). The interactive behavioral Internet program included a website that provided family-oriented nutrition education and behavior modification for parents and adolescents using counseling through email communications, weight and activity graphs for weekly self-monitoring of weight and physical activity, and self-monitoring of food intake with feedback modeled after the Traffic Light Diet. For both the intervention and control groups, the parent-child pairs were required to attend four face-to-face counseling sessions during the first 12 weeks of the program (weeks 1, 3, 6, and 12) to encourage adherence to behavioral principles, provide additional training in using their computers to participate in the Internet-based program, and solve any computer problems. Data were collected in the clinic and over the Internet at baseline and at months 6, 12, 18, and 24. Findings at 6 months showed that adolescents in the interactive behavioral program lost significantly more mean body fat and parents in that program also lost significantly more mean body weight. These weight losses, however, were reversed over the next 18 months. After 2 years, the differences in body fat for adolescents and weight for parents did not differ between the behavioral and the control groups.

While Williamson and colleagues did not observe any long-term reductions in weight outcomes of children and parents in their study, other studies show that family-based interventions can be effective in reducing the weight of children and parents in the long term. In a recent study, Collins and colleagues [57] evaluated the 24-month efficacy of a 6-month family-centered intervention, the Hunter Illawarra Kids Challenge Using Parent Support (HIKCUPS) study. Participants were 165 overweight prepubertal school-aged children in Australia who were randomized to receive one of three programs: a child-centered physical activity program (the Activity arm), a parent-centered dietary modification program (the Diet arm), or a combination of both programs (the Diet plus Activity arm). The child-centered Activity program was based on the competence motivation theory and aimed to improve children's fundamental movement-skill proficiency. The parent-centered Diet program was based on the Health Belief Model and incorporated goal setting, problem solving, role modeling, and positive reinforcement by parents to facilitate changes in eating behaviors. The Diet plus Activity arm was a combination of the diet and activity arms, with parents and children participating concurrently. Findings showed, between baseline and 24 months, that mean BMI z scores decreased significantly among children in all three intervention arms, with the highest decrease observed among children in the Diet arm, followed by the Activity arm, and then the Diet plus Activity arm. Parent weight loss was not discussed.

Another researcher who has contributed greatly to the field of family-based weight loss is Dr. Maria Golan. In a longer-term study conducted in Israel, Golan and colleagues [45] examined the effect of a 12-month family-based treatment intervention in which parents were the exclusive agents of change on weight outcomes of obese children. In this study, participants were 60 obese children aged 6–11 years from public schools in the middle-class town of Rehovot who were randomized into either an intervention or control group. In the intervention group, only parents (not children) participated in group sessions; children were not directly involved in the process of change and had no responsibility concerning the process. At group sessions, parents were taught to change the family's sedentary lifestyle, provide a prudent diet (reducing total and saturated fat and increasing monounsaturated fatty acids), decrease the family's exposure to food stimuli, apply behavioral modification strategies with the children, and practice relevant parenting skills (firm but supportive parenting practices). In the control group (child only), only the children participated in group sessions. Each child was prescribed a 6.3 MJ/day diet and attended group sessions lead by a clinical dietitian who provided information on how to follow a prudent diet, restrict energy intake, increase exercise, control food stimuli, use techniques for self-monitoring, practice problem solving and cognitive restructuring, and make use of social support (e.g., asking parents and friends for help). At the end of the 12-month intervention period, children in both groups showed a significant decrease in their degree of overweight, although the change was significantly greater in the parent-only intervention group than in the child-only control group. In addition, at 12-month post-intervention, 35 % of children who were in the parent-only group had attained a non-obese status, compared with 14 % in the child-only group. Change in the percentage of mothers classified as overweight did not differ significantly between the intervention (parent-only) group and control (child-only) group at 12-month post-intervention. However, among fathers there was a significant reduction in the percent of overweight among fathers in the parent-only intervention group, but not in the child-only control group. At a 1-year follow-up, the child-only control group had regained 7 % of their 8 % reduction in overweight, while children in the parent-only intervention group regained only 2 % of their 15 % reduction in overweight. At a 2-year follow-up, there was a mean reduction in overweight of 15 % in children in the parent-only intervention group and an increase of 3 % in children in the child-only control group.

Measurement of 50 of the original 60 children at a 7-year follow-up showed that mean reduction in percent overweight was significantly greater in the parent-only intervention group than in the child-only control group [60]. At the 7-year follow-up, 60 % of children in the parent-only group were classified as non-obese, compared with only 31 % of children in the child-only group [61, 74].

Promising Studies Underway

The importance of family-based approaches for preventing maternal and child weight obesity can also be measured by the numbers of obesity prevention efforts in the research pipeline. Developing initiatives for family-based approaches that can be implemented outside the clinic will allow easier access to difficult-to-reach populations. Seven promising studies designed for obesity prevention or treatments are currently underway: four in Australia, one in Sweden, and two in the United States (see Table 12.3).

Two studies based in Australian are targeting first-time parents. The InFANT study [75] and the NOURISH trial [76] are recruiting first-time parents and their 3–4-month-old children into an intervention that uses anticipatory guidance principles to teach parents proper feeding practices. The InFANT study is also educating parents about activity-promoting (and sedentary reduction) behaviors needed by their children during this early developmental period. Six dietitian-led programs will be held every 3 months, with measures of growth, food intake, and parenting behavior assessment to be made post-intervention and at 9-and 18-month follow-up periods. Although parent weight is not targeted per se, the intervention will focus on the parent's own obesity-preventing behaviors (healthy eating and regular physical activity) which may result in positive changes in parents' weight.

The NOURISH trial is recruiting infants born to first-time mothers at major maternity hospitals in Brisbane and Adelaide [76]. Mother-infant dyads will be randomized into usual care or the NOURISH intervention. The intervention will provide anticipatory guidance during two modules (modules implemented at ages 4–7 and 13–16 months) presented through six sessions over a 12-week period. The intervention content will emphasize healthy eating and feeding relationships for health growth – not specifically obesity prevention. Both modules promote authoritative parenting practices and feeding styles; however, physical activity (other than discouraging television viewing while feeding) is not included in the intervention material. The NOURISH trial will neither address parent weight or parental eating and activity behaviors.

In Sweden, a study is enrolling infants of obese parents (two overweight or one obese parent) at 1 year of age and following these children through age 6 [80]. The program is called STOPP, Stockholm Obesity Prevention Program, and consists of an educational component (booklets) for corresponding age groups (1–6 years) and home-based coaching

TABLE 12.3 Summary of ongoing studies focusing on family-based obesity interventions

Author	Year	Country	Design	Age of target child	Delivery channel	Intervention groups	Intervention dose
Campbell [75]	2008	Australia	RCT	3–18 months	Group sessions in community + follow-up texting and mailings	2 groups: Parents with dieticians, control group	6 sessions conducted every 3 months for 15 months conducted for parents
Daniels [76]	2009	Australia	RCT	4–7 and 13–16 months	Group sessions in community	1 group: Parents with dietician and psychologist	Fortnightly sessions divided into 2 modules at 4–7 and 13–16 months
Horodynski [77]	2011	United States	RCT	Infants younger than 4 months	Home visits + telephone contact	2 groups: Mothers with instructors, control group families with usual care by ENFEP	6 (60-min) visits reinforced with 3 telephone calls (5 min)
Horodynski [78]	2011	United States	RCT	12–36 months	Home visits + telephone contact	2 groups: Mother-toddler dyad with instructor, control group families	8 (60-min) visits reinforced with telephone contact

Skouteris [79]	2010	Australia	RCT	2–4 years	Group sessions in community	2 groups: Parent-child dyad with MEND leader, control group with delayed intervention	10 weekly sessions (90 min) for parent-child dyad combining joint active play and a 45-min parent-only education session
Sobko [80]	2011	Sweden	RCT	1–6 years	Home visits	1 group: Parents and trained coach	4 (90-min) sessions first year and 2 (60-min) sessions following years
Sacher [81]	2010	Australia	RCT	8–12 years	Group session in community	2 groups: Parent-child dyad with MEND leader, waitlist control group	18 sessions delivered over 9 weeks for child, parents, and siblings; intro and closing plus 16 PA, 8 behavioral change, and 8 nutrition lessons, with post-9-week free family swim pass

delivered by a health professional four times in year 1 and twice in each of the following years [80]. This multidisciplinary approach uses strategies informed by many disciplines to address eating, activity, and sleep by focusing on parenting skills and styles that create positive habits in the children. Again, parental weight is not a focus, but this program, similar to the other infant interventions, could easily focus on family weight management strategies.

The two US studies focus on parental feeding practices (but do not measure body weight). Important factors in obesity prevention [77, 78]. One of the studies addresses low-income, first-time mothers of infants less than 4 months of age [77], while the second study focuses on infants/toddlers between 12 and 36 months old [78]. Both these studies use the NEAT program, Nutrition Education Aimed at Toddlers. The purpose of NEAT is to assist the mothers in helping their children develop self-regulated feeding, a skill thought to be important in obesity prevention efforts. To date, no significant findings have been observed in parental feeding practices, but these low-income, rural women have improved their knowledge of appropriate feeding practices and, in general, have been receptive to the approach, offering promise for future development of the NEAT intervention. No efforts were directed toward maternal weight management, but role modeling healthy eating behaviors could be integrated into the child-based approach.

Two other promising studies are occurring in Australia, both using the MEND program (Mind, Exercise, Nutrition, Do it), a multi-community-based, healthy lifestyle program to address obesity among preschool children (MEND 2–4) [79] and children ages 8–12 years (MEND) [81]. The MEND 2–4 program is conducted for 10 weeks in community settings by MEND-trained professionals. It is offered free of change, with referrals coming from health-care providers and includes children who have poor eating habits, inactive lifestyles, obese parents, and/or a family history of related diseases (such as diabetes or high blood pressure). The MEND 2–4 study is continuing, but in the MEND program conducted with older obese children (ages 8–12 years, BMI ≥ 98th percentile), Sacher and colleagues report favorable preliminary findings, including excellent attendance by families (86%) and encouraging initial results (reduced waist circumference and BMI z-scores in the children) [81]. The MEND programs show strong promise as family-focused programs that can be implemented within community settings by professionals trained to present them. Although parental weight is not currently a focus of MEND, minor modifications could be made to expand its focus from targeting only children for behavior and weight outcomes to become a more family-focused behavioral program with weight management efforts provided for both parents and children.

Summary and Future Directions

It is clear from the studies described in this chapter that family-centered approaches are promising strategies for addressing obesity issues that might arise within families. Studies targeting newborns show positive trends for helping very young children begin life on a proper trajectory for healthy growth by teaching parenting practices (e.g., helping mothers understand how to sooth, rather than feed, babies back to sleep; importance of tummy time; use of developmentally appropriate feeding practices) [47, 49, 51, 52]. When a focus on maternal weight was added, these cognitive-behavioral strategies for child weight management resulted in weight loss for some or most of the mothers enrolled [46, 48] and, in one small study, significant short- and long-term weight loss in overweight preschoolers [50]. When weight problems are identified in school-aged children or adolescents, family-based solutions prove to be superior to child-focused strategies. Rarely are weight problems isolated to a single child within a family and risk of obesity is increased when one or more caregivers are overweight or obese. Thus, treating obesity as a family issue rather a problem of the child offers the potential for successful long-term solutions.

The majority of family-centered interventions were focused on reducing obesity in school-aged children and adolescents. Many of these family-based treatment programs were modeled after the pioneering work of Epstein [39, 54, 55] and/or Golan [40, 45]. A family-based healthy lifestyle approach characterizes Epstein's work, while that of Golan includes parent education [53]. Golan's landmark work focuses on "parent as agent of change," an approach that suggests it is parents who need to learn parenting strategies in order for children's weight to be effectively managed. Parent-based weight outcomes are included in the work of both Epstein and Golan, and data from multiple studies have noted improved weight outcomes in both child and parent.

Family-based weight management programs have been increasingly available since the mid-1970s, but the focus continues to be primarily on child outcomes, with parental weight outcomes secondary. Gan and Clark [82] in 1976 were among the first to point out that excess weight runs in families, influenced both by genetics and environment, suggesting that "...identification, therapy, and control of obesity be accomplished on a family-line basis."

Family-centered interventions have been conducted in multiple setting, including the home [47, 49, 50, 52], the clinic or hospital [59, 65], the community [62, 66], and the Internet [44]. Although family systems theories may drive these interventions, few describe the theoretical framework on which their family-centered interventions are based [48, 51, 57, 59]. Six of the interventions reviewed adapted Epstein's Traffic Light Diet [69] and these produced positive results in terms of preventing or reducing child weight outcomes [44, 56, 60, 63, 71].

While the family-based studies in this review include both the parent and child in the prevention or treatment programs, not all of the studies actually targeted and/or measured weight-related outcomes in the parent. More than half of the interventions targeting children five and younger [46–48, 50] and six of 13 in the school-aged studies [44, 56, 60, 61, 63, 64] provided a specific focus on parental weight outcomes. Only a few of those interventions that measured weight outcomes in parents actually found that the interventions had significant effects on parents' weight status, but the long-term studies by Epstein seem to underscore the importance of a family-based weight management approach [73]. Wrotniak and colleagues [83] analyzed the findings from three family-based studies in which one parent and one child (both overweight) were recruited for participation. At the 2-year follow-up, parent z-BMI change predicted child z-BMI change. Parents in the highest quartile of z-BMI change had children weight significantly greater z-BMI change than children with parents at other weight levels. Although named "family-centered interventions," none of the studies measured weight outcomes in siblings of children enrolled in the studies.

Studies conducted in the United States [73], United Kingdom [67], Israel [74], and Australia [57] show that in the long term, family-centered interventions are effective in promoting and sustaining weight reduction in children. In addition, the study by Golan et al. [45] shows that involving the parent in childhood obesity interventions results in greater improvements in weight outcomes when compared to child-only interventions.

Clinicians who care for mothers with infants should encourage a family-centered approach for healthy weight development in the young child and positive weight-related behaviors for the entire family. Mothers of children of all ages should be taught that obesity prevention is a family issue and that families should adopt nutrition and physical activity practices that result in healthy weight development for children and appropriate weight management for adult caregivers. Future research should expand family-centered obesity prevention strategies for children of all ages as a strategy for positive weight management in mothers and other family members.

References

1. Centers for Disease Control and Prevention. Reproductive health: pregnancy complications. http://www.cdc.gov/reproductivehealth/maternalinfanthealth/PregComplications.htm. Accessed 8 Oct 2012.
2. Flegal KM, Carroll MD, Kit BK, Ogden CL. Prevalence of obesity and trends in the distribution of body mass index among US adults, 1999–2010. JAMA. 2012;307(5):491–7.

3. Ogden CL, Carroll MD, Kit BK, Flegal KM. Prevalence of obesity and trends in body mass index among US children and adolescents, 1999–2010. JAMA. 2012;307(5):483–90.
4. Centers for Disease Control and Prevention (CDC). Basics about childhood obesity. Available at http://www.cdc.gov/obesity/childhood/basics.html. Accessed 22 Aug 2012.
5. Herman KM, Craig CL, Gauvin L, Katzmarzyk PT. Tracking of obesity and physical activity from childhood to adulthood: the Physical Activity Longitudinal Study. Int J Pediatr Obes. 2009;4(4):281–8.
6. Deshmukh-Taskar P, Nicklas TA, Morales M, Yang SJ, Zakeri I, Berenson GS. Tracking of overweight status from childhood to young adulthood: the Bogalusa Heart Study. Eur J Clin Nutr. 2006;60(1):48–57.
7. Whitaker RC, Wright JA, Pepe MS, Seidel KD, Dietz WH. Predicting obesity in young adulthood from childhood and parental obesity. N Engl J Med. 1997;337(13):869–73.
8. Centers for Disease Control and Prevention. Adult overweight and obesity: causes and consequences. Available at http://www.cdc.gov/obesity/adult/causes/index.html. Accessed 22 Aug 2012.
9. Olson CM, Demment MM, Carling SJ, Straderman MS. Associations between mothers' and their children's weights at 4 years of age. Child Obes. 2010;6(4):201–7.
10. Stamnes Koepp UM, Frost Andersen L, Dahl-Joergensen K, Stigum H, Naess O, Nystad W. Maternal pre-pregnant body mass index, maternal weight change and offspring birthweight. Acta Obstet Gynecol Scand. 2012;91(2):243–9.
11. Stamnes Koepp UM, Dahl-Joergensen K, Frost Andersen L, Naess O, Nystad W. The associations between maternal pre-pregnancy body mass index or gestational weight change during pregnancy and body mass index of the child at 3 years of age. Int J Obes (Lond). 2012;36(10):1325–31.
12. Olson CM, Strawderman MS, Dennison BA. Maternal weight gain during pregnancy and child weight at age 3 years. Matern Chil Health J. 2009;13:839–46.
13. Dubois L, Girard M. Early determinants of overweight at 4.5 years in a population-based longitudinal study. Int J Obes (Lond). 2006;30(4):610–7.
14. Whitaker RC. Predicting preschooler obesity at birth: the role of maternal obesity in early pregnancy. Pediatrics. 2004;114(1):e29–36.
15. Laitinen J, Jaaskelainen A, Hartikainen AL, Sovio U, Vaarasmaki M, Pouta A, Kaakinen M, Jarvelin MR. Maternal weight gain during the first half of pregnancy and offspring obesity at 16 years: a prospective cohort study. BJOG. 2012;119(6):716–23.
16. Birch LL, Davison KK. Family environmental factors influencing the developing behavioral controls of food intake and childhood overweight. Pediatr Clin North Am. 2001;48(4):893–907.

17. Davison KK, Birch LL. Childhood overweight: a contextual model and recommendations for future research. Obes Rev. 2001;2(3): 159–71.
18. McLeod ER, Campbell KJ, Diet G, et al. Nutrition knowledge: a mediator between socioeconomic position and diet quality in Australian first-time mothers. J Am Diet Assoc. 2011;111(5): 696–704.
19. Cullen KW, Baranowski T, Owens E, et al. Availability, accessibility, and preferences for fruit, 100 % fruit juice, and vegetables influence children's dietary behavior. Health Educ Behav. 2003;30:615–26.
20. Haerens L, Craeynest M, Deforche B, et al. The contribution of psychosocial and home environmental factors explaining eating behaviors in adolescents. Eur J Clin Nutr. 2008;62:51–9.
21. Hanson NI, Neumark-Sztainer D, Eisenberg ME, et al. Associations between parental report of the home food environment and adolescent intakes of fruits, vegetables and dairy foods. Public Health Nutr. 2005;8:77–85.
22. Patrick H, Nicklas TA. A review of family and social determinants of children's eating patterns and diet quality. J Am Coll Nutr. 2005;24(2): 83–92.
23. Fisher JO, Mitchell DC, Smiciklas-Wright H, Birch LL. Parental influences on young girls' fruit and vegetable, micronutrient, and fat intakes. J Am Diet Assoc. 2002;102(1):58–64.
24. Gibson EL, Wardle J, Watts CJ. Fruit and vegetable consumption, nutritional knowledge and beliefs in mothers and children. Appetite. 1998;31(2):205–28.
25. Wyse R, Campbell E, Wolfenden L. Associations between characteristics of the home food environment and fruit and vegetable intake in preschool children: a cross-sectional study. BMC Public Health. 2011;11:938.
26. Tibbs T, Haire-Joshu D, Schechtman KB, Brownson RC, Nanney MS, Houston C, Auslander W. The relationship between parental modeling, eating patterns, and dietary intake among African-American parents. J Am Diet Assoc. 2001;101(5):535–41.
27. Ray C, Roos E. Family characteristics predicting favorable changes in 10 and 11-year old children's lifestyle-related health behaviors during an 18-month follow-up. Appetite. 2012;58(1):326–32.
28. Blissett J. Relationships between parenting style, feeding style and feeding practices and fruit and vegetable consumption in early childhood. Appetite. 2011;57(3):826–31.
29. Jago R, Fox KR, Page AS, Brockman R, Thompson JL. Parent and child physical activity and sedentary time: do active parents foster active children? BMC Public Health. 2010;10:194.
30. Salmon J, Timperio A, Telford A, Carver A, Crawford D. Association of family environment with children's television viewing and with low level of physical activity. Obes Res. 2005;13(11):1939–51.

31. Barradas DT, Fulton JE, Blanck HM, Huhman M. Parental influences on youth television viewing. J Pediatr. 2007;151(4):369–73.
32. Van Zutphen M, Bell AC, Kremer PJ, Swinburn BA. Association between the family environment and television viewing in Australian children. J Paediatr Child Health. 2007;43(6):458–63.
33. Matheson DM, Wang Y, Klesges LM, et al. African-American girls' dietary intake while watching television. Obes Res. 2004;12(Suppl):32S–7.
34. Marquis M, Filion YP, Dagenais F. Does eating while watching television influence children's food related behaviors. Can J Diet Pract. 2005;66:12–8.
35. Feldman S, Eisenberg ME, Neumark-Sztainer D, et al. Associations between watching TV during family meals and dietary intake among adolescents. J Nutr Educ Behav. 2007;39:257–63.
36. Santos JL, Kain J, Dominguez-Vasquez P, Lera L, Galvan M, Corvalan C, Uauy R. Maternal anthropometry and feeding behavior toward preschool children: Association with childhood body mass index in an observational study of Chilean families. Int J Behav Nutr Phy Act. 2009;6:93. doi:10.1186/1479-5868-6-93.
37. Whitaker RC, Deeks CM, Baughcun AE, Specker BL. The relationship of childhood adiposity to parent body mass index and eating behavior. Obes Res. 2000;8(3):234–40.
38. Cutting TM, Fisher O, Grimm-Thomas K, Birch LL. Like mother, like daughter: familial patterns of overweight are mediated by mothers' dietary disinhibition. Am J Clin Nutr. 1999;69(4):608–13.
39. Epstein LH, Myers MD, Raynor HA, Saelens BE. Treatment of pediatric obesity. Pediatrics. 1998;101:554–70.
40. Golan M, Weizman A. Familial approach to the treatment of childhood obesity: conceptual model. J Nutr Educ. 2001;33:102–7.
41. Kitzmann KM, Beech BM. Family-based interventions for pediatric obesity: methodological and conceptual challenges from family psychology. J Fam Psychol. 2006;20(1):175–89.
42. Gruber KJ, Haldeman LA. Using the family to combat childhood and adult obesity. Prev Chronic Dis. 2009;6(3):1–10.
43. Lindsay AC, Sussner KM, Kim J, Gortmaker S. The role of parents in preventing childhood obesity. Future Child. 2006;16(1):169–86.
44. Williamson DA, Walden HM, White MA, York-Crowe E, Newton RL, Alfonso A, Gordon S, Ryan D. Two-year internet-based randomized controlled trial for weight loss in African-American girls. Obesity. 2006;14(7):1231–43.
45. Golan M, Weizman A, Apter A, Fainaru M. Parents as the exclusive agents of change in the treatment of childhood obesity. Am J Clin Nutr. 1998;67(6):1130–5.
46. Ostbye T, Krause KM, Stroo M, Lovelady CA, Peterson BL, Bastian LA, Swamy GK, West DG, Brouwer RJ, Zucker NL. Parent-focused change to prevent obesity in preschoolers: results from the KAN-DO study. Prev Med. 2012;55(3):188–95.

47. Harvey-Berino J, Rourke K. Obesity prevention in preschool Native-American children: a pilot study using home visiting. Obes Res. 2003;11(5):606–11.
48. Klohe-Lehman DM, Freeland-Graves J, Clarke KK, et al. Low-income, overweight and obese mothers as agents of change to improve food choices, fat habits, and physical activity in their 1 to 3 year old children. J Am Coll Nutr. 2007;26(3):196–208.
49. Paul IM, Savage JS, Anzman SL, et al. Preventing obesity during infancy: a pilot study. Obesity. 2011;19(2):353–61.
50. Stark LJ, Spear S, Boles R, et al. A pilot randomized controlled trial of a clinic and home-based behavioral intervention to decrease obesity in preschoolers. Obesity. 2011;19:134–41.
51. Wen LM, Baur LA, Simpson JM, Rissel C, Wardle K, Flood VM. Effectiveness of home based early intervention on children's BMI at age 2: randomized controlled trial. BMJ. 2012;344:e3732.
52. Wen LM, Baur LA, Rissel C, Wardle K, Alperstein G, Simpson JM. Early intervention of multiple home visits to prevent childhood obesity in a disadvantaged population: a home-based randomized controlled trial (Healthy Beginnings Trial). BMC Public Health. 2007;7:2–8.
53. Sung-Chan P, Sung YW, Zhao X, Brownson RC. Family-based models for childhood-obesity intervention: a systematic review of randomized controlled trials. Obes Rev. 2013 Apr;14(4):265-78. doi:10.1111/obr.12000. Epub 2012 Nov 9.
54. Epstein LH, Valoski A, Wing RR, McCurley J. Ten-year outcomes of behavioral family-based treatment for childhood obesity. Health Psychol. 1994;13(5):373–83.
55. Epstein LH, Wing RR, Koeske R, Valoski A. Long-term effects of family-based treatment of childhood obesity. J Consult Clin Psychol. 1987;55(1):91–5.
56. Boutelle KN, Cafri G, Crow SJ. Parent-only treatment for childhood obesity: a randomized controlled trial. Obesity. 2011;19:574–80.
57. Collins CE, Okely A, Morgan PJ, Jones RA, Burrows TL, Cliff DP, Colyvas K, Warren JM, Steele JR, Baur LA. Parent diet modification, child activity, or both in obese children: an RCT. Pediatrics. 2011;127(4):619–28.
58. Coppins DF, Margetts BM, Fa JL, Brown M, Garrett F, Huelin S. Effectiveness of a multi-disciplinary family-based program for treating childhood obesity (The Family Project). Eur J Clin Nutr. 2011;65:903–9.
59. Edwards C, Nicholls D, Crocker H, Van Zyl S, Viner R, Wardle J. Family-based behavioral treatment of obesity: acceptability and effectiveness in the UK. Eur J Clin Nutr. 2006;60:587–92.
60. Epstein LH, Valoski A, Wing R, McCurley J. Ten-year follow-up of behavioral, family-based treatment for obese children. JAMA. 1990;264:2519–23.
61. Golan M. Parents as agents of change in childhood obesity—from research to practice. Int J Pediatr Obes. 2006;1(2):66–76.

62. Gronbaek HN, Madsen SA, Michaelsen KF. Family involvement in the treatment of childhood obesity: the Copenhagen approach. Eur J Pediatr. 2009;168:1437–47.
63. Janicke DM, Sallinen BJ, Perri MG, Lutes LD, Huerta M, Silverstein JH, Brumback B. Comparison of parent-only versus family-based interventions for overweight children in underserved rural settings. Outcomes from Project STORY. Arch Pediatr Adolesc Med. 2008;162(12):1119–25.
64. Kalarchian MA, Levine MD, Arslanian SA, Ewing LJ, Houck PR, Cheng Y, Ringham RM, Sheets CA, Marsha D. Family-based treatment of severe pediatric obesity: randomized, controlled trial. Pediatrics. 2009;124:1060–8.
65. Magarey AM, Perry RA, Baur LA, Steinbeck SK, Sawyer M, Hills AP, Wilson G, Lee A, Daniels LA. A parent-led family-focused treatment program for overweight children aged 5 to 9 years: the PEACH RCT. Pediatrics. 2011;127(2):214–23.
66. Robertson W, Friede T, Blissett J, Rudolf MCJ, Wallis M, Stewart-Brown S. Pilot of "Families for Health": community-based family intervention for obesity. Arch Dis Child. 2008;93:921–6.
67. Robertson W, Thorogood M, Inglis N, Grainger C, Stewart-Brown S. Two-year follow-up of the "Families for Health" program for the treatment of childhood obesity. Child Care Health Dev. 2011;38(2):229–36.
68. Shelton D, LeGros K, Norton L, et al. Randomized controlled trial. A parent-based group education program for overweight children. J Pediatr Child Health. 2007;43:799–805.
69. Epstein L, Squires S. The stoplight diet for children. Boston: Little Brown, & Co.; 1988.
70. Boutelle KN, Cafri G, Crow SJ. Parent predictors of child weight change in family-based behavioral obesity treatment. Obesity. 2012;20:1539–43.
71. Janicke DM, Sallinen BJ, Perri MG, Lutes LD, Silverstein JH, Huerta MG, Guion LA. Sensible Treatment of Obesity in Rural Youth (STORY): design and methods. Contemp Clin Trials. 2008;29:270–80.
72. Epstein LH. Development of evidence-based treatments for pediatric obesity. In: Kadzin AE, Jr W, editors. Evidence-based psychotherapies for children and adolescents. New York: Guilford Press; 2003. p. 374–88.
73. Epstein LH, Paluch RA, Roemmich JN, Beecher MD. Family-based obesity treatment, then and now: twenty-five years of pediatric obesity treatment. Health Psychol. 2007;26:381–91.
74. Golan M, Crow S. Targeting parents exclusively in the treatment of childhood obesity: long-term results. Obes Res. 2004;1(1):357–61.
75. Campbell K, Hesketh K, Crawford D, Salmon J, Ball K, McCallum Z. The Infant Feeding Activity and Nutrition Trial (INFANT) an early intervention to prevent childhood obesity: cluster-randomised controlled trial. BMC Public Health. 2008;8:103.

76. Daniels L, Magarey A, Battistutta D, Nicholson J, Farrell A, Davidson G, Cleghorn G. The NOURISH randomised control trial: positive feeding practices and food preferences in early childhood – a primary prevention program for childhood obesity. BMC Public Health. 2009;9:1–10.
77. Horodynski M, Olson B, Baker S, Brophy-Herb H, Auld G, Egren L, Lindau J, Singleterry L. Healthy babies through infant-centered feeding protocol: an intervention targeting early childhood obesity in vulnerable populations. BMC Public Health. 2011;11:868.
78. Horodynski M, Baker S, Coleman G, Auld G, Lindau J. The healthy toddlers trial protocol: an intervention to reduce risk factors for childhood obesity in economically and educationally disadvantaged populations. BMC Public Health. 2011;11:581.
79. Skouteris H, McCabe M, Swinburn B, Hill B. Healthy eating and obesity prevention for preschoolers: a randomised controlled trial. BMC Public Health. 2010;10:220.
80. Sobko T, Svensson V, Ek A, Ekstedt M, Karlsson H, Johansson E, Cao Y, Hagstromer M, Marcus C. A randomised controlled trial for overweight and obese parents to prevent childhood obesity – early STOPP. BMC Public Health. 2011;11:336.
81. Satcher PM, Kolotourou M, Chadwick PM, Cole TJ, Lawson MS, Lucas A, et al. Randomized controlled trial of the MEND program: a family-based community intervention for childhood obesity. Obesity. 2010;18(Suppl):S62–8.
82. Garn SM, Clark DC. Trends in fatness and the origins of obesity. Pediatrics. 1976;57:433–56.
83. Wrotniak BH, Epstein LH, Paluch RA, Roemmich JN. Parent weight change as a predictor of child weight change in family-based behavioral obesity treatment. Arch Pediatr Adolesc Med. 2004;158:342–7.

Chapter 13
Obesity Screening Recommendations and Emerging Policies

Wanda Nicholson

"To Win We Have to Lose," from Weight of the Nation, Confronting America's Obesity Epidemic [1]

Abstract Screening for obesity is recommended by several expert committees and organizations, such as the United States Preventive Services Task Force, the American College of Obstetricians and Gynecologists, NIH, and the Canadian Task Force. Numerous national and regional health policies have been developed to prevent obesity and promote healthy lifestyle behaviors in adults and children. Health system-sponsored programs, community gardens, and public posting of the caloric and fat content of foods in restaurants are a sample of current efforts to stem the current epidemic of obesity.

Keywords Obesity • Screening • Recommendations • Policy • Pregnancy • Weight

---

W. Nicholson, MD, MPH, MBA
Department of Obstetrics and Gynecology,
Diabetes and Obesity Core, Center for Women's Health Research,
University of North Carolina School of Medicine,
Chapel Hill, NC, USA
e-mail: wanda_nicholson@med.unc.edu

W. Nicholson, K. Baptiste-Roberts (eds.),
Obesity During Pregnancy in Clinical Practice,
DOI 10.1007/978-1-4471-2831-1_13,
© Springer-Verlag London 2014

Introduction

Screening for obesity is a critical step in prevention and treatment. Evidence in support of obesity screening is the reduction in adverse pregnancy-related outcomes, diabetes, cardiovascular morbidity, and mortality. The United States Preventive Services Task Force [2]; the American Congress of Obstetricians and Gynecologists [3]; the National Heart, Lung, and Blood Institute [4]; and the Canadian Task Force [5] are organizations that provide recommendations for screening and management of obesity in adults. In this chapter, we focus on the individual obesity screening recommendations from committees of experts and current initiatives in the United States to facilitate lifestyle modifications among women with obesity.

The United States Preventive Services Task Force [6] is an independent, nonfederal panel of experts in prevention and evaluation of scientific evidence; scientific and logistical support for the Task Force is provided by the Agency for Healthcare Research and Quality (AHRQ). The 16 volunteer Task Force members include physicians specializing in Internal Medicine, Family Medicine, Obstetrics and Gynecology, and Pediatrics, as well as nurse practitioners and experts in behavioral health. Most members are active primary care clinicians; many are respected researchers and distinguished professors as well. The American Congress of Obstetricians and Gynecologists (ACOG) is a nonprofit national organization of obstetricians and gynecologists providing obstetrical and gynecological care to women across the life span. ACOG provides a series of practice bulletins and committee opinions on pregnancy care, gestational weight gain, motivational interviewing, and general counseling on lifestyle modifications. The National Heart, Lung, and Blood Institute is part of the National Institutes of Health. NHLBI focuses on the conduct and funding of the downstream consequences of obesity, including cardiovascular disease and the metabolic syndrome. In 1998, the NHLBI, in collaboration with the National Institute of Diabetes and Digestive and Kidney Diseases (NIDDK), and a convened expert panel, published an extensive evidence report

TABLE 13.1 Classification of overweight, obesity, waist circumference, and disease risks

	BMI	Obesity class	Disease risks[a] relative to normal weight and waist circumference	
			Men	Women
Underweight	< 18.5			
Normal	18.5–24.9			
Overweight	25.0–29.9		Increased	High
Obese	30.0–34.9	I	High	Very high
	35–39.9	II	Very high	Very high
	40 and up	III	Extremely high	Extremely high

Adapted from: National Institutes of Health [10]
BMI body mass index
[a]Disease risk for type 2 diabetes, hypertension, and cardiovascular disease (CVD)

on the identification, prevention, and management of obesity [4]. The Canadian Task Force [7], established by the Public Health Agency of Canada, develops clinical practice guidelines that support primary care providers in delivering preventive services.

Recommendations for Screening by Expert Committees

Measuring body mass index is the first step to determine the degree of adiposity. The BMI is relatively easy and reliable and correlates with percentage of body fat and body fat mass. Also, BMI is used to identify adults at increased risk for morbidity and mortality. For example, women who are overweight or obese are at increased risk of type 2 diabetes and cardiovascular disease, even within the context of a normal waist circumference (Table 13.1).

Guidelines for the screening and evaluation of overweight and obesity have been published by a number of organizations including the National Heart, Lung, and Blood Institute

Table 13.2 Summary of screening recommendations from expert committees

Expert committee	Recommendation
United States Preventive Services Task Force	Screening all adults for obesity
	Clinicians should offer or refer patients with a body mass index of 30 kg/m^2 or higher to intensive, multicomponent behavioral interventions
NHLBI	The NIH recommends screening adults for obesity with BMI, waist circumference and risk factor assessment. Subsequent intervention is then based upon overall risk assessment
Canadian Task Force	Measure body mass index and waist circumference in all adults and adolescents to determine the degree and distribution of body fat
	Measure blood pressure, heart rate, fasting glucose level, and lipid profile (total cholesterol, triglycerides, high-density and low-density lipoprotein cholesterol levels)
	Consider appropriate pharmacotherapy or referral for bariatric surgery, or both
American Congress of Obstetricians and Gynecologists	Measure BMI in all adult women presenting for any clinical visit

NHLBI the National Heart, Lung, and Blood Institute, *NIH* National Institutes of Health, *BMI* body mass index

(NHLBI) [4], the World Health Organization (WHO) [8], and the United States Preventive Services Task Force [2, 5, 9] (Table 13.2). NHLBI [10] recommends screening adults for obesity with BMI and waist circumference and risk factor assessment. Subsequent intervention is then based upon overall risk assessment [4]. The United States Preventive Services Task Force (USPSTF) recommends that clinicians screen all adult patients for obesity and offer intensive counseling and behavioral interventions to promote sustained weight loss for obese

(BMI >30 kg/m^2) adults. The Canadian Task Force on Preventive Health Care recommends measuring BMI and waist circumference in all adults. The American College of Obstetricians and Gynecologists recommends measuring BMI in all adult women as part of routine gynecologic and well woman visits [3]. Overweight or obese women should then be counseled about the healthy eating and increasing physical activity.

Current Initiatives to Prevent Obesity

Multiple national, regional, and state initiatives to promote lifestyle modifications among women and their families have grown over the past decade. These initiatives, spearheaded by the White House, CDC, healthcare organizations, and state health agencies, focus on educating adults about the adverse health consequences of obesity and the importance of healthy eating and physical activity. The long-term goal of these policy initiatives is to increase the availability of low-cost healthy foods, promote safe neighborhood venues for physical activity, and promote knowledge about the caloric and fat content of foods.

National Initiatives

The "Let's Move!" campaign [11], launched by the First Lady, Michelle Obama, combats child obesity by promoting family-centered interventions. The campaign identifies strategies to create a healthy start for children, empower parents and caregivers in setting an example of healthy eating, advocate for healthy foods in school cafeterias, increase the availability of healthy foods, and promote physical activity. Several subprograms within the Let's Move! campaign target adults through faith-based organizations and promote physical activity and regular exercise, in particularly high-risk populations, including Native Americans and Alaskan natives. The campaign ("Let's Move!

In the Clinic") promotes professional partnerships between the program and healthcare professionals.

The National Diabetes Prevention Program [12], supported by the CDC, is designed to bring to communities evidence-based lifestyle change programs for weight loss and prevention of type 2 diabetes. The program is based on the Diabetes Prevention Program research study led by the National Institutes of Health and supported by Centers for Disease Control and Prevention. The lifestyle program in this study showed that making modest behavior changes (increasing healthy food choices and physical activity to at least 150 min per week) helped male and female participants to lose 5–7 % of their body weight and reduced the risk of developing type 2 diabetes mellitus. Participants work with a lifestyle coach in a group setting to receive a 1-year lifestyle change program. Current efforts are focused on translating the program into diverse clinical settings (i.e., health departments, healthcare organizations, private clinics) and communities.

Reducing Sweetened Beverages and Posting Caloric Content

In 2012, the state of New York banned the sale of oversized sugary drinks at restaurants, street carts, and movie theaters in an effort to reduce the rising rate of obesity in the city [13]. Recent studies have shown a strong association between the number of sweetened beverages consumed, reduced physical activity, and obesity [14]. Moreover, economic models suggest that a tax on sweetened beverages would reduce the consumption of sweetened beverages by 15 % [15]. The initiative limits the containers for the sale of sugary drinks to 16 oz or less. Consumers are able to purchase larger-sized beverages if they desire, but the standard size is <16 oz.

Additionally, many cities and states have now required that restaurants post the caloric and fat content of their meals on menus and menu boards [16].

Regional- and Community-Oriented Initiatives

Ready, Set, Thrive! [17] is an example of a community-based program that is often supported by regional healthcare organizations. Sponsored by Kaiser Permanente Sacramento, the Kaiser Permanente Walk to Thrive Program is an ongoing mall walking club open to local communities and Kaiser employees in Sacramento, California. Physicians and other staff members at Kaiser host the early morning mall walking events to promote healthy habits to lower weight and blood pressure, and reduce cholesterol [17].

Conclusions

Several organizations have made recommendations for screening for obesity in adults. There are areas of emphasis that vary across organizations. For example, the Task Force's recommendation for screening is based on evidence that behavioral interventions are successful at weight reduction. In contrast, NHLBI recommends obesity screening and provides specific recommendations for lifestyle modification as well as additional clinical assessment of future medical risks. Regardless of the specific guideline that is followed, screening for obesity prior to and after pregnancy has the potential to substantially reduce the epidemic of obesity among women of childbearing age and the adverse pregnancy consequences that they may endure. Current initiatives to promote lifestyle modifications, improve health eating, and enhance venues for physical activity are gaining traction and have the potential to substantially reduce the percentage of women with obesity.

References

1. To Win We Have to Lose," from the 2013 Weight of the Nation, Confronting America's Obesity Epidemic. http://theweightofthenation.hbo.com/. Accessed on 16 Sep 2013.

2. Moyer VA, U.S. Preventive Services Task Force. Screening for and management of obesity in adults: U.S. Preventive Services Task Force recommendation statement. Ann Intern Med. 2012;157(5):373.
3. ACOG Committee on Gynecologic Practice. The role of the obstetrician–gynecologist in the assessment and management of obesity. Obstet Gynecol. 2005;106:895–9.
4. The Practical Guide: Identification E, and Treatment of Overweight and Obesity in Adults http://www.nhlbi.nih.gov.libproxy.lib.unc.edu/guidelines/obesity/prctgd_c.pdf. Accessed on 2 July 2013.
5. Lau DC, Obesity Canada Clinical Practice Guidelines Steering Committee and Expert Panel. Synopsis of the 2006 Canadian clinical practice guidelines on the management and prevention of obesity in adults and children. Can Med Assoc J. 2007;176(8):1103.
6. The United States Preventive Services Task Force Home Page. www.unitedstatespreventiveservicestaskforce.org. Accessed on 24 Sep 2013.
7. The Canadian Task Force on Preventive Health Care. http://canadiantaskforce.ca/. Accessed on 24 Sep 2013.
8. Report on Obesity. World Health Organization Technical Report Service. 2000;894:1–253.
9. Lyznicki JMYD, Riggs JA, Davis RM. Council on scientific affairs, American medical association obesity: assessment and management in primary care. Am Fam Physician. 2001;63(11):2185.
10. National Institutes of Health. Clinical guidelines on the identification, evaluation, and treatment of overweight and obesity in adults–the evidence report. Obes Res. 1998;6:515.
11. The Let's Move Campaign. America's Move to Raise a Healthier Generation of Kids. www.letsmove.com. Accessed on 24 Sep 2013.
12. The National Diabetes Prevention Program. http://www.cdc.gov/diabetes/prevention/. Accessed on 24 Sep 2013.
13. Michelle Castillo. NYC refreshes anti-sugary drink campaign with new ads. CBS News on-line. / 2013. http://www.cbsnews.com/8301-204_162-57587576/. Accessed on 24 Sep 2013.
14. Duffey KJ, Gordon-Larsen P, Steffen LM, Jacobs Jr DR, Popkin BM. Drinking caloric beverages increases the risk of adverse cardiometabolic outcomes in the Coronary Artery Risk Development in Young Adults (CARDIA) Study. Am J Clin Nutr. 2010;92(4):954–9.
15. Wang YC, Coxson P, Shen YM, Goldman L, Bibbins-Domingo K. A penny-per-ounce tax on sugar-sweetened beverages would cut health and cost burdens of diabetes. Health Aff (Millwood). 2012;31(1):199–207.
16. The Requirements to Post Calorie Counts on Menus in NYC Food Services Establishments. Section 81.50 of the New York City Code. http://www.nyc.gov/html/doh/downloads/pdf/cdp/calorie_compliance_guide.pdf.
17. The Kaiser Permanente of Sacramento "Walk to Thrive" Campaign. https://kpwalktothrive.org/. Accessed on 24 Sep 2013.

Index

A
ACOG. *See* The American College of Obstetricians and Gynecologists (ACOG)
ACPM. *See* The American College of Preventive Medicine (ACPM)
Active Mothers Postpartum (AMP), 199
ADHD. *See* Attention-deficit/hyperactivity disorder (ADHD)
Agency for Healthcare Research and Quality (AHRQ), 338
AHA. *See* American Heart Association (AHA)
AHRQ. *See* Agency for Healthcare Research and Quality (AHRQ)
The American College of Obstetricians and Gynecologists (ACOG), 20, 47, 80, 162, 185–186–188, 338, 340
The American College of Preventive Medicine (ACPM), 39–40
American Heart Association (AHA), 23
AMP. *See* Active Mothers Postpartum (AMP)
Anesthesia, 63–64
Anovulation
 adipose tissue, 15
 hypothalamic GnRH pulsatility, 15
 ovulatory cycle, 14–15
 PCOS (*see* Polycystic ovary syndrome (PCOS))
Asthma
 and obesity during pregnancy, 271, 272–277
 overweight, 271
Attention-deficit/hyperactivity disorder (ADHD), 286–287
Autism, 287

B
Bariatric surgery
 BMI, 46
 goal of, 26
 impact on fertility and pregnancy outcomes, 46, 235
 preconception care, 46

Bariatric surgery (*cont.*)
  prepregnancy interventions, 234
  restrictive and malabsorptive, 26
  tools, weight loss, 46
  for women, 46
BDI. *See* Beck Depression Inventory (BDI)
Beck Depression Inventory (BDI), 101, 102, 112
Behavioral change counseling, 42
Behavioral change models
  MI, 42–44
  SCT, 42
BIS. *See* Body image satisfaction (BIS)
Body image
  African-American women, 122–123
  and BMI, 129–130
  body image$_{current}$, 125
  body image$_{ideal}$, 125
  conceptual framework, 123–124
  figure rating exercises, 124, 125
  historical influence, 126–127
  postpartum, 142–148
  during pregnancy (*see* Pregnancy)
  social influence
    acculturation, 128–129
    maternal influence, 128
    media, 127
    opposite sex preferences, 127
  Stunkard scale, 125
  White women, 126
Body image discrepancy. *See* Body image dissatisfaction (BID)
Body image dissatisfaction (BID), 125
Body image satisfaction (BIS), 141
Body mass index (BMI)
  bariatric surgery, 46
  BMI z scores, 314–317, 319
  body fat and body fat mass, 339
  body image, 129–130
  calculation, 38
  CARDIA study, 82
  cesarean delivery, 62
  clinical assessment, health visit, 38
  definition, 11
  GDM, 5
  gestational weight gain, 246–248, 264
  and gestational weight gain, 79, 80
  high-BMI groups, 81
  male fertility, 19
  maternal prepregnancy BMI (*see* Maternal prepregnancy BMI)
  postpartum, 147, 148
  PPWR, high-BMI groups, 81
  pregnancy and postpartum, 192
  pregnancy cohorts and, 84–85
  prepregnancy, 84–85, 87
  schizophrenia, 285
  waist circumference and risk factor assessment, 340, 341
  z-BMI change, 329

C

CARDIA study. *See* The Coronary Artery Risk Development in Young Adults (CARDIA) study
Cardiovascular disease, 78, 92
CBT. *See* Cognitive behavioral therapy (CBT)
Central nervous system (CNS), 271

Cesarean delivery
  anesthesia, 63–64
  BMI, 62
  extremely obese women, 63
  obese women, 62
CNS. *See* Central nervous system (CNS)
Cognitive behavioral therapy (CBT), 149
The Coronary Artery Risk Development in Young Adults (CARDIA) study, 82, 90, 91
Cultural influences, 122–123

D

Delivery. *See also* Labor
  cesarean (*see* Cesarean delivery)
  median time, 61
  shoulder dystocia, 58
  suspected macrosomia, 58
Developmental origins of health and disease (DOHaD), 261
DOHaD. *See* Developmental origins of health and disease (DOHaD)

E

Edinburgh Postnatal Depression Scale (EPDS), 101, 102
EPDS. *See* Edinburgh Postnatal Depression Scale (EPDS)
Exercise
  ACOG guidelines, 186–188

F

Family-centered interventions
  characterization, 328
  children's dietary behaviors, 299–300
  definition, 300–301
  health-care services, 299
  infants, toddlers and preschoolers
    children's energy intake, 305
    description, 301–303
    diet activities, 305
    educational materials, 304
    home-based, 301
    introduction to solids, 301, 304
    KAN-DO, 306
    LAUNCH, 306–307
    plus obesity prevention, 304–305
    soothe/sleep, 301
    "The Healthy Beginnings Trial", 304
    weight loss program, 305
    WIC, 305
  InFANT study, 323
  long-term effects
    BMI z score, 319
    child-centered activity program, 320
    children's and parents' weight, 317
    Diet arm, 321
    Diet plus Activity arm, 321
    Epstein model, 318–319
    face-to-face counseling, 319–320
    'Families for Health", 319
    group sessions, 321
    HIKCUPS study, 320
    internet-based program, 320
    measurement, 322
    12-month post-intervention, 322
    parent-centered Diet program, 320–321
    pediatric obesity, 318
    study groups, 318
    weight outcomes, 319

Family-centered interventions (*cont.*)
  maternal and child obesity, 298–299
  MEND program, 326–327
  NEAT program, 326
  Norwegian Mother and Child Cohort Study, 299
  NOURISH, 323
  nutrition and physical activity practices, 329
  obesity prevention/treatments, 322–325
  overweight, 299
  physical activity, mothers, 300
  school-aged children and adolescents, 307–317
  STOPP, 323, 326
  weight management programs, 328–329
  weight problems, 299, 327
  z-BMI change, 329
Female fertility
  fecundity, 13, 14
  infertility treatment, 20–21
  menstrual irregularities, 14
  ovulatory dysfunction, 14
Folic acid supplementation, pregnancy, 39

G

GDM. *See* Gestational diabetes mellitus (GDM)
Gestational diabetes mellitus (GDM), 4, 20, 26, 36, 46, 54, 56, 70, 80, 92, 101, 185, 194–196, 204, 213, 233, 241, 286, 299
Gestational weight gain (GWG)
  components, 237–238
  current IOM recommendations, 237, 239
  description, 236, 263
  determinants, 238
  disproportionate risk, 264
  higher prepregnancy BMI, 264
  interpregnancy weight gain, 264
  interventional strategies, 264
  leptin production and regulation, 264
  long-term outcomes, 240
  maternal obesity, 240
  mothers and offspring, 240
  multiple linear regression models, 88
  and obesity, 263
  obesity-related maternal complications, 239
  PRAMS, 237
  prenatal interventions, 242–244
  short-term outcomes
    birth weight, 241
    maternal, 241
  US population, 237
Glucose intolerance
  definition, 13
  diet, glycemic index, 22
  PCOS, 17
Guidelines for Perinatal Care, 36–37
GWG. *See* Gestational weight gain (GWG)

H

Health
  health-care providers, 208–210
  long-term adverse, 195
  US surveillance studies, physical activity, 189, 190
"The Healthy Beginnings Trial", 304. *See also* Family-centered interventions
Hunter Illawarra Kids Challenge Using Parent Support (HIKCUPS) study, 320

I

Infant growth, maternal prepregnancy BMI and GWG, 246–248
Infertility
  anovulation (*see* Anovulation)
  definition, 12
  female fertility, 13–14
  IVF, 13
  male fertility, 18–20
  treatment, obese female patient, 20–21
  and weight loss (*see* Weight loss)
Insulin resistance
  definition, 12
  excess body weight, 15
  hyperandrogenism, 16
  insulin sensitizers, 24
  myo-inositol, 25
  PCOS, 15, 16
Interventions
  childbearing age, 234–236
  dietary, 230
  maternal weight gain, 242–244
  prenatal and postpartum periods, 241
In vitro fertilization (IVF)
  obese women, 20
  USA, 13
IVF. *See* In vitro fertilization (IVF)

K

The Kaiser Physical Activity Survey (KPAS), 193
KAN-DO. *See* Kids and Adults Now-Defeat Obesity (KAN-DO)
Kids and Adults Now-Defeat Obesity (KAN-DO), 306
KPAS. *See* The Kaiser Physical Activity Survey (KPAS)

L

Labor
  complications
    elective cesarean delivery, 57
    extensive counseling, 58
    fetal weight, 57–58
    gestational diabetes, 57
    macrosomia, 56, 58
    nondiabetic women, 56
    shoulder dystocia and birth trauma, 56, 57
    visualization, 57
  induction
    cervical ripening, 61
    cesarean delivery rate, 62
    risk-benefit ratio, 61
  management
    cardiovascular issues, 61
    cervical dilation, 60
    checklist, equipment, 59
    duration, 60
    fetal scalp electrode and intrauterine pressure catheter, 61
    overweight/obese patient, 58–59
LAUNCH, 306–307
Lifestyle interventions, 160, 162, 167
Lifestyle modification
  behavioral change models, 42–44
  randomized controlled clinical trials, 40
  structured approach, 307
  TTM, 40, 41

M

Major depressive disorder (MDD)
  decreased energy, 104
  dose-response relationship, 104
  hypothalamic-pituitary-adrenal axis, 105
  symptoms, 104
  unhealthy lifestyles, 104

Male fertility
  BMI, 19
  impaired spermatogenesis, 19
  scrotal/suprapubic lipectomy, 19
  sexual activity, 19
  weight loss, 19–20
Maternal obesity
  animal models, 288–289
  cardiometabolic, behavioral and mental health outcomes, 288
  description, 260
  developmental programming
    DOHaD, 261
    fetal origins hypothesis, 261
    and intrauterine overnutrition, 262
    maternal-fetal relationship, 262
    overnutrition hypothesis, 262
    population-based studies, 261
    pregnant obese mother, 262
    thrifty phenotype hypothesis, 261
  genetic and environmental factors, 289
  non-Hispanic blacks, 260
  offspring outcomes (*see* Offspring, long-term health)
  short-term risk in offspring, 260–261
Maternal prepregnancy BMI
  breastfeeding, 244–246
  gestational weight gain, 246–248
MDD. *See* Major depressive disorder (MDD)
Medications, weight loss
  androgen-reducing medications, 25
  anti-absorptives, 24
  antidepressants, 25
  ephedra/ephedrine, 25
  insulin sensitizers, 24
  myo-inositol, 24–25
  sympathomimetics, 24
MI. *See* Motivational interviewing (MI)
Mind, exercise, nutrition and do it (MEND) program, 326–327
Motivational interviewing (MI)
  behavioral change, 43
  description, 42–43
  OARS acronym, 43
  patient-provider relationship, 44

N
The National Diabetes Prevention Program, 342
The National Heart, Lung and Blood Institute (NHLBI), 338–340
NELIP. *See* Nutrition and Exercise Lifestyle Intervention Program (NELIP)
Neurodevelopmental outcomes
  CNS, 271
  mental health disorders in children, 271
Newborn health, 231, 234
NHLBI. *See* The National Heart, Lung and Blood Institute (NHLBI)
NOURISH, 323
Nutrition and Exercise Lifestyle Intervention Program (NELIP), 214–215
Nutrition Education Aimed at Toddlers (NEAT) program, 326

O

Obese pregnant woman
  counseling, 36–37
  gestational diabetes, 36
  Institute of Medicine weight gain, pregnancy guidelines, 35, 36
  maternal and fetal complications, 35
Obesity
  description, 7
  fertility
    female (see Female fertility)
    male, 18–20
  maternal, 79–80, 89
  MDD, 103–105
  midlife, 82
  perinatal intervention studies, 109–112
  and PND
    antenatal MDD, 106–107
    conceptual model, 106
    lifestyle factors, 106
    psychosocial factors, 105
  postpartum, 90
  pregnancy (see Pregnancy)
  prepregnancy, 86
  reclassification, 4
  transgenerational cycle, 4
  USA, 13
  US trends, women, 79
Obesity prevention
  family issue, 329
  KAN-DO, 306
  LAUNCH, 306–307
  NEAT, 326
  plus, 304–305
  STOPP, 323–324
  treatments, 323
Offspring, long-term health
  ADHD, 286–287
  asthma, 271, 272–277
  autism, 287
  childhood and adolescent obesity, 262
  gestational weight gain, 263–264
  neurodevelopmental outcomes, 271, 278–284
  obesity risk, 263
  pregnancy and offspring cardiometabolic risk, 265–270
  schizophrenia, 285–286
Overweight
  Affordable Care Act, 249
  anesthesia, 63–64
  child, 232–233
  childbearing age, 234–236
  and GWG (see Gestational weight gain (GWG))
  interventions, 249
  labor (see Labor)
  maternal prepregnancy BMI (see Maternal prepregnancy BMI)
  mother, 233–234
  postoperative and postpartum complications, 67–68
  pregnancy status, 248
  pregnant women (see Obese pregnant woman)
  surgical issues
    cesarean delivery, 65
    intrapartum and postpartum hemorrhage, 65
  VBAC, 68–69
Overweight, postpartum care
  ACOG Resource Guide, 162, 163–165
  NICE recommendations, 162, 163–166
  obesity, 166
Ovulatory dysfunction
  decreased fertility, obese, 14
  definition, 12, 14

P

Parenting Eating and Activity for Child Health (PEACH), 317
PCOS. *See* Polycystic ovary syndrome (PCOS)
PDSS. *See* Postpartum Depression Screening Scale (PDSS)
PEACH. *See* Parenting Eating and Activity for Child Health (PEACH)
Perinatal depression (PND)
   EPDS, 101, 102
   maternal suicide and infanticide, 101
   prevalence, 100–101
   screening, 101
Perinatal obesity, 6, 8
Physical activity and obesity. *See also* Obesity
   ACOG, 185–186
   cesarean delivery, 189
   clinical practice, 216
   contraindications to aerobic exercise, 186, 187
   description, 185
   diabetes risk, 215
   GDM and non-GDM women, 214
   health outcomes, 213–214, 216
   Hispanic women, 215
   moderate-intensity, 186
   NELIP, 214–215
   ongoing interventions, 212–213
   overweight, 189 (*see also* Overweight)
   Physical Activity Guidelines for Americans, 186
   positions, 187, 188
   pregnancy (*see* Pregnancy and postpartum)
   pregnancy complications, 186
   theoretical based interventions, 214
   transtheoretical model, 215
   US Children's Bureau, 185
   USDHHS, 186–187
   warning signs to terminate exercise, 186, 188
PND. *See* Perinatal depression (PND)
Polycystic ovary syndrome (PCOS)
   description, 16
   lean women, 16
   management, 17–18
   obesity, 16
   significance, 16–17
Postpartum
   African-American women, 147
   Australian study, 146
   BMI, 147, 148
   body image, 142, 143–145
   clinical trials and public health reports, 161
   description, 160–161
   dissatisfaction, body image, 146
   evidence-based models, 161–162
   feeding, 146–147
   insurance coverage, 161
   normal/prepregnancy size, 142, 146
   overweight (*see* Overweight, postpartum care)
   physiological changes, 161
   pregnancy, 148–150 (*see also* Pregnancy and postpartum)
   socioeconomic status, 161
   weight loss (*see* Weight loss, postpartum care)
Postpartum depression (PPD)
   and obesity, 107
   postpartum weight retention, 112
   prepregnancy BMI, 108
   research, 110–111
   and weight retention, 112–113

Postpartum Depression
    Screening Scale
    (PDSS), 101, 102
Postpartum weight retention
    (PPWR)
  average, 83
  BMI and gestational weight
    gain, 79, 80
  childbearing cohorts, 81–83
  fat accumulation and body
    composition
    changes, 90
  GWG, 88
  high-BMI groups, 81
  hormonal adaptations, 78
  overweight/obese after
    pregnancy, 87
  pregnancy and visceral fat
    changes, 91
  pregnancy cohorts and
    high BMI, 84–85
    predictors, 86
    US cohorts, 86
    variability, estimates, 83
  pregnancy weight gain, 89
  prepregnancy body size,
    87–88
  reproductive maturation
    and timing,
    pregnancy, 89
  self-report, prepregnancy
    weight, 81
PPD. *See* Postpartum depression
    (PPD)
PPWR. *See* Postpartum weight
    retention (PPWR)
Pre-and postnatal periods,
    184, 204
Preconception care
  approaching, patient, 37
  clinical assessment, health
    visit
    BMI, 38
    folic acid
      supplementation, 39
    screening, 39–40
    type 2 diabetes and lipid
      screening, 38–39
    WHR, 38
  definition, 34–35
  interventions, lifestyle
    modifications
    behavioral change models,
      42–44
    randomized controlled
      clinical trials, 40
    TTM, 40, 41
  obese pregnant woman (*see*
    Obese pregnant
    woman)
  research, 48
  tools, weight loss
    bariatric surgery, 46
    contraceptive options,
      45–46
    dietician, 44
    lifestyle modification, 44
    low-fat diets, 45
    physical activity, 45
    weight gain, during
      pregnancy, 46–48
Prediabetes, 13, 22
Pregnancy
  abdominal shape change, 138
  African-American women,
    137
  Black and White women, 139
  body distortion, 139
  body image, 130, 131–136
  childbearing, 138
  complications, 5
  GDM, 5
  GWG, 5
  Institute of Medicine (IOM),
    137
  insulin sensitivity, 5
  outcomes
    bariatric surgery, 46
    childbearing age, 48
    exercise, 47
    overweight and obese
      women, 54

Pregnancy (*cont.*)
　phase, 130
　physical activity, 141–142
　positive maternal identity, 130
　postpartum, 148–150
　prepregnancy (*see* Prepregnancy)
　psychological factors, 141
　transgenerational obesity, 6
　women's adaptation, 137–138
Pregnancy and postpartum
　accelerometry, 191
　aerobic fitness, 199
　AMP, 199
　BMI, 192
　complex interactions, 211
　critical gaps, 200
　dietary intervention, 200
　dissemination, 210–211
　environmental enablers, 194
　GDM (*see* Gestational diabetes mellitus (GDM))
　GWG (*see* Gestational weight gain (GWG))
　health behaviors, 209
　health-care providers, 208–209
　household activities, 192
　information, 210
　interventions, 204–208
　KPAS, 193
　measurement, 200–201
　moderate and vigorous, 191
　National Health and Nutrition Examination Survey, 189
　nonpregnant patients, 212
　nulliparous women, 193
　overweight/obese women, 198–199, 201–203
　partner's/husband's participation, 193–194
　preeclampsia, 196–197
　program components and intervention strategies, 211–212
　qualitative and quantitative studies, 194
　social desirability, 191
　sociodemographic factors, 193
　trimester, 191–192
　US surveillance studies, self-reports, 189, 190
Prepregnancy
　body image, 139–140
　eating behaviors, 140
　obesity
　　antenatal MDD, 107
　　and PPD, 108
　weight status, 140

R
Racial/ethnic disparities, 122
RE-AIM framework
　application, 161
　Chronic Disease Model, 175
　postpartum interventions
　　adoption, 177–178
　　Chronic Care Model, 178, 179
　　Diabetes Prevention Program, 176
　　efficacy, 178
　　evaluation parameters, 175–176
　　implementation, 178
　　PREMIER, 176
　　theoretical approach, 178
　　Weight Loss After Delivery (project), 176, 177
　　weight retention and gain, 179
Recommendations
　ACOG guidelines, 186–188
　health-care providers, 208–210
　physical activity guidelines, 208–210
　Physical Activity Guidelines for Americans, 186
Reproductive maturation, 89

Resting metabolic rate (RMR)
  daily caloric intake, 22
  definition, 13

S
Schizophrenia
  adult offspring, mothers, 286
  and birth weight, 285
  gestational diabetes, 286
  inflammatory cytokines, 286
  maternal infection, 286
  mother offsprings with
    pregnancy BMI, 285
  neurodevelopmental and
    metabolic conditions,
    285
  paucity, 285
School-aged children and
    adolescents
  behavioral weight control
    program, 316
  BMI z scores, 314–317
  description, 307, 308–312
  Epstein Traffic Light Diet
    protocol, 313–314
  intensive phase, 316, 317
  lifestyle modification
    approach, 307
  parent-plus-child group, 313
  PEACH, 317
  pre-post design study, 316
  Project STORY, 314
  randomized controlled
    trial, 313
Screening
  ACOG, 338
  AHRQ, 338
  Canadian Task Force, 339
  description, 338
  lifestyle modifications, 343
  national initiatives, 341–342
  NHLBI, 338–339
  obesity prevention, 341
  recommendations
    classification, 339
    guidelines, 339–340
  NHLBI, 340
  USPSTF, 340–341
  regional-and community-
    oriented initiatives, 343
  sweetened beverages and
    caloric content, 342
  USPSTF, 338
Scrotal/suprapubic lipectomy, 19
SCT. *See* Social cognitive
  theory (SCT)
Sensible treatment of obesity in
    rural youth (STORY)
    project, 314
SES. *See* Socioeconomic status
    (SES)
Shared decision making
  anesthesia, 63–64
  cesarean delivery, 62–63
  description, 55
  labor
    complications risk, 56–58
    induction, 61–62
    management, 58–61
  postoperative and postpartum
    complications, 67–68
  surgical issues
    first-generation
      cephalosporin, 65
    intrapartum and
      postpartum
      hemorrhage, 65
  VBAC, 68–69
Social cognitive theory
    (SCT), 42
Socioeconomic status (SES), 122
Stockholm obesity prevention
    program (STOPP),
    323, 326
STOPP. *See* Stockholm obesity
    prevention program
    (STOPP)

T
"The Healthy Beginnings
    Trial", 304
Transgenerational obesity, 4, 6

Transtheoretical model (TTM), 41
TTM. *See* Transtheoretical model (TTM)
Type 2 diabetes, 78, 92

U

The United States Preventive Services Task Force (USPSTF), 338, 340–341
United Status Department of Health and Human Services (USDHHS), 186–187
USDHHS. *See* United Status Department of Health and Human Services (USDHHS)
The US Preventive Services Task Force (USPSTF), 39–40
USPSTF. *See* The United States Preventive Services Task Force (USPSTF)

V

Vaginal birth after cesarean (VBAC), 68–69
VBAC. *See* Vaginal birth after cesarean (VBAC)

W

Waist to hip ratio (WHR), 38
Weight control, 124
Weight loss. *See also* Preconception care
  behavioral intervention, 114
  counseling, 27
  diet, 21–22
  exercise, 21, 23
  male fertility, 19–20
  medications (*see* Medications, weight loss)
  postpartum care
    African American women, 174
    Centers for Disease Control and Prevention (CDC), 167
    diet and exercise interventions, 167–174
    large-scale studies, 175
    NHLBI, 167
    PREMIER, 166
    statistically significant, 174–175
    WISEWOMAN, 166–167
  sexual quality, 20
  surgery, 25–26
WHR. *See* Waist to hip ratio (WHR)
WIC. *See* Women infants and children (WIC)
Women infants and children (WIC), 305

MIX
Papier aus verantwortungsvollen Quellen
Paper from responsible sources
FSC® C105338

If you have any concerns about our products,
you can contact us on
ProductSafety@springernature.com

In case Publisher is established outside the EU,
the EU authorized representative is:
**Springer Nature Customer Service Center GmbH
Europaplatz 3, 69115 Heidelberg, Germany**

Printed by Libri Plureos GmbH
in Hamburg, Germany